Histological Laboratory Methods

Histological Laboratory Methods

Brenda D. Disbrey
F.I.M.L.T., A.I.S.T.

Chief Histological Technician,
John Bonnett Clinical Laboratories,
Addenbrooke's Hospital, Cambridge

J. H. Rack
M.A., M.B., B.Chir., M.R.C.Path.

Consultant Pathologist,
Norfolk and Norwich Hospital, Norwich.
Formerly Senior Assistant Pathologist to
Addenbrooke's Hospital, Cambridge

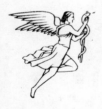

E. & S. LIVINGSTONE
EDINBURGH AND LONDON, 1970

SBN 443 00694 6

Printed in Great Britain

To the memory of
ARTHUR MAX BARRETT
(1909-1961)
who showed us
that knowing how
comes from asking why

Preface

THIS book contains reliable histological methods with particulars of how and why they are used. The methods will satisfy all the needs of a general histological laboratory and have been written in sufficient detail to be understood by those with little or no previous experience.

It is hoped that the book will appeal to three groups of readers. First, the younger technicians in routine histological laboratories attached to medical, veterinary, industrial and academic organizations. Secondly, workers in other fields who occasionally need to employ histological techniques: this group includes school biology teachers as well as a wide variety of research workers. Thirdly, those who need to know something about histological techniques without being called upon to practise them: this group comprises trainee pathologists and students of such sciences as biology and agriculture.

The preparation of a histological specimen usually calls for the combination of several techniques, which are carried out in sequence. For convenience, the book has been divided into chapters, each dealing with one stage of preparation or one group of techniques. As far as possible, these chapters have been written so that they may be read in any order, and each is furnished with appropriate cross-references to other parts of the book.

No attempt has been made to prepare a comprehensive list of all available methods. Those selected have almost all been in routine use in the John Bonnett Clinical Laboratories for many years and have given consistently reliable results, even in relatively inexperienced hands. When no single method satisfies all requirements, it has been necessary to recommend two or more, with an indication of the merits and drawbacks of each. In making a selection, a number of perfectly good alternatives have doubtless been omitted because of personal preference or unfamiliarity.

With many methods, experience has shown that certain stages commonly present difficulties or require unusual care if good results are to be obtained. Particularly detailed guidance is given for these stages, although it must be appreciated that a written account can never take the place of practical instruction. Stress has also been laid on certain theoretical aspects of the subject which often present problems to the beginner. An attempt has been made to forestall some of the questions and correct some of the misconceptions encountered in discussions with a wide variety of scientific workers requiring advice about histological techniques, and whilst teaching and examining candidates for Institute of Medical Laboratory Technology or National Certificate examinations.

Some methods have been in use for many years and have undergone modifications with the passage of time. For this reason, as well as for those who wish to pursue the subject further, a comprehensive list of references has been included, all of which have been seen by one author or both, either in the original or in photographic copy. A list of books for further reading is included in the first chapter.

It is a pleasure to thank the very many student technicians and trainee pathologists whose persistent questions stimulated us to write this book.

We are ever grateful to those who taught us, and especially to the late Dr Max Barrett, University Morbid Anatomist and Histologist to Addenbrooke's Hospital, whose understanding of technical methods matched his skill as a pathologist and was surpassed only by his kindness as a man.

For items of practical advice we are indebted to so many colleagues and authors that it would be impossible to thank each individually.

We have drawn on the services of many libraries. In Cambridge we have made extensive use of those in the departments of Anatomy, Physiology and Zoology and the University Library, as well as using many other departmental libraries; in addition we have made use of the libraries of the Norfolk and Norwich Hospital and the Royal Society of Medicine. We are grateful to all these institutions and librarians for their help, but we owe a special debt of gratitude to Miss Carole Cousins, Assistant Librarian to the Cambridge University Department of Pathology, for tracing and obtaining many of the older periodicals.

For undertaking the considerable task of typing the manuscript, we are grateful to Miss Jean E. Claydon.

Our thanks are due to Mrs Christine M. Colmer, A.I.M.L.T., for scrutinizing the proofs.

Messrs Hopkins and William Ltd., kindly supplied information on which the table of dyes is based.

One of the most satisfying aspects of writing this book has been to watch it take shape in the hands of our publishers, Messrs E. & S. Livingstone, from whose staff we have learned to expect skilled help and complete co-operation.

1970 THE AUTHORS

Contents

Throughout this book, the following conventions are used:

Alcohol. The word is used as an abbreviation for Industrial Methylated Spirit 74° O.P. On the rare occasions when pure ethyl alcohol ('absolute alcohol') is necessary, the word ethanol is used.

Distilled water. This term is used for water distilled in an ordinary metal still. De-ionized water may be substituted for it. In methods that demand glass-distilled water, this fact is stated; de-ionized water may not be satisfactory for these methods.

Formalin. This is a saturated solution (37–40 per cent) of formaldehyde gas in water. All formulae are expressed in terms of formalin, not formaldehyde.

Mixtures of fluids. Percentages refer to the volumes of the fluids mixed (v/v), not their weights.

Solutions. Percentages refer to the weights of solids and the volumes of liquids (w/v). Thus, 5 per cent means 5 g. per 100 ml.

CHAPTER 1

Histology in Perspective

General notes. The basic technique. Common variants. Special techniques. The uses of histology. Future trends. Further reading.

HISTOLOGY originally meant the science of tissues, but the meaning has become restricted so that the word histology is now usually taken to mean the study of the fine structure of animal tissues and organs. The histologist's basic tool is the optical microscope, and most of the work of the histological laboratory is the preparation of specimens for microscopical examination at magnifications of ×40 to ×400, and occasionally as much as ×1000. Transmitted light is almost always used, since this reveals the detailed structure of cells and tissues, whereas reflected light would merely provide information about the surface of the specimen. For use with transmitted light, however, very thin preparations are necessary, because they must be translucent and must reveal fine details which would be obscured by structures above or below them. Thin preparations may be obtained by squashing or smearing tissue, or by cutting thin slices from it. Although both of these methods are used in the histological laboratory, thin slices or *sections* are much the commoner since they show the various components that make up the tissue and also how one component is related to another. Squashed or smeared preparations, on the other hand, demonstrate only the nature of the components and not their distribution. When smears or sections have been made, they are usually stained to show structures of special importance or interest.

It must be emphasized that the finished product differs in many ways from the original tissue, being a multicoloured and unevenly distorted two-dimensional representation. Provided that the colours and the distortion are consistent from one specimen to another they are capable of being interpreted, so that the essential purpose of a histological laboratory might be described as the production of consistently deformed specimens. It is equally important for those examining the preparations to

B

appreciate that they are seeing no more than a distorted likeness of the original structure of the tissue. The best they can hope for is a likeness that will be distorted in precisely the same way on every occasion.

The basic histological technique

All technical methods demand a certain amount of scientific knowledge combined with considerable skill and experience. Newcomers to a histological laboratory will undoubtedly be bewildered by the many processes in operation, some of which may be performed by automatic machines. They are, however, recommended to bear in mind that most of the activity is directed towards the objectives mentioned above; namely, the preparation of suitably thin sections and their staining.

This is not the place to enter into technical details, which are to be found in the chapters that follow; it may, however, be helpful at this stage to follow a typical specimen through the various processes necessary for the preparation of a section.

If the specimen is large, it is necessary to cut one or more representative pieces from it; if small, the whole specimen is used. At this stage a ticket is prepared from stiff paper or thin card with an identifying number written on it. This will accompany the piece through the ensuing processes; therefore the number must be written in black pencil or India ink which withstand solvents. The correct identification of specimens is of paramount importance, especially in hospital laboratories dealing with many similar specimens from different patients.

Before proceeding further the piece must be *fixed*. This may have occurred before the specimen was received or may take place in the laboratory. Fixation is the stabilization of the important constituents of the tissue (especially proteins) so that they will not be dissolved, displaced or distorted during subsequent procedures. As far as possible this stabilization is achieved without altering the character or distribution of the tissue constituents.

After thorough fixation, the piece is subjected to increasingly strong alcohol until all the water has been replaced. When this has been done, the alcohol is in its turn replaced by a fat solvent or *clearing agent*. The piece is then transferred to molten paraffin wax which is miscible with the clearing agent and replaces it. When the wax cools, it not only encases the piece of tissue, but also occupies all the space that originally contained water, so that the tissue itself is sufficiently hard for thin sections to be cut.

The tissue is cut by means of a *microtome*, which is of necessity a precision instrument since the average section is about one two-hundredth part of a millimetre in thickness. After it has been secured to a microscope slide, the section is stained by haematoxylin which colours nuclei and then by eosin which colours cytoplasm. Finally a thin coverslip is stuck over the section by means of a colourless and transparent adhesive with the same refractive index as glass.

The common variants

Tissue components are demonstrable by a wide variety of methods. Most of these make use of coloured dyes although a few depend on opaque precipitates such as metallic silver. The choice of a suitable method is governed by the type of tissue examined and the particular component sought. In many cases it may be necessary to use different methods on several sections from the same specimen. Sometimes it is necessary to know that a particular feature is absent from the tissue, and sections are stained to show whether it is present or not. For this purpose, it is more important than usual to employ a consistently reliable method. As a further precaution, a *control section* (in which the particular feature is known to be present) should be stained by the same method.

Paraffin wax is not the only satisfactory embedding medium. The commonest alternative in general use is nitrocellulose, which may be used instead of wax or in combination with it.

An entirely different way of hardening tissue sufficiently for thin sections to be cut, is to freeze it solid. The frozen sections produced by this method are valuable when time does not permit the preparation of paraffin wax sections, or when the purpose of the section is the demonstration of substances that are lost when wax is used (e.g. lipids). Frozen sections are suitable for a wide variety of staining methods. Smears, likewise, can be stained by many alternative methods after they have been adequately fixed.

Since the ordinary histological section is a two-dimensional slice through a three-dimensional piece of tissue, it cannot provide complete information about structure. When three-dimensional information is important, it will be necessary to prepare many sections from the same piece of tissue. For full information, *serial sections* must be prepared (i.e. every section must be cut, stained and examined). Often enough information can be obtained from sections cut from the tissue at intervals.

The great majority of tissues and organs can be examined by most if not all of the techniques outlined above. A few specimens, however, present special problems and require either unusual care or a modification of routine practice. These include pieces of brain and spinal cord, eyes, calcified tissues, and unusually tough tissues.

Special techniques

Beyond the basic technique and the common variants there are many special techniques. These may be used occasionally in the general laboratory; they account for most of the work of some specialist laboratories.

The preparation of sections for electron microscopy is fundamentally similar to the basic histological technique for the optical microscope. The details, however, are quite different, requiring special methods of fixation, embedding, and section cutting.

Autoradiography is a method of recording the radioactivity of tissue components in sections or smears of specimens from experimental animals or, occasionally, from human patients. It makes use of photographic emulsion which is closely applied to the section or smear and is sensitive to radioactivity.

Histochemistry is a word used to describe the accurate localization of tissue components by a chemical reaction. It is true that almost all histological staining methods depend on some kind of chemical reaction, but in many of them the chemistry is not fully understood. Many histological staining methods are entirely reliable, even though it is not clear precisely what kind of chemical bond is formed between the dye and the tissue, or what kind of molecular configuration in the tissue attracts the dye. A method is said to be histochemical when the chemistry of the reaction is completely understood, so that the kind of chemical bond and the nature of the reacting groups in the tissue are precisely defined in chemical terms. Some methods in constant use in the histological laboratory are fully understood and may therefore be classed as histochemical reactions; many other histochemical methods are available for special laboratories and for occasional use in general laboratories. Among the many uses of histochemistry are the detection of traces of metals or other foreign substances and the localization of enzymes by marking the products of their activity.

The preparation of museum specimens often falls within the scope of the histological laboratory because the type of specimen and the techniques of preparation are in general similar to those used for histological examination.

Other special techniques are mentioned below in the section concerned with possible future developments of histology.

The uses of histology

As a method of examination, histology may be applied to normal or abnormal tissues from man or animals. In addition to their use as research methods for the discovery of new facts, histological techniques are extensively used in teaching centres. Although originally concerned exclusively with structure, histology also sheds light on function by providing information about the minute organization of cells and tissues to supplement the sciences of physiology and biochemistry which deal with the nature and activity of the tissue components rather than their localization.

Histology is extensively used in the study of abnormal tissues. It provides invaluable information about natural human and animal diseases, so that histological laboratories play a vital part in the diagnostic service of every hospital. Histology is an essential part of much experimental work: this includes not only experiments concerned with the production of abnormalities, but also the protracted experimental studies that are necessary before new drugs, cosmetics, and food-additives can be regarded as safe for human use. Investigations of methods of food preservation make use of histology to assess changes in stored meat. In terms of size and number, the most important histological laboratories are those in hospitals, teaching centres, and organizations making experimental toxicity tests of new drugs.

Although all histological laboratories make use of similar techniques, the detailed organization will vary from one laboratory to another according to the type of work it does. Thus, a laboratory that prepares large numbers of identical sections for teaching purposes will probably make use of automatic tissue processing machines and staining machines, whereas a research laboratory in which no two specimens are alike will often prefer manual methods.

The purpose of the laboratory also governs the rate at which it must work. A hospital diagnostic laboratory must provide results quickly, whereas a research laboratory concerned with the investigation of fine structure can afford to take more time. One of the fundamental practical problems of the histological laboratory is the incompatibility of speed with perfect quality. According to its type of work, each individual laboratory will choose which of the two to sacrifice or will compromise by losing a little of both.

Future trends

The following suggestions about possible developments in histological techniques are written with hospital laboratories primarily in mind. Many of the predictions are likely to be proved wrong by the passage of time and, in any case, the expansion of hospital diagnostic services depends in part on the demands of clinical medicine and in large measure on the availability of funds.

Changes will be of two kinds: new ways of using old techniques, and the introduction of entirely new ones. Old techniques are continually being modified, and the tendency will be to make use of modifications that provide results sooner or with less effort. Labour-saving devices such as knife-sharpeners and pre-formed individual embedding moulds for wax are likely to become universally used. The need for quicker schedules will favour the use of very rapid processing machines, unless the pressure for speed is so great as to eliminate paraffin sections altogether and replace them with frozen sections prepared in the cryostat for immediate diagnosis of routine surgical specimens.

Staining methods will become more precise, with the gradual replacement of empirical histological methods by specific histochemical ones. It is likely that improved knowledge of the chemistry of tissues, fixatives and dyes will put some of the reliable empirical histological methods in current use on a respectable chemical basis.

The ordinary optical microscope is unlikely to undergo any striking changes, but special forms of optical microscopy will be more widely used. It is likely that fluorescence microscopy will become more popular and that there will be a wider range of fluorescent substances (fluorochromes) with specific affinities for tissue components. Fluorescence microscopy is particularly suitable when a search must be made for objects that are small or few. The phase-contrast microscope is rarely used in the routine laboratory, but is likely to make a larger contribution if specimens are received fresh and unfixed for the preparation of cryostat sections.

New requirements are harder to foresee, but it seems likely that more attention will be directed to the cytoplasm, which receives almost no consideration from the routine methods in current use, whereas the nucleus has been regarded as diagnostically important for more than a century.

Although electron microscopy has already provided a great deal of information about cytoplasm and other tissue constituents, it is not yet of much value as an aid to diagnosis. It seems likely, however, that when more information has been collected about the ultrastructure of cells in health and disease, the electron microscope will be increasingly useful for solving diagnostic problems.

Histochemistry has already advanced to the stage where it is comparatively simple to identify enzyme activity in individual cells, whereas formerly it was difficult to do more than recognize its presence in the tissue or organ as a whole. Much of this advance is due to the use of cryostat sections. Since the cryostat is now widely distributed in hospital laboratories, it is likely that enzyme histochemistry will be found to be of practical use in the diagnosis of disease.

Tissue culture may remain the preserve of virologists and research cytologists. It is, however, possible that cultures of cells from individual tumours may, in the future, be used for an assessment of their sensitivity to cytotoxic drugs. If these drugs become more numerous and more specific, it might be necessary to study the effect of a whole series of them on tumour tissue cultures in much the same way that a range of antibiotics is tested against bacteria.

Likewise, it is possible that new developments in the study of immunity may call for the widespread use of immuno-fluorescence techniques, in which sites of antigen-antibody reaction are demonstrated with fluorescent antiglobulin reagents.

It is difficult to see how computors could be employed in diagnostic histology. If, however, a scanning device could be perfected, it is quite probable that it would prefer histological preparations of an entirely different type from those favoured by the human eye. This, in turn, might lead to the introduction of a range of new technical methods.

There will, no doubt, be other new techniques, of which we have at present no suspicion. So far as the routine laboratory is concerned, however, the most likely developments will come from the wider use of techniques that are at present the preserve of the specialist. If this is so, it should be possible to obtain a glimpse of the general laboratory of tomorrow by studying the special laboratories of today.

Further reading

The following list contains a careful selection of books about histological techniques and kindred subjects. Each of them has been found useful. Titles and publishers are mentioned in the list of references (p. 379). An attempt has been made to distinguish between books for inexperienced readers, and more advanced books suitable for consultation.

For general accounts of histological techniques, the following are comparatively simple and easily read: Drury and Wallington (1967), Culling (1963), and McManus and Mowry (1960). Although limited in scope, Clayden (1962) is particularly straightforward and easily understood by the beginner.

For consultation about all aspects of general histological techniques, Lillie (1965) is indispensable except for readers of German, who may prefer Romeis (1968). The theoretical basis of histological techniques is clearly explained in two books by Baker (1958 and 1966), and the properties and behaviour of biological stains by Conn (1961).

Many books have been written about particular parts of

general histological technique, or about special techniques. Histochemistry has a large literature of its own. The books by Chayen *et al.* (1969), Bancroft (1967), and Casselman (1959) are comparatively straightforward, so that any of them may be read as an introduction to histochemistry. Lillie (1965) should be consulted for specific methods, and Pearse (1960 and 1968) for detailed theoretical information. Readers of French will do well to consult Lison (1960). For an unusually comprehensive list of references, see Barka and Anderson (1963).

The following will be found useful for particular aspects of histological technique. Steedman (1960) gives a good theoretical and practical account of waxes and microtomy. Brain (1966) deals with the theory and practice of decalcification. For practical guidance in handling specimens of brain and spinal cord, Russell (1939) and Anderson (1929) should be consulted.

For technical methods that lie beyond routine histological preparation, it will be profitable to consult Rogers (1967) on autoradiography and Paul (1965) on tissue culture. The preparation of sections for the electron microscope is dealt with in a simple and straightforward way by Mercer and Birbeck (1966), or in more detail by Kay (1965) and Pease (1964). For the mounting of museum specimens, Edwards and Edwards (1959) should be consulted; for more elaborate methods of specimen preparation see Tompsett (1956).

No laboratory worker can afford to be ignorant of the toxic and inflammable hazards of the chemicals he handles. Gaston (1964) provides comprehensive information on this neglected subject together with practical advice about necessary precautions. Anyone concerned with radioactive substances is recommended to study the *Code of Practice for the Protection of Persons Exposed to Ionising Radiations in Research and Teaching* (1964) issued by H.M.S.O. Those handling experimental animals will obtain useful guidance from the *UFAW Handbook on the Care and Management of Laboratory Animals* (1967).

For mathematical and chemical tables, as well as much miscellaneous information, *Documenta Geigy* (1962) is invaluable for any laboratory. Silverton and Anderson (1961) also provide tables and factual information of particular relevance to medical laboratories. Gray (1954) is a source book of histological formulae with a comprehensive reference list.

For an introductory account of optical microscopy, Casartelli (1965) is recommended. Clearly written but slightly more advanced books on the same subject are Hartley (1962) and Barer (1968). For a fascinating, but in places advanced, account of the contribution of several physical methods to biological investigation, Chayen and Denby (1968) should be consulted.

For the study of normal histology, the book by Cruickshank, Dodds and Gardner (1968) is confined to human tissues, but presents an easy introduction because of the many excellent colour photographs. For more detailed study, Ham (1965) is recommended. At the electron microscopic level, Haggis (1966) presents a well-illustrated simple account.

A good simple textbook of human anatomy and physiology is Sears (1958). Those wishing to acquire simple basic information about pathology may use Cater (1953) as an introduction, or proceed directly to the rather more detailed books by Perez-Tamayo (1961) and Wright (1958). For diagnostic cytology, Hughes and Dodds (1968) will provide a comprehensive introduction, and Koss (1968) may profitably be used as a work of reference.

Since many histological techniques are of considerable antiquity, it is of historical interest to consult the older textbooks. Moreover, it is often profitable to do so, since they not infrequently include points of practical guidance that have been overlooked by later authors. Of the foremost importance in this respect is *The Microtomist's Vade-mecum* (early editions by Lee; later editions by Gatenby and others—see list of references). Other works in English that should not be overlooked are Mallory (1938) and the first three editions of Carleton's *Histological Technique* (1926, 1938 and 1957) which differ in many respects from the fourth edition. For readers of French, Langeron (latest edition 1949), and for readers of German, Schmorl (latest edition 1934), will be worth consulting.

CHAPTER 2

Fixation

General notes. Properties of an ideal fixative. Chemicals available. Fixation in practice. Individual fixing fluids: Formalin-saline; Neutral buffered formalin solution; Mercuric-chloride-formalin; Heidenhain's Susa; Bouin's fluid; Carnoy's fluid; Helly's fluid; Flemming's fluid; Alcohol; Acetone; Alcoholic formalin.

EXCEPT in special instances, the first step towards the production of a histological section is *fixation*. The exceptions are the relatively uncommon fresh frozen sections which are discussed later (p. 274). As the word implies, fixation confers stability upon tissue. Not only does the tissue resist deterioration, it also withstands the subsequent processes that are necessary for the production of sections. Until fixed, many tissues are too soft to be handled easily (hence fixation was referred to as hardening by many early writers). Unfixed tissue is subject to attack by bacteria and by the enzymes that are present within the cells themselves, the former process being named *putrefaction*: the latter *autolysis*.

Since the most important constituents of tissue are composed wholly or partly of proteins, fixation is directed primarily towards the preservation of proteins by making them insoluble. On rare occasions it is important to preserve other tissue constituents such as lipids, carbohydrates, or mineral deposits. It may then be necessary to employ unusual fixatives which are not ideal for proteins. The mechanisms whereby proteins are fixed vary from one fixative to another. This problem is dealt with in two books of Baker (1958 and 1966) to which the reader is recommended for clearly expressed information about all the theoretical aspects of fixation. Baker classifies fixatives according to their ability to coagulate a soluble protein; he uses the terms *coagulant* and *non-coagulant* to describe the two categories. Some other authors have used the terms precipitant and non-precipitant in the same sense. Coagulation may be brought about when a fixative (e.g. mercuric chloride) combines with protein to make an insoluble compound. Some fixatives, however, coagulate protein by denaturing it without entering into combination (e.g. alcohol). Non-coagulant fixatives (e.g. formalin) invariably form addition compounds with proteins.

Properties of an ideal fixative

An ideal fixative would react rapidly and completely with the tissue, fixing all the constituents without removing any part of any of them. It would penetrate rapidly and deeply, without impeding its own progress by causing hardening or shrinkage of the outer layer. Tissue would not be distorted by swelling or shrinkage during fixation, and would be stabilized sufficiently to withstand the chemicals used at later stages of processing. Tissue would be made hard enough to be handled with ease at later stages but not over-hardened. The full range of staining methods would be possible after its use. An ideal fixative would show no tendency to deteriorate before or after the tissue was placed in it. There would be no rigid upper limit of fixing time beyond which damage was caused. It should not be necessary to apply any after-treatment to correct unwanted side-effects. If an ideal fixative could be created, it would also, doubtless, be cheap, non-toxic, non-inflammable, and non-irritant.

Chemicals available

In the past, many chemicals have been used for fixing tissue. Those in common use have stood the test of time and are few in number. Some may be used singly but a better result is often obtained when two or more fixatives are mixed. In suitably chosen mixtures, each fixative makes good the deficiencies of the others.

It is unfortunate that the word fixative may be used in two different senses. First, it may refer to the pure chemical substance; secondly, it may mean a dilution or mixture that can be used to fix tissue. Sometimes it is hard to know how the word is being used. In order to make a clear distinction, throughout this book we have used the word fixative only in the first sense—i.e. to denote the chemical agent. When we wish to mention a dilution or mixture that is of practical use for fixing tissue, we refer to it as a *fixing fluid*.

Before giving details of satisfactory fixing fluids, it is necessary to list the individual chemical agents in common use, and to note the special qualities of each.

Formalin. A saturated solution (40 per cent) of formaldehyde gas in water. Irritant to nose, eyes, and skin. Undergoes slow spontaneous oxidation to formic acid. May throw a precipitate of paraformaldehyde in the cold; this redissolves on warming.

A non-coagulant fixative. Penetrates well without undesirable hardening or shrinkage. Sometimes gives rise to a fixation deposit, especially in tissue that contains much blood.

It is important to note that a formula may be expressed either in terms of formalin or of formaldehyde (e.g. 4 per cent formaldehyde means the same as 10 per cent formalin). In this book all formulae are given in terms of *formalin.*

Mercuric chloride (mercury perchloride; corrosive sublimate). Soluble in water to about 7 per cent. Corrosive to skin and very poisonous. Attacks almost all metals.

A coagulant fixative. Penetrates moderately well, without undesirable hardening or shrinkage. Usually gives rise to a fixation deposit. Is radio-opaque, and therefore interferes with subsequent radiological tests (e.g. for decalcification). Enhances staining by some methods (e.g. trichrome) by virtue of its mordanting effect.

Potassium dichromate. Dissolves slowly in water. Usually used as a 2–3 per cent solution. May cause damage to skin.

A non-coagulant fixative unless used in acid solutions below pH 3·4 when it reacts in the same way as chromic acid. Tissue is coloured yellow and needs prolonged washing after fixation. Never used alone; always in conjunction with other fixatives. Causes no hardening or shrinkage. Enhances staining by phosphotungstic acid haematoxylin. Forms pigmented compounds with chromaffin tissue. Used in some methods for the demonstration of myelin (Marchi; Weigert-Pal).

Chromic acid. An aqueous solution of chromium trioxide. Usually used as a 1-3 per cent solution. Causes damage to skin.

A coagulant fixative. Penetrates slowly, causing hardening but little shrinkage. After fixation, tissue needs prolonged washing.

Picric acid. Soluble in water (up to 1·5 per cent) or alcohol (up to 8 per cent). Picric acid is explosive, as are some picrates (Greenbury, 1966). The crystals must not be allowed to become dry.

A coagulant fixative which forms picrates with many proteins and some carbohydrates. Tissue must not be transferred to an aqueous fluid, since some of these picrates are soluble until treated with alcohol. Penetrates very poorly. Causes shrinkage but does not harden or distort. Tissue is coloured yellow which makes it easy to identify during processing and section cutting. Picric acid enhances some staining methods (e.g. trichrome).

Acetic acid. Coagulates nucleoproteins but otherwise has little or no fixing effect. Used in several mixtures because it causes considerable swelling of tissue and so counteracts the shrinking effect of other constituents. Penetrates well and causes no hardening.

Trichloracetic acid. Deliquescent crystals. Corrosive to skin. A coagulant fixative which causes swelling of tissue and is never used alone. May remove minerals (e.g. calcium, iron, or copper) from tissue.

Osmium tetroxide. Obtained in sealed ampoules of crystals or aqueous solution. Unstable in air. Should be freshly made up whenever possible. Stored solutions should be kept in brown glass bottles and stabilized by the addition of one drop of saturated aqueous mercuric chloride solution to every 10 ml. of solution. Irritant to eyes. Expensive.
   A non-coagulant fixative which penetrates very poorly, causing little hardening or shrinkage. Forms insoluble compounds with lipids. Tissue needs prolonged washing after fixation. Interferes with most staining methods. Widely used for electron microscopy.

Alcohol and *acetone.* Coagulant fixatives used only for special purposes (p. 24).

Fixation in practice

It is unlikely that any single fixing fluid will fulfil all needs. On the other hand, it is plainly necessary to limit the number of fluids in everyday use. The methods that are described in detail below will satisfy all the ordinary requirements of a routine laboratory. Some will be used infrequently; others are virtually interchangeable and will be used or not according to personal preference. For some purposes the best results are obtained if tissue is fixed in two fixing fluids, one after the other. The first fluid is then said to provide *primary fixation* and the second fluid *secondary fixation*. In many laboratories, formalin-saline (or neutral buffered formalin solution) is used almost exclusively, but there is much to be said for providing a quick-acting fixing fluid as an alternative for urgent biopsy fragments. If this is supplied in small containers, it will not be used for unsuitably large specimens. For many years we have provided operating theatres with small containers of Heidenhain's Susa. This has given good results but we are prepared to believe that Bouin's fluid or mercuric-chloride-formalin would be equally satisfactory.

If a fairly rapid section is needed from a large specimen, another approach must be followed, since no rapidly acting fixing fluid will penetrate well. When a suitable fragment may be cut from the fresh specimen, this can be fixed in Susa or a similar fluid. If, however, the specimen is already partly fixed in formalin-saline or neutral buffered formalin solution, it is not wise to transfer a piece from it to Susa; although Bouin's fluid or mercuric-chloride-formalin may be used as a secondary fixative with good results.

Whatever fixing fluid or combination of fluids is preferred, it is important to ensure that an adequate volume is used (about 20 times the volume of the tissue in it). Economy at this stage is one of the four common causes of bad fixation. The others are: too short a time for full fixation, the use of poorly penetrating rapid fixatives for large pieces, and allowing a specimen to settle to the bottom of a container so closely that fluid cannot circulate between the tissue and the glass.

Individual fixing fluids

Most of the formulae given below are of great age. In some cases a number of closely-related formulae exist, but in each case we have given details of one that we have found satisfactory for its purpose. One or another of these methods will suffice for any ordinary specimen but details of certain fixing fluids used exclusively for special methods are given elsewhere (e.g. in the chapters that deal with the nervous system and cytology).

Formalin-Saline
(Formol-saline; formal-saline)

A simple fixing fluid suitable for almost any specimen. Rarely interferes with subsequent staining; suitable for museum specimens. Duration of fixation not critical.

Formalin   100 ml.
Sodium chloride   9 g.
Distilled water   900 ml.

Fixation for 12-48 hours will suffice for an average-sized block of tissue, which may then be transferred to 50 per cent alcohol.

Merits

(i) After fixation, tissue may be processed and embedded in paraffin, special waxes, or nitrocellulose, or may be used for frozen sections.

(ii) Decalcifying methods work well after formalin-saline.

(iii) Any routine staining method may be used after this fixing fluid, although some (e.g. trichrome stains) may not give their most brilliant results.

(iv) Penetration is good, so that formalin-saline may be used to fix large specimens. For this reason it is suitable for museum specimens, and also because colours may be restored after its use. (This is impossible when any fixative other than formalin is used.) It may also be useful to restore colour before photographs are taken. The time needed to fix a large specimen will depend on its size and density.

(v) Tissue does not become unduly hard in formalin-saline, even after many months.

(vi) Tissue may be transferred from formalin-saline to a wide variety of other fixing fluids for special purposes (secondary fixation). Examples include mercuric-chloride-formalin for trichrome stains and potassium dichromate for chromaffin granules.

Drawbacks

(i) Fixation is slow, so that formalin-saline is unsatisfactory for some purposes (e.g. urgent biopsy work).

(ii) Sections from tissue fixed in formalin-saline show evidence of considerable shrinkage. This is not due to the fixing fluid (which actually causes slight swelling) but to the dehydrating alcohols which cause more shrinkage after formalin than after other fixatives.

(iii) Formaldehyde reacts with haemoglobin to form acid formaldehyde haematin. This shows itself as a brown deposit in sections from tissue fixed in formalin-saline, especially if the tissue contains much blood. A method is available for the removal of this deposit from sections (p. 84) but it is not applicable before every stain. The deposit is less conspicuous in tissue fixed for shorter periods, or fixed in a buffered fluid (see below).

(iv) Formalin-saline becomes acid on storage as the formaldehyde is oxidized to formic acid. This process is slow, but tissue stored for several months will often fail to yield good staining results.

Neutral Buffered Formalin Solution

Similar to formalin-saline but with advantages (Lillie, 1948).

Formalin	100 ml.
Sodium dihydrogen phosphate (monohydrated)	4 g.
Disodium hydrogen phosphate (anhydrous)	6·5 g.
Distilled water	900 ml.

Dissolve the salts in some water with gentle heat, then mix with the rest of the water and the formalin.

Merits

This fluid has all the merits of formalin-saline, and may be interchanged with it. The buffer salts stabilize the pH, conferring two additional merits:

(i) Fixation deposit (acid formaldehyde haematin) is less conspicuous.

(ii) Tissue may be stored for longer periods without loss of staining quality and without the loss of such tissue constituents as iron, calcium, and copper.

Drawbacks

Fixation is slow, and shrinkage is considerable (see Drawbacks i and ii in formalin-saline above).

Mercuric-Chloride-Formalin

(Formal-sublimate; Lendrum's fixative)

A quicker fixative than formalin-saline. Suitable for most purposes. The proportion of mercuric chloride varies in different published formulae but we have used this one for many years with satisfactory results.

Mercuric chloride (sat. aqueous solution)	900 ml.
Formalin	100 ml.
1% aqueous acid fuchsin	a few drops

A thin piece of tissue will be fixed in 6 hours but may be left for longer without deterioration (up to a few weeks). Fixed pieces may be transferred to 80 per cent alcohol. The acid fuchsin tints tissue, making it conspicuous in the paraffin block;

C

if dye is not added, the tissue is hard to see because mercuric chloride whitens it.

Merits

(i) Provided that pieces are thin (2–3 mm.), fixation is much more rapid than in formalin-saline with no greater distortion of the tissue.

(ii) The rapid hardening effect is particularly useful when dealing with unusually soft tissue (e.g. pieces of a gelatinous tumour).

(iii) Whole specimens are fixed in formalin-saline rather than mercuric-chloride-formalin, but pieces from such specimens may be transferred to the latter fluid, to hasten fixation or to improve particular special stains.

(iv) Nuclear chromatin is more distinct than after formalin-saline.

(v) Connective tissue may be demonstrated particularly well after mercuric-chloride-formalin (e.g. by trichrome methods or elastic stains).

Drawbacks

(i) Poor penetration makes this fixing fluid unsuitable for thick pieces of tissue or for any uncut surgical specimens larger than biopsy fragments.

(ii) A fixation deposit is almost invariable after this fixing fluid. This must be removed from the sections (p. 84).

(iii) Mercuric-chloride-formalin is not suitable if frozen sections are required. The hardening effect makes tissue difficult to cut by this method. Moreover, the mercury salts take the edge off a microtome knife.

(iv) Silver impregnation methods are possible after this fixing fluid but the results are mediocre.

(v) This fixing fluid does not suit lymphoid tissue (lymph nodes, spleen, tonsils, Peyer's patches, etc.). Unlike other tissues, these become finely fissured during sectioning. Although at a glance the damage appears insignificant, the detailed histological picture may be ruined.

(vi) Like any other fluid that contains mercuric chloride, this should not be allowed to come into contact with metal other than a special mercury-resistant stainless steel. When mercuric-chloride-formalin is used at the first stage of an automatic processing machine, suitable tissue containers must be chosen.

Heidenhain's Susa

An excellent rapid fixing fluid for small specimens such as surgical biopsy fragments (Heidenhain, 1916).

Stock solution

Mercuric chloride	45 g.
Distilled water	800 ml.
Sodium chloride	5 g.
Trichloracetic acid	20 g.
Glacial acetic acid	40 ml.

Dissolve the mercuric chloride in the distilled water, using heat. When cold add the other reagents. This stock solution may be kept indefinitely.

For use

Stock solution	80 ml.
Formalin	20 ml.

This fluid begins to deteriorate after about a month or two. Small fragments will be well-fixed in 3-4 hours and may then be transferred to 80 or 90 per cent alcohol, or even to undiluted alcohol.

Merits

(i) Particularly suitable for small surgical fragments because fixing time is short and tissue is transferred directly to a high-grade dehydrating alcohol.

(ii) The moderate hardening effect makes it easy to cut suitably orientated pieces from fixed specimens and is also of considerable assistance during section cutting.

(iii) This rapid method is recommended for use in laboratories where the routine fixing fluid is formalin-saline on its own or formalin-saline followed by mercuric-chloride-formalin. After fixation in Susa, sections resemble those from tissue fixed in formalin-saline or mercuric-chloride-formalin. The architectural appearances are similar since Susa causes little distortion. Staining qualities are also similar provided that care is taken not to overstain with acidic dyes (e.g. eosin). Nuclear fixation is better than by formalin-saline, but red blood corpuscles are often distorted and rendered refractile.

(iv) Unlike most fixing fluids that contain mercuric chloride, Susa produces little or no fixation deposit.

(v) Most staining methods work well after Susa. Inadequate results, however, may be obtained with some trichrome stains and silver impregnation methods. The fixing fluid is also unsuitable if iron, calcium or copper salts are being sought, since it may remove small deposits of these substances from tissue.

Drawbacks

(i) Only thin pieces may be used since penetration is relatively poor.

(ii) Tissue left in Susa for longer than 24 hours becomes unduly hard. After fixation, the fluid should be replaced by 80 per cent alcohol, in which the tissue may be stored for several months without deterioration.

(iii) Mercury salts attack metals. Susa, therefore, shares this drawback with mercuric-chloride-formalin (see Note vi above).

Bouin's Fluid
(P.F.A.)

An alternative to Susa, although not quite so rapid (Bouin, 1897).

Picric acid (sat. aqueous solution)	75 ml.
Formalin	25 ml.
Glacial acetic acid	5 ml.

Small fragments will be well-fixed in 6 hours but may be left indefinitely without deterioration. Fixed pieces must be transferred to 70 per cent alcohol; washing in water will cause damage.

Merits

(i) A fairly rapid method.

(ii) The fluid causes little distortion and does not produce undue hardness even after a long period.

(iii) Staining methods, including trichrome stains, work well. The fluid has been recommended for the preservation of glycogen but it is better to use an alcoholic picric acid fixative (p. 152).

(iv) The bright yellow colour makes tissue easy to see during embedding and section-cutting.

Drawbacks

(i) Penetration is relatively poor.

(ii) Frozen sections for fat are unsatisfactory after this fluid since water dissolves the protein-picrate complexes on which fixation largely depends.

(iii) Sections of kidney fixed in Bouin's fluid are unsatisfactory; for this particular tissue another fixing fluid should be used.

Carnoy's Fluid

Occasionally used in routine laboratories when very rapid paraffin sections are required (Carnoy, 1887).

Alcohol	60 ml.
Chloroform	30 ml.
Glacial acetic acid	10 ml.

Provided that thin (2 mm.) pieces are used, fixation will be complete in 90 minutes. This time can be reduced to 45 minutes at 56°C if a thinner piece (1 mm.) is sliced off after 15 minutes when the surface is hard. (If a very thin piece of fresh tissue is placed in the fluid in the first instance, it will be likely to curl.) Fixed tissue may be transferred directly to undiluted alcohol.

Merits

(i) The most rapid fixing fluid that is suitable for paraffin sections.

(ii) One of the few fixing fluids that contains no formalin. Suitable, therefore, for certain protein staining methods, such as the oxidized tannin-azo method (Dixon, 1959).

(iii) Does not dissolve glycogen.

Drawbacks

(i) Although nuclear detail is excellent, cytoplasm is poorly preserved and may be largely stripped from the cells. Red blood corpuscles are either lysed or coagulated into amorphous brown masses.

(ii) Tissue suffers severe shrinkage, becoming hard and brittle so that fragmentation is apt to occur during section cutting.

(iii) Because of these effects, tissue should not be left in the fluid for more than a few hours at room temperature (or 24 hours at 4°C). To store the tissue for longer periods, the fluid should be replaced by 80 per cent alcohol.

(iv) The fixing fluid dissolves lipids.

Helly's Fluid

(Formol-Zenker; Zenker-Formalin)

A tedious method which may, nevertheless, be worthwhile when fine cellular detail is required (Helly, 1903).

Stock solution

Potassium dichromate	25 g.
Mercuric chloride	50 g.
Sodium sulphate	10 g.
Distilled water	1000 ml.

Dissolve all the salts together with gentle heat. This solution will keep indefinitely.

For use

Stock solution	100 ml.
Formalin	5 ml.

Do not mix these two solutions until the fixing fluid is required since the mixture begins to deteriorate at once. Thin pieces of tissue (2-3 mm.) will be well-fixed in 24-36 hours. They may be left in the fluid up to a total of 36-48 hours but longer periods should be avoided. Tissue is transferred from fixing fluid to running tap water for 6-12 hours and then to 50 per cent alcohol. For delicate specimens running tap water should be avoided; it is better to use many changes of formalin-saline during 24 hours. For longer storage than 48 hours, transfer the tissue to formalin-saline.

Merits

(i) This fluid is excellent for nuclear and cytoplasmic detail. It is therefore, recommended for tissues such as bone marrow.

(ii) Tissue architecture is well preserved with minimal distortion. The fluid produces a useful amount of hardening.

(iii) Helly's fluid may be used as a secondary fixing fluid for tissue that has been partly fixed in formalin-saline. The results obtained by using this sequence of fixing fluids are similar to those obtained with Helly's fluid above. It is said that sometimes they may be even better (Wallington, 1955).

(iv) Decalcifying fluids work well after Helly's fluid.

Drawbacks

(i) The fixed pieces need to be washed. This is tedious and delays processing. Unless washing is thorough, a yellowish brown precipitate forms within the tissue; removal of this precipitate (p. 86) is difficult.

(ii) Ribbons of sections cut from tissue fixed in Helly's fluid may be difficult to handle because they are more liable to become charged with static electricity than other ribbons. When this occurs, the sections also tend to wash off the slides during staining.

(iii) The instability of the fixing fluid is an inconvenience, particularly when it is used outside the laboratory.

(iv) Since it contains mercuric chloride, this fluid will produce a fixation deposit which must be removed from the sections (p. 84).

(v) The mercuric chloride in Helly's fluid also attacks metals except for a special mercury-resistant stainless steel.

Note

We have preferred to use the name Helly's fluid because it avoids the possibility of confusion which is apt to occur when the name

Zenker is introduced. Zenker (1894) published a fixing fluid with the following formula:

Distilled water	100·0 ml.
Mercuric chloride	5·0 g.
Potassium dichromate	2·5 g.
Sodium sulphate	1·0 g.
Glacial acetic acid	5·0 ml.

It will be noted that this original formula contains acetic acid, so that it is quite unnecessary for the word acetic to be added (Zenker-acetic; acetic-Zenker) as is frequently done nowadays.

Helly (1903) published his formula several years later. He described it as a modification of Zenker's fixing fluid, and recommended it for lymphoid tissue. The only changes that he made to Zenker's original formula were the omission of acetic acid and the addition of formalin; all other constituents remained in similar proportions. Nevertheless, these changes completely alter the character of the fixing fluid, since the action of strongly acidified dichromate (in Zenker's fluid) is identical with that of chromic acid, whereas Helly's fluid contains unaltered dichromate ions which produce a quite different effect (Baker, 1966).

Flemming's Fluid

(Flemming's strong fluid)

A fluid which enables lipid to be demonstrated in paraffin sections. Otherwise less satisfactory than the fluids already described. Used infrequently in routine laboratories. (Flemming, 1884.)

Chromic acid (1% aqueous)	15 ml.
Osmium tetroxide (2% aqueous)	4 ml.
Glacial acetic acid	1 ml.

Mix immediately before use. Very thin pieces of tissue (about 1 mm.) will be well-fixed in 12 hours and must then be washed thoroughly in running water before transfer to 50 per cent alcohol. Tissue should not be stored in the fluid but may be stored in 80 per cent alcohol after washing and then treating with 50 per cent alcohol.

Merit

When tissue that contains lipid droplets is treated with osmium tetroxide, a black precipitate forms in the droplets. This is not dissolved by alcohol, chloroform, benzene, or paraffin wax; the lipid droplets are therefore demonstrated as black granules in paraffin sections. The precipitate is, however, slightly soluble in xylene or toluene (Baker, 1958) so that these solvents should not be used for clearing or dewaxing, although we have found D.P.X. to be a satisfactory mounting medium.

Drawbacks

(i) Penetration is poor and fixation is uneven, so that the method can only be useful when fine detail is wanted: it would be quite useless for assessment of general tissue structure.

(ii) Few staining methods give good results after Flemming's fluid. Unstained sections are satisfactory if lipid droplets are the only requirement. Nuclei are demonstrable by Heidenhain's iron haematoxylin (p. 105), and other tissue components may be stained tolerably well by the picro-Mallory trichrome method (p. 117).

(iii) The fluid is unsatisfactory for routine use because of its poor keeping qualities and the high cost of osmium tetroxide.

(iv) Thorough washing is needed after fixation.

Alcohol

Used only for a few special purposes. Thin pieces of tissue (1-2 mm.) in undiluted alcohol will be fixed in 2-3 hours; they should not be left for longer than 6 hours. Tissue in 80 per cent alcohol will be fixed equally quickly and may be left in the fluid indefinitely.

Merits

(i) The only satisfactory fixative for some histochemical methods.
(ii) Glycogen is not dissolved.
(iii) Preserves Nissl substance in neurones.
(iv) Suitable for smears (p. 323).

Drawbacks

(i) Penetration is poor.
(ii) Alcohol causes excessive hardening and shrinkage.
(iii) Lipids are dissolved.

Acetone

Used only for a few special purposes. Thin pieces of tissue (1-2 mm.) will be fixed in 1-2 hours at room temperature or in 24 hours at 0-4°C. The tissue is dehydrated in several changes of acetone and may then be cleared in benzene.

Merits

(i) The only satisfactory fixative for some histochemical methods.
(ii) Has been used as a fixative when very rapid paraffin sections are required although we have had much better results with Carnoy's fluid.

Drawbacks

    (i) Acetone causes excessive hardening and shrinkage.
    (ii) Nuclear chromatin is poorly preserved.
    (iii) Lipids are dissolved.

Alcoholic Formalin

Usually used for secondary fixation after formalin-saline. Occasionally useful for primary fixation for special purposes.

Formalin	100 ml.
Alcohol	800 ml.
Distilled water	100 ml.

Thin pieces (2-3 mm.) of fresh tissue will be fixed in 6-8 hours. When the fluid is used for secondary fixation, tissue should first be fixed for 12-24 hours in formalin-saline and then transferred to alcoholic formalin for about 12 hours. Beyond 18 hours no further improvement is likely. Fixed tissue is transferred to 80 per cent alcohol.

Merits

    (i) When alcoholic formalin is used for secondary fixation, tissue becomes harder than after formalin-saline alone. Sections are easier to cut and staining is more precise. The improved quality of sections from necropsy material and non-urgent surgical specimens fully justifies the additional trouble. The results are as good as those produced by secondary fixation in mercuric-chloride-formalin although they differ in appearance. Alcoholic formalin is much cheaper: mercuric-chloride-formalin is quicker.

    (ii) Although rarely suitable for primary fixation, alcoholic formalin may be used for carbohydrates, Nissl substance, or metals (calcium, iron and copper), which it preserves better than aqueous fluids. Undiluted alcohol probably preserves these substances even better, but causes much more distortion and will only be used in special circumstances.

Drawbacks

    (i) Alcoholic formalin dissolves most lipids.

    (ii) If used for primary fixation, alcoholic formalin does not penetrate well. Fortunately this is not so when it is used for secondary fixation.

    (iii) Hardening and shrinkage are too great when alcoholic formalin is used for primary fixation. For secondary fixation after formalin-saline, however, the hardening effect is not great and actually improves the tissue, which also shows less evidence of shrinkage.

CHAPTER 3

Dehydration and Clearing

General notes. Notes on dehydration. Notes on clearing. Automatic processing machines. Processing schedules. Common errors.

IN ORDER to cut sections, it is necessary to make the tissue completely rigid. This may be done by freezing it (p. 274) or by impregnating it with, and surrounding it by, a solid substance. Occasionally a solid wax is used that is miscible with water (p. 36) but for routine work it is usual to use paraffin wax.

Since paraffin wax will not mix with the water which forms a large proportion of all animal and plant tissues, it is necessary to remove that water before replacing it with wax. For special purposes this may be done by freeze-drying or freeze-substitution, but these methods are beyond the scope of routine laboratories, which must make use of chemical methods. Ideally the replacement of water by wax would be accomplished by an intermediary which was freely miscible both with water and with wax; such substances exist (an example is dioxane) but they are not widely used.

The popular and long established method is to use two intermediaries between water and wax. The first of these is freely miscible with water and capable of replacing it; this is therefore known as a *dehydrating agent*, and the process whereby it replaces water as *dehydration*. In practice one of the lower alcohols is nearly always used as a dehydrating agent and the choice for routine purposes is governed by expense. In Britian the cheapest is commercial ethyl alcohol (ethanol) but in other countries isopropanol is cheaper. For special purposes, butanol or cellosolve (ethylene glycol monoethyl ether) may be used.

The second intermediary must be freely miscible with paraffin wax, and will therefore be chosen from amongst the relatively inexpensive fat solvents. The solvent chosen must obviously be freely miscible with the dehydrating alcohol; it should also cause a minimum of distortion of the tissue. It is, perhaps, unfortunate that the name clearing agent continues to be used for this fat solvent. The process was, reasonably enough, referred to as *clearing* at a time when the solvents in routine use (xylene and cedarwood oil) rendered the piece of tissue translucent, but many of the so-called clearing agents in routine use nowadays have by no means such a striking effect.

Notes on dehydration

As already mentioned, the dehydrating agent in common use is ethanol; it is, however unnecessary to use the chemically pure reagent. Throughout this book the name *alcohol* is used to denote industrial methylated spirit (74° O.P.),which is quite satisfactory for dehydration and for almost every other laboratory purpose; the name *ethanol* is reserved for chemically pure ethanol (sometimes known as absolute alcohol). When dilutions of alcohol are mentioned, these are made according to volume, but in any case there is no need for great precision in the preparation of dilutions. It is, however, preferable to use distilled water for making dilutions, since the subsequent staining results are unsatisfactory in some regions when tap water is used.

During dehydration, tissue is liable to suffer distortion. This can be minimized by transferring the fixed tissue to dilute alcohol and from there to stronger and stronger concentrations until it reaches undiluted alcohol. The liability to distortion is greater after some fixing fluids than others. Moreover, some fixing fluids have the merit that tissue may be transferrred from them directly into a strong concentration of alcohol. The total time taken for dehydration and the starting point will therefore depend to a large extent in the method of fixation that has been used. The schedule will also depend upon the size of the piece, and whether the tissue is compact or loose textured. It is not, however, wise to use unnecessarily slow dehydrating schedules since dilute alcohol makes tissue soft and strong alcohol has an undesirable hardening effect. If tissue has to be left for any length of time (e.g. overnight), it is possible to steer a middle course by using alcohol of moderate strength (70-90 per cent) in which the tissue may be left indefinitely.

Notes on clearing

The transfer of tissue from alcohol to clearing agent is not as likely to cause distortion as the transfer from fixing fluid to alcohol. Some specimens, however, seem to be particularly sensitive to sudden changes; these include organs that are partly dense and partly soft (e.g. eyes; bone with marrow), laminated structures (e.g. thrombus), and pieces of brain. For these specimens especially, it is wise to make the change less abrupt by introducing a mixture of equal parts of alcohol and clearing agent. We use such a mixture whenever possible during the routine processing of every kind of tissue.

The time taken for complete clearing depends on the agent used and also on the compactness of the tissue and the size of the piece. Specific recommendations will be found in the schedules of dehydration and clearing that appear in this chapter. Not all clearing agents produce their effects at the same rate so that one of them should not be substituted for another in any schedule without careful thought. Moreover, some agents produce unwanted distortion; this might be disastrous if they were applied to particularly sensitive tissues. Whichever agent is used, it is essential that the process of clearing be thorough; incompletely cleared tissue cannot be impregnated by paraffin wax. Thorough clearing does not, however, demand absolute purity of the chemical agent used; commercial grades are as effective as pure reagents which would be many times more expensive.

The following list includes the clearing agents in common use and their most important qualities.

Xylene. The most rapid agent in common use. Causes great distortion and hardening. Goes milky when incompletely dehydrated tissue is added; this information may be valuable in urgent cases. Inflammable. Non-toxic but may cause dermatitis. Cheap. Suitable only when speed is essential. Unsuitable for tissue that contains much blood or collagen, for brain and for specimens made up of hard and soft elements (e.g. eyes).

Toluene. Similar to xylene although slightly slower and causing a little less hardening and distortion. Inflammable.

Benzene. Relatively quick-acting but less so than xylene or toluene. Causes less distortion although this may still be considerable. May be used as a routine clearing agent for most tissues. Unsuitable for brain or eyes. Toxic. Inflammable.

Chloroform. Much slower than the agents already mentioned. Causes far less distortion and hardening. Expensive. Non-inflammable. Toxic and stupefying. Must not be subjected to great heat. Suitable for routine use for any type of tissue when quality rather than speed is important and cost is irrelevant.

Carbon tetrachloride. ⎱ As good as chloroform in routine use and
Trichloroethylene. ⎰ much cheaper. Carbon tetrachloride is toxic whereas trichloroethylene is merely stupefying; both are non-inflammable. Neither must be subjected to great heat; trichloroethylene must not be subjected to direct sunlight.

Cedarwood oil. A very slow clearing agent, used only for special purposes. Causes no hardening or distortion however long the tissue spends in it. Tissue may be transferred from 95 per cent alcohol. Very expensive. Especially suitable for large pieces and for sensitive tissues (e.g. embryos, brain, eyes).

Automatic processing machines

Dehydration and clearing may be carried out by machines more readily than any other process in the routine histological laboratory. All that is required is a mechanism for transferring the pieces of tissue through a series of containers in accordance with a predetermined time schedule. Many schedules for dehydration and clearing need more hours than are available in a single working day. Automatic processing machines can be left to work overnight and consequently the processes are completed sooner. The incorporation of a mechanism that agitates the pieces of tissue whilst they are in the various fluids reduces the time still further.

Sometimes the first stage of the machine is occupied by a container of fixing fluid; if this arrangement is used it is necessary to ensure that the tissue containers are not attacked by the fixing fluid when the latter contains mercuric chloride (p. 18). At the other end of the process it is almost universal practice to put containers of molten paraffin wax at the last two stages of the machine, so that when the tissue is removed it is already impregnated. (An account of impregnation may be found in the next chapter.)

What fluids are used at the other stages will depend in part on the method used for fixation. It would be pointless to list all the possible schedules that could be devised by the permutation and combination of various dilutions of alcohol with various clearing agents. Our own schedules are set below, but there is no reason why everyone should not design his own. When doing so it is worth trying to arrange for the tissue to spend a short time in several containers of undiluted alcohol and clearing agent rather than a longer time in a single container of each of these fluids. The time spent at each stage is governed by the size of the specimens. These times need not necessarily be equal, but if the machine is equipped to carry two or more batches of tissue in series there is much to be said for using equal times at every stage.

To renew the fluids in the containers of an automatic processing machine, it is not necessary to replace all of them. If the first container of undiluted alcohol is discarded and each of the succeeding ones moved back one place, it is only necessary to put fresh fluid in the last container to obtain satisfactory results. Exactly the same procedure is followed for the containers of clearing agent and paraffin wax.

Processing schedules

The following schedules have been found to be sufficient for the common requirements of a routine laboratory. For extraordinary requirements, suitable schedules may be found elsewhere (large pieces, p. 303; brain, p. 228; eyes, p. 312; extra-rapid paraffin methods, p. 308).

Manual processing schedule I

A routine schedule for use after formalin-saline, neutral buffered formalin solution, or Helly's fluid. If used after other fixing fluids, one or more of the early stages are omitted. Thus after Bouin's fluid start at stage 2, after mercuric-chloride-formalin or alcoholic formalin at stage 3, after Heidenhain's Susa at stage 4 or 5. Satisfactory for pieces up to 4 mm. thick; unnecessarily slow for very small pieces fixed in rapid-acting fixatives. Chloroform or carbon tetrachloride may be used in place of trichloroethylene.

1. 50% alcohol, 2–3 hours.
2. 70% alcohol, 2–3 hours.
3. 80% alcohol, 2–3 hours.

4. 90% alcohol overnight.
5. Alcohol I, 2–3 hours.
6. Alcohol II, 2–3 hours.
7. Alcohol III, 2–3 hours.
8. Trichloroethylene overnight.
9. Molten paraffin wax I, $1\frac{1}{2}$–$2\frac{1}{2}$ hours.
10. Wax II, $1\frac{1}{2}$–$2\frac{1}{2}$ hours.
11. Wax III, $1\frac{1}{2}$–$2\frac{1}{2}$ hours.
12. Embed in fresh wax.

Manual processing schedule II

A quicker schedule which should only be used for thin pieces (up to 2 mm. thick). Particularly suitable for tissue that can be transferred directly from fixing fluid to fairly strong alcohol (e.g. after Bouin's fluid). Tissue from mercuric-chloride-formalin or alcoholic formalin starts at stage 2, from Susa or Carnoy's fluid at stage 4. If the tissue were fixed in formalin-saline, neutral buffered formalin solution, or Helly's fluid, it would need 1–$1\frac{1}{2}$ hours 50 per cent alcohol before stage 1. Chloroform or carbon tetrachloride may be used in place of trichloroethylene.

1. 70% alcohol, 1–$1\frac{1}{2}$ hours.
2. 80% alcohol, 1–$1\frac{1}{2}$ hours.
3. 90% alcohol, 1–$1\frac{1}{2}$ hours.
4. Alcohol I, 1–$1\frac{1}{2}$ hours.
5. Alcohol II, 1–$1\frac{1}{2}$ hours.
6. Alcohol III, 1–$1\frac{1}{2}$ hours.
7. Trichloroethylene overnight.
8. Molten paraffin wax I, 1–$1\frac{1}{2}$ hours.
9. Wax II, 1–$1\frac{1}{2}$ hours.
10. Wax III, 1–$1\frac{1}{2}$ hours.
11. Embed in fresh wax.

Automatic processing schedule IA

The automated counterpart of Manual schedule I above. The same modifications may be made according to the fixing fluid used, and the same alternative clearing agents may be substituted.

1. 50% alcohol, 2 hours.
2. 70% alcohol, 2 hours.
3. 80% alcohol, 2 hours.
4. 90% alcohol, 2 hours.
5. Alcohol I, 2 hours.
6. Alcohol II, 2 hours.
7. Alcohol III, 2 hours.
8. Trichloroethylene I, 2 hours.
9. Trichloroethylene II, 2 hours.
10. Trichloroethylene III, 2 hours.
11. Molten paraffin wax I, 2 hours.
12. Wax II, 2 hours.

Tissue is then removed from the machine into a third container of wax and is subsequently embedded in fresh wax. The third container of wax may be at reduced atmospheric pressure (see next chapter).

Automatic processing schedule IB

We have preferred to use this processing schedule for routine use. It is a variant of IA above, suitable for tissue that has undergone secondary fixation in alcoholic formalin after primary fixation in neutral buffered formalin solution. The provision of two containers of 90 per cent alcohol enables two batches of tissue to be loaded onto the machine in series without awaiting the first change.

1. 90% alcohol, 2 hours.
2. 90% alcohol, 2 hours.
3. Alcohol I, 2 hours.
4. Alcohol II, 2 hours.
5. Alcohol III, 2 hours.
6. $\begin{cases} \text{Alcohol} \\ \text{Trichloroethylene} \end{cases}$ equal parts, 2 hours.
7. Trichloroethylene I, 2 hours.
8. Trichloroethylene II, 2 hours.
9. Trichloroethylene III, 2 hours.
10. Molten paraffin wax I, 2 hours.
11. Wax II, 3 hours.

Tissue is then removed from the machine into a third container of wax, and subsequently embedded in fresh wax.

Automatic processing schedule II

The automated counterpart of Manual schedule II above. The notes to that schedule apply equally well to this one.

1. 70% alcohol, 1½ hours.
2. 80% alcohol, 1½ hours.
3. 90% alcohol, 1½ hours.
4. Alcohol I, 1½ hours.
5. Alcohol II, 1½ hours.
6. Alcohol III, 1½ hours.
7. $\begin{cases} \text{Alcohol} \\ \text{Trichloroethylene} \end{cases}$ equal parts, 1½ hours.
8. Trichloroethylene I, 1½ hours.
9. Trichloroethylene II, 1½ hours.
10. Trichloroethylene III, 1½ hours.
11. Molten paraffin wax I, 2 hours.
12. Wax II, 2 hours.

Tissue is then removed from the machine into a third container of wax, and subsequently embedded in fresh wax.

Common errors in dehydration and clearing

(i) If attempts are made to dehydrate and clear thick pieces of tissue quickly, the fluids do not penetrate the middle of the pieces and the wax blocks will be soft.

(ii) A similar result occurs when tissue has been in close contact with the bottom of a vessel, or with another piece of tissue. The latter occurs when too many pieces are processed in one container.

(iii) After use, the tissue containers of an automatic processing machine are covered with wax. If this is not removed from the perforations, it will prevent free diffusion of fluid when the container is used again.

(iv) If the alcohol and clearing agent on an automatic processing machine are not renewed often enough, dehydration and clearing will be inadequate.

(v) All the tissue on an automatic processing machine must be immersed in fluid at each stage. This requires practice in applying Archimedes' principle if flooding is to be avoided.

(vi) Automatic processing machines occasionally develop faults such as failure of the agitating mechanism or of the heaters which maintain the wax in a molten state. The usual cause is fracture of an electric cable due to frequent handling but sometimes wax contaminates electrical contacts and interrupts the current. Solidification of

D

wax in a container usually results in a batch of tissue becoming dried up and irrevocably damaged.

More rarely the machine fails to follow its expected schedule of changes. This is almost always due to carelessness in setting the programming mechanism, but may on occasions be brought about by a severe drop in the voltage of the mains supply. In our experience it is exceptionally rare for the machine itself to be at fault if it has been properly maintained.

CHAPTER 4

Wax Embedding

General notes. Paraffin wax. Hardened paraffin wax. Impregnation. 'Vacuum embedding'. Embedding. Trimming. Wax blocks. Schedules. Common errors.

TISSUE is embedded in wax to make a block sufficiently rigid for uniformly thin sections to be cut. The block may be made harder by cooling it, but for practical purposes it is necessary to use a wax that is solid at room temperature. In addition to encasing the piece of tissue, wax must penetrate it, replacing the fluid in which it is saturated (usually a clearing agent). This process is called *impregnation* and takes place more rapidly if the molten wax is hot. However, heat will cause considerable deterioration of tissue, so that a wax must be chosen which has as low a melting point as is consistent with solidity at room temperature. A series of sections cut from a wax block adhere to each other to form a ribbon. These sections are easier to handle than single sections so that, in this respect, waxes have a decided advantage over other embedding media such as nitrocellulose.

Ideally a piece of tissue embedded in wax should remain unchanged for long periods; for this reason an inert and stable wax is preferable.

In practice the customary embedding medium for many years has been paraffin wax. This may be improved by various additives, some of which are freely obtainable although others are incorporated only in proprietary waxes of unpublished formula. A comparative study of these waxes has been made by Headden and McWilliams (1968).

Although the classical embedding medium is paraffin wax (long-chain aliphatic hydrocarbons), there are many other organic substances with large molecular weight which have similar properties. Among these, esters have been used as embedding media; a wax of suitable qualities can be made from a mixture of esters and is therefore known as ester wax (Steedman, 1960). This is soluble in alcohol so that clearing agents are not required; it also makes harder blocks than paraffin wax of the same melting-point.

Polyethylene glycols of sufficiently high molecular weight also have a waxy consistency. These are miscible with water and are therefore called water-soluble waxes. Tissues embedded in water-soluble wax does not need preliminary dehydration and clearing. For routine use, however, this merit is more than offset by two drawbacks: first, it is difficult to find a fluid which does not dissolve the wax and which is therefore suitable for spreading the sections before they are mounted onto slides. Secondly, the waxes are hygroscopic so that blocks prepared from them are difficult to store. The use of water-soluble waxes is described in detail by Steedman (1960), who also provides useful information about every kind of embedding medium.

Paraffin wax

Paraffin waxes are not pure chemicals; they are mixtures of hydrocarbons. Many different mixtures are available and each is known by its melting-point. For histological use in a temperate climate, a wax is usually chosen that has a melting-point in the region of 52-56°C. Where it is possible to segregate soft samples of tissue (e.g. liver; kidney), better results are obtained by using wax of lower melting-point (45-50°C), thus avoiding unnecessary distortion due to heating the tissue. Such wax is not, however, rigid enough for all tissue (especially fibrous or muscular tissue).

Crude commercial paraffin wax was long used for histological purposes. This, however, is inconsistent in behaviour, so that it is better to use waxes that have been prepared expressly for histological use. Waxes of this type may be obtained in bulk from oil refining companies or their agents, or may be purchased from histological suppliers.

It is unnecessary to filter new wax of this type, although when pieces are used for a second time they will need filtering. The most convenient arrangement is a wax dispenser which incorporates heating elements and a temperature control as well as a filter. If a wax dispenser is not available the well-heated molten wax may be poured through coarse filter paper such as is used for bacteriological media (e.g. Hyduro 904½). If only a small quantity is required, this may be obtained by putting broken pieces of solid wax in a filter funnel and filtering in an incubator.

Hardened paraffin wax

Tough tissue that contains much collagen requires a harder embedding medium than tissue that is composed predominantly of cells. So also do pieces of brain and, above all, specimens that are made up partly of tough tissue and partly of cellular tissue. For specimens like these it is worth while using waxes that are harder than ordinary or modified commercial paraffin wax. Such waxes are also helpful when sections thinner than 5 μ are required.

Among the substances that have been added to paraffin wax to harden it are beeswax, rubber, dental impression wax, asphalt, and bayberry wax. We have used 10 per cent beeswax as an additive with satisfactory results; others have preferred 6 per cent dental impression wax (Alston No. 2 Toughwax), or a combination of 0·3–1 per cent rubber and either 0·1 per cent asphalt or 1–5 per cent beeswax. Silverton and Anderson (1961) quote several formulae for hardened waxes. Most of these are obtainable ready-made from specialist suppliers who also market proprietary waxes, the formulae of which remains a trade secret. Popular waxes of this kind are: Fibrowax, Paramat, and Paraplast, all of which are suitable for routine work. An even harder (and more expensive) wax is Ralwax, which has the added merit that sections can be cut with little or no freezing. We have used Fibrowax and Ralwax I (formerly known as V.A.5) for special purposes with satisfactory results, although the lack of translucency (especially of Ralwax) is a nuisance when sections have to be cut from blocks that contain multiple tissue fragments or irregular pieces.

Impregnation

The change from clearing agent to wax causes less damage to delicate tissue than the change from alcohol to clearing agent. Most routine specimens withstand the transition well enough to give acceptable results. Nevertheless, when unusually sensitive tissues (e.g. embryos or eyes) are processed, it is helpful to use an intermediate mixture of equal parts of clearing agent and wax. This mixture is only fluid if warm, and is usually used at the temperature of the wax incubator, so that the container must be tightly closed to avoid evaporation of the clearing agent.

Solid blocks can only be obtained if virtually every trace of clearing agent is replaced by wax, although cedarwood oil is an exceptional clearing agent in this respect and does not need to be replaced entirely. With any of the usual routine clearing agents, if removal is not complete the centre of the piece will be unsupported when sections are cut. Specimens of cellular tissue will give incomplete sections with holes in their centres. If the tissue contains collagen or muscle fibres, these will be raised by the microtome knife, some being detached while others stand up on the surface of the block giving it a furry appearance. Sections from such blocks show poorly-stained bundles of tissue separated by cleft-like spaces.

The use of a large excess of wax for a long period would result in replacement of the clearing agent, but in practice it is far quicker and easier to use several small volumes. It is usual to treat tissue with three separate baths of wax.

Tissue suffers considerable distortion when it is subjected to high temperature. Moreover, it seems that wax should not be too fluid or distortion is increased. For these reasons, it is best to impregnate tissue at a temperature 1–2°C above the melting-point of whatever wax is used, rather than at any arbitrary temperature.

'Vacuum embedding'

This name is almost universally used for the technique of impregnating tissue with paraffin wax under reduced pressure. It is an unfortunate name, since the process is one of impregnation rather than embedding, and the reduction in pressure comes nowhere near a total vacuum. The basis of the method is that volatile clearing agents leave the tissue quicker when the surrounding pressure is low. Moreover, any air that might be dissolved in the clearing agent or wax is also removed and thus has no chance to form bubbles within the tissue. The process has been particularly popular for tissues that contain tiny cavities (e.g. lung), but is not infrequently used for every kind of tissue in routine laboratories. It is true that time may be saved by vacuum embedding, since each treatment with wax need only last $\frac{1}{2}$–1 hour instead of the routine 1–3 hours, but we have not found the time saved worth the complications involved; we have done without vacuum embedding for many years and have

found it possible to produce satisfactory sections of every kind
of tissue (including lung). In any case, it is not usually possible
to use reduced pressure on an automatic processing machine, so
that even the laboratories that make use of vacuum embedding
do so only for the third treatment with wax.

Vacuum embedding equipment is available in several forms,
but the following general description includes the essential
components of all of them.

1. A container with a thermostatically controlled heating device
(usually in a water-jacket around the whole container) and a tight-
fitting lid or door.

2. A connection from the container to a vacuum line. This is
usually a water-pump, in which case a trap-bottle must come
between the pump and the container so that any water that might
reflux from the pump cannot enter the container.

3. A valve to close the connection between the container and the
source of vacuum. This is usually a metal clamp on a thick-walled
rubber tube.

4. A vacuum gauge connected to the container. This may be either
a mercury manometer or an aneroid gauge with a dial.

5. A valve to allow air to re-enter the container at the end of the
process.

The apparatus is used at a temperature 1–2°C above the
melting-point of the wax. It is loaded with one or more vessels
containing the tissue in molten wax. The lid is closed and the
vessel evacuated until the negative pressure reaches 400-500 mm.
(16–20 in.) of mercury. When this pressure is reached, the
valve 3 is closed and impregnation allowed to continue for
$\frac{1}{2}$–1 hour. Air is then admitted slowly through the valve 5,
and the tissue is removed. The whole cycle may then be
repeated with fresh wax.

Embedding

After thorough impregnation, the piece of tissue needs to be
encased in a piece of paraffin wax of suitable size and shape for
sections to be cut from it. This process is known as embedding,
and is nothing more than placing the tissue in a mould that
contains molten wax, and then cooling it to solidify the wax.
The tissue is then encased in wax as well as being thoroughly
impregnated with it. At this stage it is usual to remove it from
the mould although it is possible to obtain special moulds

(Tissue-Tek) which are only partly removed since a piece of the mould also acts as a block-holder during subsequent section cutting. These are unlikely to be favoured in routine laboratories because they are expensive and require additional storage space for blocks.

Conventional moulds are of two types: those that are used repeatedly, and those that are used once and then discarded. Disposable moulds can be made from paper or metal-foil to whatever size is suitable; they can be stripped from the solid block. Cardboard or thin plastic moulds can also be broken and discarded, but these are almost always obtained ready-made so that it is not practicable to use moulds of precisely the right size. For a discussion of recent developments in embedding procedure, the reader is recommended to Orchin (1967). For repeated use, metal or strong plastic moulds are usually used; watchglasses have been used for tiny fragments. Since these moulds cannot be broken from the solid wax block, it is important to smear them liberally with a layer of glycerol before use, to prevent the wax sticking to the mould. Moulds may be made from two right-angled metal pieces, each the shape of a letter L (Leuckhart's embedding pieces). These can be placed on a glass slab and their position varied to make blocks of varying sizes. It is, however, very difficult to cool the blocks rapidly by immersion in water. For many years we have used shallow flat-bottomed tins (about three inches diameter) that are sold for baking buns or small tarts.

In practice it is convenient to start with wax at a temperature about 10°C higher than its melting-point. Sufficient is poured into the mould to make a block about one-quarter of an inch (or a half-centimetre) thicker than the piece of tissue. The tissue is then taken in a pair of warmed (not heated) forceps, and placed in the mould with the face to be sectioned at the bottom of the mould. Usually it is immaterial which face is sectioned, and the tissue will be embedded with the flatter of the two downwards. When it is important to cut sections from a particular face, an indication is often given by a V-shaped groove cut in the unimportant face; this grooved face would then be left uppermost. When a specimen needs to be embedded on edge (e.g. a thin piece of cyst wall), it is better to wait until the lower layers of wax solidify before introducing the tissue which will quickly be gripped by the solidifying wax and held upright.

When a specimen consists of multiple small fragments (e.g. curettings), these should be packed close to one another so that a single compact block will be obtained. When the mould is considerably larger than the pieces of tissue to be embedded, several separate blocks may be cut from one cake of wax. If this is done, it is necessary to ensure that the space between the pieces is sufficient to give an adequate margin to each block. Moreover, care must be taken to avoid distributing the pieces of tissue in the wax in a way that would make cutting between them difficult.

When the lower layers of wax begin to solidify, they lose their translucency, so that a skin appears to form on the bottom of the mould. At this stage, the mould should be floated on cold water. As soon as a skin forms across the top of the wax, the whole mould should be submerged. The value of controlled cooling is that small crystals of wax ('micro-crystals') are formed, and the block will produce satisfactory sections. Slow cooling would allow large crystals to form so that the block would be liable to fragmentation during section cutting. Excessive cooling (e.g. by ice-water) produces a similar effect. Ordinary cold tap water (about 10–12°C) gives satisfactory results. When the block is solid, the mould is removed. If glycerol was used, the blocks will be slippery to handle unless they are left in water for a few moments.

Trimming

After embedding, it is nearly always necessary to remove surplus wax. It is often necessary to separate several blocks that have been cast together in one mould. The object is to leave a rectangle in which the tissue is bordered by about 3–5 mm. of wax. Solid wax is hard to cut, so that large pieces of wax are best removed by making deep score marks and then breaking the wax cake like a block of chocolate. The same manoeuvre is used to separate several wax blocks that have been cast in one mould. When small amounts of wax need to be removed, these are shaved from the edge of the block. The best instrument for both of these purposes is a heavy knife such as an old microtome knife of small size. On no account should flimsy blades be used.

Wax blocks

When blocks have been trimmed, the next step is usually to attach them to block-holders so that sections can be cut. Material can, however, be stored indefinitely in wax blocks and, in any case, the blocks will usually be stored after sections have been cut. There are certain hazards to guard against when storing blocks. These include: confusion of one with another, excessive heat, mould growth through damp, and destruction by rodents, cockroaches, and other insects.

The best storage systems make use of boxes or packets, each of which contains the blocks from one specimen only. Small cardboard boxes may be filed conveniently in numerical order in office filing drawers. Alternatively, boxes or packets may be filed numerically in larger boxes. When space is limited, or blocks are not often re-used, it is common practice to file a dozen or more in a single small box, packet, or plastic bag. When this is done, blocks from several specimens will go into the same box, so that accurate labelling of each block is particularly important.

Laboratories that use processing machines make use of tickets at an earlier stage. When tissue is processed by hand, it will be kept in labelled bottles until embedded in wax, at which stage a ticket will be needed. In either case the ticket should be made of tough paper or thin card; information should not be recorded with water-soluble ink or ball-point pens. Fairly black graphite pencils (e.g. 2B) and India ink are satisfactory. Tickets are sealed to the wax block by heating the latter with a hot iron. Obviously the face away from the tissue must be used. When blocks are segregated for filing, so that only those from a single specimen are filed in each box or packet, it is unnecessary to secure the ticket to the block. It is, however, wise to file the ticket inside the box or packet since it may prove very helpful at a later date if confusion is suspected.

Schedules

No hard and fast times can be given for impregnation. It is usual to treat tissue with three separate baths of molten wax before it is embedded. For most pieces of tissue, each treatment should last for $1\frac{1}{2}$–3 hours. When a 'vacuum embedding' apparatus is used, these times may be reduced to $\frac{1}{2}$–1 hour.

Since impregnation and embedding are the last stages of a series of treatments, it is usual to draw up a complete schedule of dehydration, clearing and impregnation. Our suggested schedules for routine use may be found in the previous chapter (pp. 30–33). For special problems, information may be sought elsewhere (large pieces, p. 302; eyes, p. 310; extra-rapid paraffin methods, p. 307).

Common errors in impregnation and embedding

(i) Blocks are occasionally encountered with white opaque centres which yield when compressed. This softness of the centre is particularly noticeable after the surface has been cut off by the microtome, when it may also be possible to smell the clearing agent in the block. Sections cut from these blocks are usually incomplete, lacking a centre.

Blocks that show these faults are insufficiently impregnated. At first sight it would seem obvious that inadequate impregnation was due to *deficient treatment with wax*. Unfortunately the problem is not as simple as this, and it may be necessary to look for the explanation at an earlier stage of processing. Impregnation will obviously be inadequate if tissue spends insufficient time in wax, or is treated with too small a volume of wax, or with too few baths of fresh wax. But wax can only impregnate tissue that is saturated with clearing agent; if any other fluid remains in the tissue, it will prevent impregnation. Thus, *inadequate clearing* will leave alcohol in the tissue to prevent wax from penetrating it thoroughly. Furthermore, *inadequate dehydration* will leave water in the tissue to prevent proper clearing and, in turn, proper impregnation.

When faced with a badly impregnated piece of tissue, it may, therefore, be necessary to review the whole schedule of dehydration, clearing, and impregnation. Sometimes it will be found that the wrong fluid was used at some stage; sometimes pieces of tissue in close contact make a mass too thick to be penetrated by the various fluids; sometimes a piece of tissue contains too much lipid for the clearing agent to remove, so that tissue lipid blends with the wax to soften it. If another piece of tissue from the original specimen is available, the simplest solution is to start afresh with it. When, however, the tissue cannot be replaced, it should be taken step by step through several baths of fresh clearing agent to alcohol, then thoroughly dehydrated and, finally, returned through clearing agent to wax.

(ii) Severe shrinkage of tissue may occur. When it does, the blocks are usually too hard to cut properly. Both the blocks and the sections appear translucent (a few kinds of tissue such as thyroid normally have this appearance). Sections from such tissue are fragmented by close-set lines parallel to the edge of the knife.

This damage is caused by *overheating*, which may occur either during impregnation, or at the time of embedding. Some tissues (e.g. lymphoid tissue and brain) are particularly sensitive, and may be damaged if left in molten wax at relatively low temperatures (58–60°C) for many hours. The same effect is produced if tissue is allowed to dry between clearing agent and wax.

(iii) Sometimes the tissue is found to be too far from the bottom of the wax. This is inconvenient when the block is mounted on a microtome, since it becomes difficult to ensure that the surface of the tissue is parallel to the edge of the knife. Moreover, unnecessary wear is caused to the knife edge and time is wasted in removing the excess of wax.

This fault occurs when the bottom of the wax is allowed to solidify before the tissue is placed in position. Either the wax was too cool to start with, or the delay before embedding the tissue was too great.

(iv) Careless handling of moulds that contain tissue in molten wax is apt to cause a tight collection of fragments to disperse, making an unwieldy block. Any pieces embedded in special positions (e.g. on edge) may fall over.

(v) Blocks occasionally have a coarse crystalline structure, showing an appearance like a mosaic or crazy paving, and they tend to break up, especially when sections are being cut. These blocks have either been cooled too slowly or (rarely) too quickly.

(vi) If glycerol was not washed off the surface of wax blocks, they will be slippery. This adds an unnecessary hazard to subsequent processes that require sharp instruments such as trimming knives and microtomes. Moreover, if glycerol is allowed to remain on the wax, it will cause softening of the block after a day or so.

CHAPTER 5

Microtomes and Knives

General notes on microtomes. Cambridge rocker. Sledge. Rotary.
Freezing. Care of microtomes. Knives. The knife edge. Tilt.
Slant. Sharpening: Honing; Automatic sharpeners; Regrinding;
Stropping.

A MICROTOME is a machine for cutting thin sections from a piece
of tissue. Many different varieties of microtome are available,
but all of them consist of four basic components:

1. A knife held in a firm support;
2. A device for holding the piece of tissue firmly;
3. A mechanism for moving the tissue across the knife blade
(or the knife across the tissue);
4. A mechanism for advancing the piece of tissue a very small
and accurately measured distance so that a section of suitable
thickness can be cut.

Sections cut from tissue embedded in paraffin wax are usually
about 5 μ thick (μ standing for micron and signifying one-
thousandth part of a millimetre). Given ideal conditions it
would therefore be possible to cut 200 sections from a piece of
tissue one millimetre in thickness, or about 5,000 from a piece
one inch thick. It is obvious that any machine producing sections as thin as this needs to be precisely made.

The mechanical problem to be overcome in the design of a
successful microtome is the combination of easy running with
stability. The knife must be clamped rigidly enough to prevent
vibration, and the moving parts must be made in such a way that
minor degrees of wear (which are inevitable) do not cause loose-
ness. Any unwanted freedom of movement will result in sections
of uneven thickness.

The following brief notes indicate the particular merits and
the common defects of the types of microtome in general use;
these notes are not intended to serve as detailed descriptions of
individual instruments, for which the suppliers (p. 398) should
be consulted. Nor is any attempt made, at this stage, to give an
account of section cutting: that will be found in the next
chapter.

Cambridge rocker microtome

The block is attached to a pivoted arm and moves across the edge of the knife in an arc. At each stroke, the tissue is automatically advanced horizontally towards the knife. This type of microtome is simple and convenient in use; it is suitable for the preparation of serial sections. It is not, however, suitable for large or unusually hard blocks. Sections are cut from a slightly curved surface on the block; this is no disadvantage unless more sections are needed at a later date when it will be found difficult to match the original position. In everyday use the rocker microtome gives little trouble; the cord that operates the mechanism may break with consequent damage to the block or knife. The working parts show little wear after years of use; the first part to wear out is usually the ratchet pawl that works the advancing mechanism; this pawl is easy to replace.

Sledge microtome with moving block

Sledge microtomes (sometimes known as sliding microtomes) have a carriage which moves on rails. On some microtomes the knife is attached to the moving carriage (see below), but more commonly the block of tissue is attached to the carriage; this is then pushed under the knife, which is fixed above it in a suitable position. The carriage incorporates a mechanism for raising the block by suitable steps; adjustments are also included for varying the orientation of the block in case the tissue is not embedded parallel with the base of the block-holder.

This type of microtome has become increasingly popular in the last few decades, often replacing the Cambridge rocker microtome in routine laboratories. Sledge microtomes are straightforward to use, requiring less experience than the rocker microtome, although the effort needed to operate them is greater. It is easy to rest a piece of ice on the block without removing it from the microtome; this avoids any difficulty about orientation of the block such as occurs if the block has to be removed for cooling. Another reason for the popularity of sledge microtomes of this type is their versatility; not only are they suitable for any kind of paraffin block (including unusually hard or large ones), but they can also be used with simple attachments for frozen sections. They incorporate an adjustment of knife slant, and are therefore suitable also for nitro-cellulose sections.

The commonest defects in use are wear of the ratchet pawl and the return spring in the advancing mechanism. After prolonged use the runners show signs of wear, with consequent instability of the carriage. When this occurs, sections will be uneven; either individual sections are irregular in thickness or, more often, alternate sections are thick and thin. Harder blocks of tissue show this fault before others.

Sledge microtome with moving knife

In this type of microtome the tissue is stationary and the knife, which is attached to a carriage, moves across its surface on rails. The advancing mechanism raises the block. Although theoretically this type of microtome could cut any type of section, in practice the movement of the knife precludes cutting ribbons of sections. The sledge microtome with moving knife is, in fact, used almost exclusively for cutting nitrocellulose blocks and for preparing frozen sections. Since the knife is clamped at only one point, it is possible to vary the angle of slant easily; this is useful for nitrocellulose blocks. For frozen sections it is helpful to have a fixed block to which the cooling mechanism can be attached.

The microtome is easy to operate but the knife may lift and fail to cut blocks of hard tissue. The knife is also subject to more vibration than that of microtomes with two knife clamps. Exceptional care is needed in use, since the knife has a long unguarded edge. Moreover, the knife is not in a constant position and therefore cannot be avoided by the instinct that every microtomist rapidly develops when using a machine with a stationary knife.

Rotary microtome

The basic principle of the rotary microtome is the same as that of the sledge microtome with moving block. The block is attached to a carriage which moves on rails. In this instance the carriage travels up and down, and is moved by turning a handle. The knife is fixed with its edge upwards. The advancing mechanism pushes the block forward automatically as the carriage completes its movement.

Although it is possible to use the rotary microtome for cutting nitrocellulose, it is really designed for paraffin blocks, and is particularly suitable for cutting serial sections or for the preparation of large numbers of sections from each block (e.g. for teaching). The design is less convenient when only one or two sections are needed from a large number of blocks, because it is not as easy to remove and replace the blocks as it would be with a sledge or rocker microtome. The rotary microtome is also less satisfactory for hard blocks that need to be cut with more than usual force; the gearing is such that it is harder to apply force through the handle than by the direct action of a sledge microtome.

Freezing microtome

The block is stationary, and the block-holder incorporates a cooling mechanism which may be a thermo-electric module or a carbon dioxide expansion chamber. The knife-holder is pivoted at one end and supported at the other by a rest which moves in an arc of a circle on a hard metal quadrant. The advancing mechanism is automatic, and is usually graduated in steps of 5 μ.

Freezing microtomes are designed exclusively for cutting frozen sections and are unsuitable for any other kind of block. They are easy to operate, although uneven sections will be produced unless constant pressure is applied to the handle. This type of microtome will not cut large sections; if large frozen sections are needed, a freezing attachment should be used with a sledge microtome.

The practical aspects of the preparation of frozen sections are dealt with in Chapter 19 (p. 274).

Care of microtomes

It is essential to keep microtomes free from rust and grit. Rust is particularly likely to affect sledge microtomes, since these are often used with pieces of ice above the level of the rails. After use, therefore, all the working parts of a sledge microtome need to be thoroughly cleaned with rags. Scraps of wax are best removed with a rag soaked in xylene; this will also remove old oil and grease from rails and other working parts. Freezing microtomes also become wet because of condensation. Rocker microtomes and rotary microtomes need less extensive cleaning since most of the working parts do not become contaminated with moisture or with fragments of wax. It is necessary, therefore, to clean only the region of the knife clamps and block-holders after use; the other working parts should be cleaned and lubricated periodically (e.g. once a week for a microtome in daily use). The lubricants in common use for microtomes are light machine oil and thin grease. Oil should be used for all advancing mechanisms. Grease is better than oil for adjusting screws and securing bolts for knives and blocks. Rails and carriages are often lubricated with oil but grease may be preferred for heavy sledge microtomes. Grease is certainly better if the microtome is not likely to be used again soon. In that case it is also wise to protect the microtome from dust.

Knives

Microtome knives are manufactured in a wide variety of sizes and shapes. Some microtomes, such as the Cambridge rocker, use knives of one particular size and shape; others, however, will accept a wider variety, so that it may be important to provide an accurate specification when ordering new knives or replacements. A short description of size includes the length of the blade (without handle), the width of the blade, and the thickness of the broadest part of the back of the knife. It is worth remembering that repeated sharpening and grinding will reduce the width of the blade (and, in a few cases, will very slightly reduce its thickness). Examples of common knife sizes are: $100 \times 32 \times 7\frac{1}{2}$ mm. for freezing microtomes, and $240 \times 32 \times 13$ mm. for many types of sledge microtome.

Shapes of microtome knives are more difficult to classify. Some blades have flat (plane) surfaces; others have concave surfaces; sometimes one surface is flat and one concave. The degree of concavity may be great or only slight. In practice, two types are widely used: these are knives with two flat surfaces, and knives with two slightly concave surfaces. The knife with two flat surfaces is commonly referred to as the *wedge knife* because of its shape. It is universally used on freezing micro-tomes, and is the commonest shape used on rotary microtomes and sledge microtomes with a moving block. The merits of the wedge knife are its ability to cut hard objects, and the relative

E

absence of vibration at the knife edge. The knife needs to be sharpened less frequently than other types of knife, although the sharpening process is longer because more metal has to be removed to produce a new edge.

The knife with two slightly concave surfaces is usually described as *biconcave*. This type of knife is used on the Cambridge rocker microtome, and is sometimes chosen for cutting nitrocellulose sections on a sledge microtome. The edge does not withstand hard blocks and needs frequent sharpening.

The two shapes of knife described above will satisfy all routine needs. If, however, a laboratory handles enough nitro-cellulose blocks to justify additional equipment, it may be worth investing in special knives for this purpose. These knives have one surface greatly concave and the other flat; they are referred to as *plano-concave* knives.

Most microtome knives have detachable handles. The handle is not necessary when the knife is clamped on to a microtome; in fact it would interfere with the operation of some types of microtome. The handle must also be removed when a knife is sharpened on an automatic sharpening machine. In all other situations, however, a knife is safer with a handle on it; and it is essential to use a handle if the knife is sharpened by hand. In the interests of safety, the rule should be that all knives retain their handles until clamped on to a microtome or sharpening machine, or put into their cases. Only when the knife is firmly at rest in one of these situations, should the handle be unscrewed. Most handles are interchangeable, so that it is not necessary for every knife to have a separate handle.

Since the microtome knife is one of the greatest hazards in a histology laboratory, it is wise to institute a few other rules about the handling of knives. Microtomes with knives clamped on to them should never be left unattended; the knife must be either removed or securely covered. When not in use, knives should be in their cases and not left to lie on a bench (where their edges are likely to suffer damage as well as being a danger). A knife ought to be carried in its case, but if carried without one, the edge of the knife should be towards the person carrying it, since he is more aware of the hazard than anyone else. Everyone who handles knives must be taught the necessity of suppressing the instinct to catch one if it should fall; the only safe policy is to step sharply backwards and leave the knife to fall to the ground. When wiping a knife, it is obviously safe to do so from the back towards the edge; it is not safe to smother the blade in cloth and then draw it through longitudinally.

The knife edge

The process of sharpening a knife consists of removing metal from the blade until a new edge has been produced which is free from imperfections. With a wedge knife, it would be theoretically possible to remove a thin layer from the whole of each surface of the blade to do this; but such a process would be extremely laborious and slow. In practice a small amount of metal is removed from the cutting edge only. Thus a small part of the blade close to the cutting edge has a *bevel* on each side. The edge angle (Fig. 1; *a*) is considerably greater than the blade angle (*b*) of the knife as a whole.

Knife tilt

In order to avoid compressing the block, the back of the bevel must be clear of the face of the block when the edge is cutting a

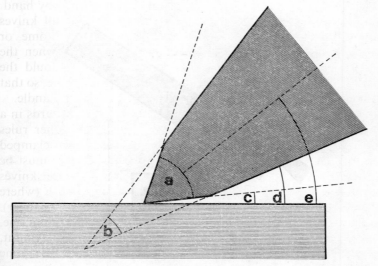

Fig. 1

section. That is to say there must be a clearance angle between
the bevel and the block (Fig. 1; *c*). Since the bevel is a very
narrow strip, it would be quite impossible to measure the
clearance angle directly, and so it is common practice to measure
the inclination or tilt of the knife as a whole. It is nowadays
customary to measure this angle of inclination or angle of tilt
between the face of the block and an imaginary line that joins
the edge to the midline of the back of the knife (Fig. 1; *e*). We
would, however, caution readers that the same term has been
used to describe the angle between the face of the block and the
surface of the knife that is adjacent to it (Fig. 1; *d*). Although this
latter meaning is used by some current manufacturers' catalogues,
as well as by important authors such as Apáthy (1897a and b),
we prefer to use the term angle of tilt to refer to angle *e*, which
can also be applied to biconcave knives, and which is favoured
by most modern writers including some manufacturers'
catalogues.

In any event it is rarely necessary to know the precise angle
of tilt of a knife. Many microtomes include a scale which is
marked in arbitrary units; this is a perfectly adequate guide for
all routine purposes.

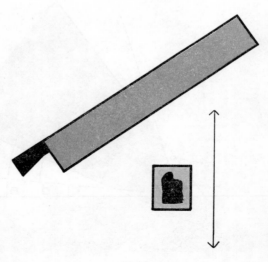

Fig. 2

Knife slant

This term refers to the relationship of the edge of the knife to the edge of the block. It is entirely independent of the angle of tilt. For most purposes the knife is not slanted; thus the whole front edge of the block meets the knife edge at the same time. However, for special purposes, such as nitrocellulose sections, the knife is slanted (Fig. 2). The edge of the knife is then not parallel with the edge of the block, and one corner is cut first. The greater the slant, the further the knife will cut into one corner before it even enters the other front corner. The slanted knife is not so liable to vibration during section cutting. Its edge is also effectively sharper since the angle of an oblique section through a wedge is smaller than that of a transverse section (Fig. 3). On the other hand, it is obviously extremely difficult to produce a ribbon of paraffin sections if a slanted knife is used.

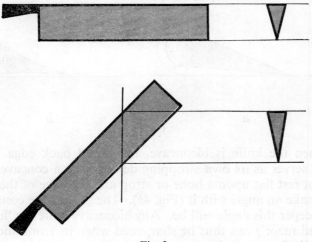

Fig. 3

Although they might appear to be the same at first glance, there is, in reality, no similarity between a slanted knife and a slanted block (i.e. a block placed diagonally on its holder). Altering the alignment of the knife is useful for particular purposes: setting the block diagonally is never justified.

Sharpening

In order to sharpen a knife edge (i.e. to renew the bevel

described above), the edge must make an angle with the hone or strop. When the blade is flat (a wedge knife), the bevel is produced at the edge by raising the back of the blade to an accurately measured height above the level of the hone or strop. It is important that this height (and therefore the angle between the blade and the hone or strop) should be the same each time the knife is sharpened, otherwise the bevel will be difficult to renew without excessive removal of metal from the edge. If a sharpening machine is used, it is easy enough to record the height of the back of the blade above the hone. However, when a knife is sharpened by hand, it is not possible to ensure that this height remains constant unless each knife is provided with its own attachment of suitable width. This attachment (known as a *stropping device* or, more often, as a *back*, Fig. 4a) clips on to the broad edge of the knife in order to raise it to a constant height above the hone or strop.

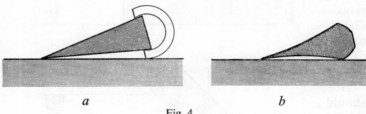

a   b

Fig. 4

When the knife is biconcave, the broad back edge of the blade serves as its own stropping device since a concave blade cannot rest flat upon a hone or strop and the edge of the blade will make an angle with it (Fig. 4b). The greater the concavity, the steeper this angle will be. Any biconcave knife (or 'hollow-ground razor') can thus be sharpened when its front and back edges lie flat on the hone or strop.

The sharpening of any delicate edge-tool requires two processes. The first, known as *honing*, consists of the removal of metal from the edge until minute imperfections are smoothed out and the edge is restored to a straight line. The second process, known as *stropping*, is designed to polish the edge once the straight line has been produced. Honing inevitably requires an abrasive surface since metal is removed. Moreover, in order to avoid folding the edge over, the knife must be pushed across the abrasive surface of the hone rather than pulled. On the other hand, stropping needs a soft surface across which the knife must obviously be pulled.

Honing

In many laboratories, knives are honed by machines (see below). However, it is still prudent for everyone who handles microtome knives to be able to hone them by hand. Many natural and synthetic sharpening stones have been used for this purpose (Arkansas stone, Belgian yellow stone, Carborundum, etc.), but most laboratories now use pieces of plate glass, which have two advantages: they can be cut to whatever size is suitable, and they can be made more or less abrasive to suit each particular need. The piece of glass should be perfectly flat (mirror glass used to be chosen); it can be obtained ready-ground, or can be ground in the laboratory with carborundum powder (Silicon carbide, No. 120) and another sheet of glass. The carborundum powder is made into a thick paste with either water or oil. Grinding should continue until the surface is uniformly and finely ground. When the surface has been prepared, all traces of carborundum powder should be removed. This can easily be done with a jet of hot water.

Hones must always be kept clean when not in use; stones should be wiped with well washed (non-fluffy) rag; glass hones should be washed with hot water and then dried. Hones must be stored out of the way of dust and grit.

In use, every hone must be damped. This may be done with water or soapy water, but usually a light machine oil is preferred. When a glass hone is used, it is necessary to add abrasive powder to the oil (or water) to make a thin paste. The abrasive used will depend on the amount of sharpening that a knife needs. A badly nicked or worn edge would justify a coarse powder (Aloxite aluminium oxide, No. 2F). Following a coarse powder, or when only moderate damage has been done to the edge, a fine powder (Aloxite optical smoothing powder, No. 50) is used. After these relatively coarse powders, the knife should be honed with a polishing powder which has very little abrasive effect (White Bauxilite, micro size 1200). Polishing powder on its own will be enough to restore an edge that has been slightly used and is relatively undamaged.

As already stated, a knife is honed by pushing the edge
across the hone rather than pulling it. The best edge is obtained
if the blade is moved obliquely across the surface of the hone,
not pushed across it in an axis perpendicular to the blade (Fig.
5). This is just as well, because many blades are much too long
to be sharpened by a simple transverse movement unless an
enormous hone were available. In addition to the oblique
direction of movement, the knife should be slanted on the hone
so that the end nearest the handle (the heel) precedes the far end
(the toe).

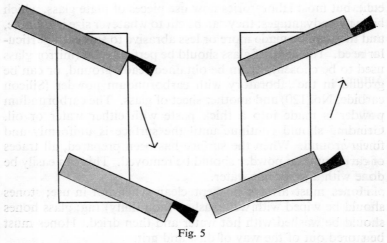

Fig. 5

Honing requires no added pressure; the weight of the blade on
the hone is enough. It is of the utmost importance that pressure
on the whole edge is uniform; on no account should the heel
be allowed to fall below, or rise above, the toe. Provided that
the honing paste (or oil) is of uniform consistency and is evenly
dispersed, the edge should pick it up in such a way that it covers
the blade to a consistent breadth. This will also show that the
edge is in contact with the hone and not riding above it. At
the end of each movement, the knife is turned on its back and
repositioned; it is not necessary to lift the back of the knife
from the hone, but if the whole knife is lifted the edge must
always be raised before the back and the back must be replaced
before the edge if a proper bevel is to be maintained. The edge
should never fall hard on to the hone.

When a knife is badly damaged, it will need to be honed until the edge is restored. Otherwise it is not possible to lay down precise rules, but about 100 complete to-and-fro movements with each grade of honing paste (or each grade of stone) are usually sufficient. Each complete movement should be slow and deliberate, taking about 4 seconds.

After the knife has been honed, it will need to be stropped (see below). It is generally agreed that a knife edge should be allowed to settle down after it has been honed; it is not wise to try to cut sections with it on the same day. Some people believe that knives should always be kept with their edges aligned in a magnetic north-south direction. However, provided that knives are honed and stropped properly, they will be found to be satisfactory whatever compass bearing they rest at.

Automatic knife sharpeners

These consist in essence of a knife-holder and a honing-plate with a mechanism for moving one relative to the other and a mechanism for turning the knife blade at intervals. It is possible to vary the height of the knife above the plate so that a consistent angle of bevel is obtained for each knife. A separate honing-plate should be used for each length of blade. The honing-plate needs to be roughened at frequent intervals (preferably after each knife has been sharpened). Automatic knife sharpeners save much time and labour. They have the additional merit that the edge remains straight, in contrast to that of a hand-honed knife which is worn away more in the middle than at the ends until it becomes curved. Moreover, hand-honing causes wear on the stropping device which develops flats where it is ground away, with consequent gradual alteration of the bevel angle.

The following notes refer to the Elliott automatic knife sharpener, although in the main they are also applicable to all automatic sharpeners. Before fixing the knife it is wise to verify that the correct honing plate is on the machine and that it is set at the right height for the knife in question. Powder is added and made into a fine paste with oil. The knife is then clamped on to the machine in such a way that it is suspended near to its point of balance; without this precaution one corner is liable to descend on to the plate before the rest of the blade.

The time switch is set to a suitable length of time for sharpening (30 minutes with each grade of powder is usually satisfactory).

The abrasive powders used on automatic sharpeners are the same as those that we have already recommended for hand honing. Similarly, it is common practice to follow coarse or medium powder with fine. To do this it is not necessary to remove the knife from the machine; it is sufficient to raise it above the honing plate and wipe the blade. The plate, however, should be removed, washed with hot water, dried, replaced, and covered with fine powder and oil which are then mixed into a thin paste. When the finest grade of powder has been used, the knife is removed and washed under hot water to remove any abrasive particles. It is then wiped dry and is ready for stropping.

The rough surface of the honing plate is restored by a lapping bar and coarse abrasive powder (Aloxite 2F) mixed with oil. The machine is usually run for 30 minutes with the lapping bar, after which the honing plate should be washed and dried.

Regrinding

In due course a knife will need to be reground. For this purpose it should be returned to the supplier. A knife needs to be reground if the edge has been badly nicked; otherwise it is only necessary after many months (if sharpened by hand) or several years (if sharpened by machine).

Stropping

As already mentioned a knife is stropped in order to polish the cutting edge. Stropping will therefore be needed after a knife has been honed. It is a usual practice to strop again before cutting sections; if many blocks need to be cut it is also helpful to strop the knife several times during the day. Although stropping can never restore the edge to a worn knife, it will restore the keenness to an edge that has become slightly dull in use.

Several forms of strop are available. Whatever pattern is chosen, it is important that the leather should be of good quality and properly dressed. When a strop becomes dry, or loses its bite, it will need to have its dressing renewed. To do this the surface of the leather is scraped with a sharp edge (such as a glass slide) to remove the old dressing and accumulated wax.

Fresh dressing is then applied and rubbed in with the fingers. It is of the utmost importance that strops be kept away from dust and grit.

The two types of strop that are suitable for microtome knives are the flexible (or hanging) strop, and a strop mounted on a board. If mounted, the base may be solid or slightly springy (saddleback type). In theory a hanging strop should be unsatisfactory, since it might turn the edge of the knife. In practice, however, the hanging strop is widely used and gives excellent results so long as it is pulled hard enough to remain flat. A secure wall-mounting is obviously essential. Hanging strops are supported by canvas; this canvas may profitably be used as a coarse strop (without any dressing) before using the leather surface.

Stropping does not require pressure; the weight of the knife is enough. A stropping device must be fitted to a wedge knife and this (or the back of a concave knife) must not be lifted from the strop. The edge is pulled, not pushed, over the strop, and should be pulled obliquely rather than in an axis perpendicular to the edge (Fig. 6). The knife is turned on its back, never on its

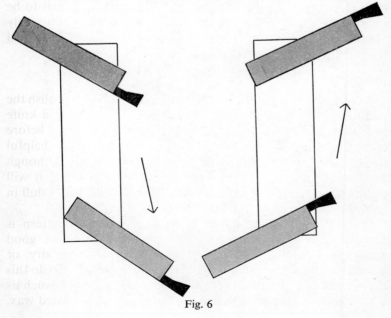

Fig. 6

edge. About 30 complete strokes (to-and-fro) on the canvas side and 50 on the leather side should be sufficient. In order to avoid the possibility of injury, the strop handle should be gripped with the whole hand, the thumb remaining close beside the forefinger. If the thumb is separated by the handle from the other fingers, it is much more liable to injury from the turning knife.

CHAPTER 6

Cutting and Mounting Sections

Block-holders. Cutting sections. Mounting sections. Adhesives for sections. Slides and coverslips. Common errors.

Block-holders

Paraffin wax blocks are almost always attached to block-holders which are attached in turn to the microtome. As already mentioned, it is possible to use special moulds that also do duty as block-holders (Tissue-Tek). It is even possible to cast extra-thick blocks which can be clamped to the microtome without a block-holder; these are satisfactory only when the tissue is easy to cut.

Block-holders are usually rectangles of hard material with one surface deeply grooved to make a good joint with molten wax. They may be made from metal or hard wood, but even better block-holders are made from resin-bonded compressed textile (e.g. Carp). Some types of microtome have clamps that accept only block-holders of a special shape. It is, however, possible to obtain adaptors for these microtomes to enable them to be used with rectangular block-holders if those are preferred.

Wax blocks are attached to block-holders by heat. This is applied by means of a metal palette knife or large spatula. Even better results are obtained by using an iron disc (about 30×5 mm.) on an iron stem mounted in a wooden handle. The metal is heated in a flame and applied to the block-holder. At the same time the wax block is held against the other face of the hot metal. As soon as the wax begins to run, the hot iron is withdrawn and the block pressed firmly onto the block-holder. The seal can be improved by running the edge of the hot iron around the periphery of the block where it is in contact with the block-holder.

Whenever possible, the block-holder should be at least as large in area as the wax block. If the piece of tissue is large it will need a block-holder that is too wide for the microtome clamp. For such pieces, it is worth having a stepped block-

holder with one side wide enough to accept the block and the
other just narrow enough to fit the microtome clamp.

If metal block-holders are used, care must be taken to remove
condensation water before they are used. If this is present, the
block will not remain attached.

Blocks are removed from block-holders with a rigid knife,
such as a small old microtome knife. Deep cuts are made into
each edge of the wax block close to the block-holder. At the
same time, gentle leverage is applied. Usually it is only necessary
to cut two or three sides before the block separates abruptly. If
too much leverage is used, it may be propelled some distance.
It is not necessary to clean traces of wax from the block-
holder; these form a useful base for the next block that will be
attached. When a sledge microtome is used, the block can
conveniently be removed from its holder whilst still in the
microtome clamp. With other types of microtome, the block-
holder is removed from the clamp before the block is separated.

Cutting sections

Before attempting to cut sections, it is essential to ensure that
the knife is sharp, securely clamped, and tilted to a suitable
angle. The block must be attached firmly to the block-holder
which must itself be securely fastened to the microtome. It is
then necessary to remove surplus wax from the face of the block
until the whole area of tissue is exposed. This is done by
removing coarse shavings (15–50 μ). It may be necessary to
alter the tilt of the block in order to expose the whole of the
tissue. The front and back edges of the block are given a final
trim and one corner may be removed. The block is then cooled
with ice; this may be done on the microtome or the block may
be removed and placed on ice.

Although some people cut paraffin sections one at a time, it is
preferable to cut them in *ribbons*. When this is done, the
sections can be handled more easily with less damage (except at
the ends of the ribbons). The only drawback to cutting ribbons
is the need to use an unslanted knife: in practice this does not
present any difficulties so long as the knife has been properly
sharpened. In order to obtain good ribbons, the front and back
edges of the block should be trimmed parallel to each other; if
not, the ribbon will be curved (Fig. 7). The edges must also be

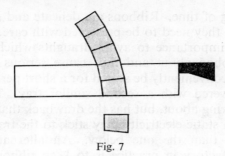

Fig. 7

parallel to the knife, otherwise the sections will not adhere to one another.

Sections are usually cut at a thickness of 5 μ. These ribbon well. Thicker sections can be produced in ribbons, up to a limit of about 12 μ. Beyond this thickness the sections do not adhere properly to one another. Sections thinner than 5 μ will form satisfactory ribbons provided that they can be cut at all. The preparation of extra-thin sections depends chiefly upon the rigidity of the microtome, the sharpness of the knife, and the hardness of the paraffin wax. With attention to these points, it should be possible to cut ribbons of sections as thin as 2 μ.

It is virtually impossible to teach section cutting except by demonstration. Therefore the following account should be regarded as no more than a general guide; it should be supplemented by practical instruction

The best sections are produced by cutting slowly. However, many tissues will disintegrate unless cut fairly rapidly; this is particularly true of hard tissues. Thus, in practice, the best sections are those cut as slowly as is possible from that particular block. It will usually be found easier to begin by cutting two or three sections rapidly. These adhere well and can be picked up. The rest of the ribbon is then formed by cutting as slowly as possible. It is helpful to breathe on each section as it is cut; this flattens the sections, preventing wrinkles. When the ribbon is long enough, it is detached from the knife. Before another ribbon is cut, it is essential to ensure that both faces of the knife are thoroughly clean and dry. After cutting sections, they may be mounted on slides at once. Often, however, it is more convenient to keep the ribbons until a number of blocks have been cut; the ribbons can then be mounted one after another with a saving of time. Ribbons are delicate and susceptible to heat, so that they need to be preserved with care. It is also of the greatest importance to avoid draughts which might blow pieces of ribbon about and thus cause serious mistakes. A ribbon may conveniently be stored for a short period on a slide tray and covered with a second similar tray. This prevents sections blowing about, but has the drawback that any sections charged with static electricity may stick to the tray that covers them rather than the one below. An alternative that has proved satisfactory in practice is to keep ribbons in shallow boxes. The cardboard boxes in which slides are supplied are suitable if their lids are torn off. A ribbon is lowered gently and folded as many times as necessary; if it is tossed carelessly into the box, it may attach itself by static electricity and become tangled. Ribbons in these boxes are safe from minor draughts, and keep well so long as the surrounding temperature is not too high. If ribbons need to be preserved for more than a few hours, they should be put into a box with a lid and kept cool (4°C).

Mounting sections on slides

There are two ways of doing this and each has its particular advantages. Individual sections may be mounted onto slides on a hot-plate, or ribbons of sections may be spread on warm water before mounting. An adhesive (e.g. albumin) is commonly used; methods for applying such adhesives will be found below, also general notes about slides and coverslips.

The advantage of spreading sections on hot water is that the method is quicker. It is particularly suitable when several sections need to be mounted from a single ribbon. The water should be free from dissolved air, otherwise bubbles will form on the sections; distilled or recently boiled water should be used. The water should be changed daily to avoid the growth of fungi and to dispose of fragments of tissue from sections previously mounted. When tap water is used, this should be collected from a fast-flowing tap, avoiding the first few drops since water taps not infrequently harbour acid-alcohol-fast bacteria. If these become attached to sections they may lead to mis-diagnosis (Carson et al., 1964).

The best container is a thermostatically controlled bath with a matt black surface. For occasional use, an enamel bowl will serve, especially if the inside is painted black. In use, the bath or bowl is filled with water, and the temperature is adjusted until it is 2–5°C below the melting-point of the wax. If an adhesive is used, it is convenient to add it at this stage. The container is then tapped sharply to dislodge any bubbles clinging to its sides.

A suitable length is broken from the ribbon and picked up by one end with a pair of forceps. The free end is then placed on the water and the remainder lowered onto the surface. When lowering the ribbon, it is important to stretch it gently to remove creases; this can be done either by making the movement quickly, or by stabilizing the free end by gentle pressure of a finger. The shiny side of the ribbon should be downwards, since it is easier to remove creases when this is so. Creases are removed by gentle stretching wth fine forceps, using the edges rather than the points of the forceps blades; this can be done by holding the forceps with the fingers curled around the handle. The ribbon is then broken into suitable lengths for mounting. These will usually be single sections, although several sections from a tiny block are often easier to handle than single sections and are therefore mounted together. The ribbon is broken with the forceps which should be kept dry: if they are dipped into the water the sections will stick to them. Any damaged sections (usually the end ones) are discarded.

A selected section is mounted onto a slide (prepared with adhesive if this is used) by dipping the slide into the water and moving it squarely up to the end of the section. The slide should not be vertical in the water but should be held obliquely with its upper end overhanging the floating section. As soon as the slide and section touch, the slide is withdrawn without altering its angle. If the slide is vertical or tilted away from the section, too much water will be collected and the section will tend to shift its position on the slide. If several slides are prepared from one ribbon, the sections should all be aligned similarly; subsequent examination may be less easy when some are mounted endways and others sideways. The slides must then be dried thoroughly in an incubator or in a current of warm air. The temperature should not exceed 65°C so long as any water remains on the slide.

F

The alternative method of mounting sections makes use of a hot-plate rather than a water-bath. The plate is operated at a temperature 2–5°C below the melting-point of the paraffin wax in use, and should have a thermostatic control. The slide is placed on the hot-plate and flooded with distilled water. If an adhesive is used, this will already have been smeared on the slide or added to the water. A suitable piece of the ribbon is detached with a scalpel and transferred gently, shiny side downwards, onto the wet slide. Creases are removed by gently stretching. Once the section is quite flat, excess water may be removed with a pipette or a piece of filter paper. The slides are then dried in an incubator as already described, or may be left on the hot-plate until thoroughly dry.

The hot-plate is slower in use than a water-bath. It will, however, be more convenient when the number of sections is small. It may also be preferred for sections of tissues that are particularly susceptible to wrinkles during mounting. Examples of such tissues are arteries, eyes, cartilage, and embryos, all of which are better mounted on a hot-plate if perfect results are to be obtained.

Adhesives for sections

Although it is not essential to use any adhesive when mounting sections on slides, there are good reasons for doing so. The duration of drying of mounted sections can be reduced to an hour or less; if no adhesive were used they would need to be dried for many hours to prevent the sections from washing off during staining. Some tissues (e.g. brain, lymph nodes, and spleen) are particularly liable to wash off if no adhesive has been used, especially during a prolonged staining method or one that includes the use of an alkaline solution. On the other hand, adhesives should not be used for sections that are to be stained by specific methods for proteins, and are best avoided when very fine cytological or histochemical detail is to be demonstrated.

In practice, the adhesive in common use is egg albumin. This is used in the form of a mixture of equal parts of albumin and glycerol with a small crystal of thymol added as a preservative. The albumin may be obtained from fresh eggs or by reconstituting dried egg albumin (5 g. of albumin added to 100 ml. of distilled water). In any case, the egg-white (or reconstituted egg-white) should be beaten to remove lumps. The thymol is then dissolved in a small volume of water (using heat); this and the glycerol are added and, after thorough mixing, the solution is strained through several layers of damp muslin and stored in small bottles at $-20°C$. As an alternative, the ready-prepared mixture may be obtained from laboratory suppliers who sell it as Mayer's egg albumin (Mayer, 1883).

Other substances have been used as adhesives, including starch, gelatin, and serum. Steedman (1960) lists several formulae.

As has already been indicated, the adhesive may be either smeared on the slide, or added to the water that is used for floating the sections. To treat slides, all that is necessary is to dip a finger into the adhesive and wipe it over the slide, leaving a thin film over the whole of the surface. Slides so treated should be kept away from dust, and should be used within a few hours. One disadvantage of this method is the likelihood that the smear will be too thick in parts, and may stain with eosin or similar dyes. There is also a tendency for keratinized squames from the finger to be left on the surface of the slide.

Neither of these drawbacks applies if the adhesive is added to the water used for floating the sections. When a hot-plate is used, a few drops of adhesive are added to the water that floats the sections. When a water-bath or bowl is used to float ribbons of sections, approximately 1 ml. of adhesive is added to each litre of water. Although this would be wasteful of adhesive if only occasional sections were handled, we have found in routine use that the absence of squames is a considerable advantage, and that the film of adhesive produced is entirely unobtrusive whatever staining method is subsequently used.

Slides and coverslips

For all ordinary purposes, sections are mounted on slides. However, if the sections are small and numerous (e.g. class teaching sets) they may be mounted on coverslips rather than on slides. The advantage of this procedure is that large numbers can be stained together with uniform results. When the finished sections are to be examined with special precision, it is better to mount them on coverslips of suitable thickness. This nullifies the effect of variation in thickness of the layer of mounting medium (Aumonier and Setterington, 1967).

Whichever is used will need to be cleaned before use. For routine use it is sufficient to polish the slides and coverslips with a fluff-free duster. When they are very dirty, or when specially good results are required, the slides and coverslips should be cleaned in alcohol or acid alcohol (1 per cent hydrochloric acid in 70 per cent alcohol) before being polished.

The slides in common use measure 76×25 mm. (3×1 in.) and are usually $1-1\cdot2$ mm. thick. Larger slides are available in stock size of 76×32 mm. ($3 \times 1\frac{1}{4}$ in.), 76×40 mm. ($3 \times 1\frac{1}{2}$ in.), and 76×50 mm. (3×2 in.).

For very large sections it is easier to use photographic lantern coverplates 82×82 mm. ($3\frac{1}{4} \times 3\frac{1}{4}$ in.) or old photographic plates from which the emulsion has been removed.

Coverslips also are made in a wide variety of sizes. The optical quality of the coverslip is more important than that of the slide, and so it is not surprising that the coverslip will often be the more expensive of the two. Either circular or rectangular coverslips may be used: for routine use the rectangular are more popular, but when sections are mounted on coverslips rather than slides, the circular shape is often preferred. The size of coverslip used depends on the type of section prepared. The majority of sections can be covered by slips of 22×22 mm., 22×32 mm., or 22×40 mm., but many laboratories will occasionally need larger sizes, such as 22×64 mm., 64×48 mm., 76×41 mm., 76×64 mm., or 79×60 mm. If necessary, large coverslips may be cut to a special size. This is done with a glass-writing diamond, using a large glass slide as a firm base to prevent the coverslip from yielding, and the edge of a second slide as a ruler.

The most useful size of circular coverslip is 22 mm. diam., but larger and smaller sizes are available (from 6 mm. to 76 mm. diam.). Several thicknesses are also available. The thinnest are very fragile, whereas the thickest ones do not suit the correction of most microscope objectives (they may altogether prevent the use of high power oil-immersion lenses). The most popular coverslips are No. $1\frac{1}{2}$ thickness ($0\cdot155-0\cdot185$ mm. thick). The more viscous the mounting medium used, the thinner the coverslips should be.

Common errors

Mistakes in cutting and mounting sections may not always become apparent until the sections are mounted and stained. Nevertheless, this is an appropriate place to summarize the common faults in sections, together with the errors that cause them.

(i) *When the microtome is operated repeatedly, the block does not make contact with the knife.* This is due to a defect of the advancing mechanism of the microtome. It should not, of course, be confused with contraction of the block caused by ice, when the microtome may need to be operated two or three times before the block advances to the plane of the knife edge.

(ii) *The block strikes the knife but is not cut by it.* The usual reason is insufficient knife tilt, so that there is no clearance angle (Fig. 1c, p. 51) and the block strikes the back of the bevel rather than the knife edge. This causes a greater resistance to movement than is felt when the knife is cutting normally. Similar resistance is encountered on the return movement, when the block again strikes the knife. A block that has been subjected to this treatment has a highly polished surface, lacking any knife marks, but sometimes showing dull smears along its surface.

More rarely sections are not cut because the knife or block are insecurely clamped.

(iii) *The block strikes the knife, but broken fragments are produced instead of entire sections.* This occurs when the wax is not homogeneous. Either large wax crystals have formed, or water is incorporated in the solidified wax.

Large crystals are often recognizable because the block resembles crazy paving; it may crumble into fragments when attempts are made to cut it. Commercial wax is particularly liable to this fault; wax modified for histological purposes is only likely to show it when it has been cooled unusually slowly or unusually quickly.

When water is included in the wax, the blocks show a cloudy opalescence. Such wax is unsuitable for histological use and should be discarded or returned to the supplier.

(iv) *Sections are produced, but fail to adhere to one another to form ribbons.* This is a very common problem for which there are many possible causes, so that the solution may be hard to find. One common cause is careless trimming of the front and back edges of the block: sections will not ribbon when these edges are ragged, or when either of them is too close to the tissue in the block, or when the edges are not approximately parallel with one another and with the knife edge. Sections will not form ribbons if the wax is too hard because a wax of high melting-point has been used or the block has been cooled too much. A blunt knife is a fairly common cause.

Fragments of wax from previous sections on either side of the knife edge may prevent ribbons from forming, as also may droplets of water on the knife or block. If attention to all these details fails to cure the fault, it is worth experimenting with different angles of tilt.

(v) *Sections roll up instead of lying flat.* This is usually due to a blunt knife. Other causes are too much knife tilt and unusually thick sections.

(vi) *Ribbons are formed but are curved instead of straight.* Usually the front and back of the block are not parallel (Fig. 7). A similar result may sometimes be produced by a knife of uneven sharpness.

(vii) *The unstained mounted sections are incomplete.* Likely causes are careless handling of the sections with forceps, careless separation of individual sections from the ribbon, and incomplete removal of wax from the surface of the block before sections are saved.

(viii) *The stained sections are incomplete.* In addition to the causes just mentioned (vii), sections may detach themselves in whole or part during staining. This is apt to occur when the amount of adhesive has been insufficient, or the duration of drying too short; it is particularly common when sections have been allowed to dry at room temperature rather than in an incubator or on a hot-plate.

(ix) *The sections have small oval holes in them.* These holes occur when the block is cut down in big steps. When superfluous wax is removed from the surface of the block in order to expose the whole face of the tissue, the last few shavings should not be thicker than 15–20 μ, otherwise there is a risk that some of the underlying tissue may be plucked out to leave small deficiencies in subsequent sections. Lymphoid tissue and brain are particularly liable to this fault.

(x) *Small round patches of the section fail to adhere to the slide.* These can usually be recognized by a difference in staining intensity; on examination under high power they are in a different plane of focus to the rest of the section; sometimes the loose patch has a crack around it, or it is folded back, or a part is missing.

This fault occurs when bubbles of air are trapped between the section and slide. Bubbles are common if ordinary tap water is used for mounting sections; they may also be caused if sections are allowed to fall flat onto the water rather than being lowered by one end first.

(xi) *The section is traversed by innumerable cracks.* These cracks are somewhat similar to those in dried mud. Some tissues (e.g. brain) are particularly susceptible.

The fault is caused by the use of excessive heat during the handling of the tissue. This may, of course, occur before the sections are cut. It will also occur, however, if sections are mounted from water that is too hot, or are dried at a high temperature.

(xii) *Sections are produced and ribbons are formed, but the sections are corrugated.* There are several possible causes for this fault which is a common one and which makes subsequent handling of the sections difficult since sharp folds may be almost impossible to flatten on the mounting water and in any case are apt to trap air beneath the sections.

The commonest causes are a blunt knife, an insufficiently cooled block, and an excessively fast speed of cutting. The fault may also appear when the mounting water is too cold, or the sections are placed on the water upside-down, or they fall flat onto the water instead of being lowered by one end.

(xiii) *The sections are marked by parallel tears or scratches at a right angle to the knife edge.* This is usually caused by a damaged knife edge. It will also occur when there are gritty particles in the tissue or wax. Occasionally fragments of cotton-wool, paper, or hair on the surface of the tissue are responsible.

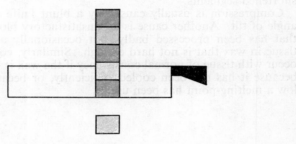

Fig. 8

(xiv) *Sections are unequal in thickness, being alternatively thick and thin* (Fig. 8). This is usually due to insecure clamping of the knife or block-holder or to inadequate mounting of the block on its holder. With blocks of very hard tissue it may occur if there is any wear of the rails (or pivots) of the microtome.

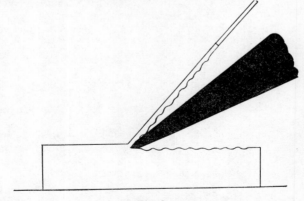

Fig. 9

(xv) *Individual sections are uneven in thickness.* There is usually a regular alternation of parallel thick and thin bands producing a ribbed or rippled effect (Fig. 9). These ripples are often referred to as 'knife-chatters'. They may occur when a concave knife is used with a very hard block even if the microtome is otherwise perfect. Usually, however, they are due to one of the mechanical faults listed in Note xiv above.

(xvi) *Stained sections show amorphous stainable material around their edges* and within any spaces (e.g. blood vessels). This effect is produced by the use of too much adhesive.

(xvii) *Sections are smaller than the block.* This reduction in size is caused by compression, and occurs only in the axis at a right angle to the knife edge. Thus the ribbon is of full width but is made up of shortened segments.

Compression is usually caused by a blunt knife or an incorrect angle of tilt. Another cause is an unsatisfactory block, usually one that has been processed badly, but occasionally a piece of hard tissue in wax that is not hard enough. Similarly, compression may occur with tissue of normal consistency if the wax is too soft; either because it has not been cooled sufficiently, or because wax of too low a melting-point has been used.

CHAPTER 7

Theoretical Basis of Staining

General notes. Dyes. How tissues are coloured. Mordants. Lipid stains. Metachromasia. Accentuators. Progressive and regressive staining. Counterstains.

AN OBJECT can only be seen when it gives out light. The object may be the source of the light, although more commonly it acts merely as a reflector or transmitter of light from elsewhere. Because an object is *visible*, it does not necessarily follow that it will be *distinguishable* from its surroundings; in fact it can only be distinguished if the light leaving the object differs in intensity or wavelength from that leaving the surroundings. Histological techniques that depend on differences of light *intensity* include the silver (and other metal) impregnation methods, phase contrast, and the use of polarized light. By each of these techniques, objects are made to appear black or white or intervening shades of grey. Most histological methods, however, make use of differences in *wavelength*, so that the light leaving the object is different in colour from that leaving the surroundings.

Histologists sometimes refer to any technique that demonstrates particular structures as a *staining method*. No one would criticize this name when a coloured dye is attached to the structures in question. In some methods, however, a colourless substance is allowed to react with a part of the section to produce a coloured compound (e.g. Perls's method for ferric iron). Many authors prefer not to apply the name stain to reactions of this kind since no dye is used. Nor is it correct to use the name stain for methods that demonstrate structures by the deposition of metal (e.g. silver impregnation methods for reticulin fibres). It is often possible to avoid ambiguity by using the word *dye* rather than stain when referring to a coloured substance that can be attached to tissue components to demonstrate them.

Dyes

These play a part in almost every method and so deserve a

brief general description. Theoretical notes about some of the other methods (those that do not make use of dyes) are included with the method in question; for silver impregnations see Chapter 16.

The two essential qualities of every dye are: it must be a coloured substance; it must attach itself to the tissue. Sometimes these two properties reside in different parts of the dye molecule, in which case the word *chromophore* is used to describe the coloured part, and the word *auxochrome* is used for the part that attaches to the tissue.

A dye (like any other coloured object) absorbs light of particular wavelengths. When white light falls on it or passes through it, those wavelengths are lost and the light that leaves the dye is coloured. A red dye appears *red* because it absorbs the *green* component of white light, and so on. Light is selectively absorbed by a dye because of a particular group of atoms in the dye molecule or a particular arrangement of double bonds within the molecule. Other molecules that include the same group of atoms or arrangement of double bonds are likely to be coloured (not necessarily the same colour). Hence it is possible to classify many dyes into families, each of which is characterized by a particular chemical group or molecular structure. Anyone interested in the theoretical aspects of dyes and their action on tissues is strongly recommended to read the relevant chapters in the small book by Baker (1966) or those in the larger book by the same author (Baker, 1958). For information about the chemical and physical properties of dyes, the book by Conn (1961) should be consulted.

The original histological dyes were of natural origin, being derived from plants (e.g. haematoxylin; orcein; alizarin) or animals (e.g. carmine). A few of these are still used, but they are exceptions, since almost every dye in current use is a synthetic organic chemical substance. Most of them are manufactured because of their dyeing qualities, and often they are in commercial use as textile dyes.

How tissues are coloured

The precise chemical or physical reaction that occurs when a dye becomes attached to a tissue is not always known. Some of the methods in common use are completely obscure in this respect. These continue to be used because the results are consistent and useful; they are often known as *empirical* methods.

Sometimes, however, the reaction between dye and tissue is understood in general terms. It is usually obvious which chemical group in the dye molecule enters into the reaction, and it is often possible to deduce which are the reactive groups in the tissue, but it is unusual to be able to discover the precise localization of those groups within the tissue. On the rare occasions when this localization is complete, the method may be classified as *histochemical*, and can be used as a precise analytical technique.

Many of the dyes in common use appear to become attached to tissue because they are acidic or basic. The basic dyes stain acidic tissue, and vice versa. Common acidic components of tissue are nuclei (which contain phosphoric groups), mucus and cartilage (which contain sulphuric groups), and some proteins which contain more free carboxylic than amino groups. Because these acidic tissue components attract basic dyes, they are often referred to as *basophil* (sometimes written basiphil). The affix *phil* has the meaning 'fond of' as in eosinophil (attracting eosin), and philharmonic (fond of harmony). The word basophil (and its opposite acidophil) cause confusion unless it is clearly understood that *basophil means acidic*, and *acidophil means basic*. Common instances of acidophil tissue components (which are basic because of a relative excess of free amino groups) are red blood corpuscles and eosinophil leucocytes.

It should be appreciated that the term acidic refers only to the acidic groups (sulphuric, phosphoric, carboxylic, etc.) on the protein or dye. The term basic has precisely the opposite meaning. In neither case does the term refer to the pH of the fluid that bathes the tissue or dissolves the dye. Thus an acidic dye may be used at an alkaline pH, or a basic dye at an acid pH (e.g. basic fuchsin in the Ziehl-Neelsen method). A few dyes and many proteins contain both acidic and basic groups; these substances behave as acidic in alkaline solutions, and as basic in acid solutions. This is a result of the suppression of ionization of acidic groups of dye or protein in an acidic environment leaving an excess of ionized basic groups. The reverse occurs in an alkaline environment. Such dyes and proteins are known as *amphoteric*. In each instance it is possible to find a pH at which the charge on the ionized acidic groups is exactly balanced by that on the ionized basic groups. This pH is known as the iso-electric point.

Mordants

In many histological methods the dye is used with a mordant. A mordant is a substance that has a strong affinity for the dye and also for a tissue component. Mordants used in histological dyeing methods include compounds of aluminium, iron, tungsten, molybdenum, chromium, and mercury. In each case it is the metal that provides the link between dye and tissue.

Sometimes the tissue is treated with the mordant at some stage before it is dyed. Examples of this sequence include many trichrome stains (which are improved by fixing the tissue in mercuric chloride solutions), the Weigert-Pal method (where tissue is transferred from the fixing fluid to a chrome solution before it is processed), and Heidenhain's haematoxylin (where the section is treated with iron alum before it is dyed). Often, however, it is satisfactory to add the mordant to the dye solution. Common instances of this combination include: Harris's and Ehrlich's haematoxylin, and Verhoeff's elastic stain.

Because dye is attached to the tissue by means of an intermediary metal compound, methods that make use of mordants are often classified as *indirect*, in contrast to the *direct* methods in which no mordant is used. A term which is sometimes used for the combination of dye and mordant is *lake* or *dye-lake*. Once the full combination tissue-mordant-dye has taken place, the bonds are not easily broken; they are, for instance, resistant to water and alcohol. The resistance of these bonds has two important practical applications. If an excess of a mordanted dye needs to be removed, it will be necessary to select a suitable agent (e.g. acid alcohol for the differentiation of haematoxylin in the haematoxylin and eosin methods). Secondly, water or alcohol may be used for the removal of the excess of an unrelated dye that is attached directly to tissue, without disturbing a mordanted dye that had previously been used (e.g. 50 per cent alcohol for the differentiation of eosin in the haematoxylin and eosin methods).

Lipid stains

Some histological techniques do not depend on chemical bonds and are therefore not dyeing methods in the strict sense. These methods are used for the demonstration of lipid in frozen sections. Lipids are coloured red by Sudan IV (otherwise known as Scharlach R) because the Sudan IV is more soluble in tissue lipid than in the solvent (e.g. 70% alcohol). This means that Sudan IV leaves the solvent and becomes fairly strongly concentrated in the tissue lipid. The same principle applies to Sudan III, Sudan black, and oil red O. Because the colouring agent is dissolved in the lipid and not chemically combined, it is possible to obtain a deeper colour by using a mixture (e.g. Sudan III and Sudan IV) since the second colouring agent can dissolve even when the lipid is saturated with the first.

Metachromasia

Sometimes a dye will demonstrate special components of the tissue in a colour that is different from that of the dye itself. Thus toluidine blue is itself blue and colours most tissue blue, but will demonstrate certain components (e.g. mast cell granules) as purple. This phenomenon is known as metachromasia (or metachromasy) and occurs even when the dye is chemically pure; it is not due to a coloured impurity. By no means every dye is metachromatic, in fact the property is limited to relatively few basic dyes. Furthermore, only a few tissue components may be demonstrated by metachromatic staining. It has been suggested that metachromasia occurs when polymerized dye becomes attached to certain tissue components, while the rest of the tissue is coloured by dye in single molecules.

Accentuators

Some histological techniques include the use of a substance which is neither dye nor mordant and yet improves the staining. Such a substance is known as an *accentuator*. It does not enter into any lasting combination with the dyed tissue and its mode of action is usually completely obscure. In some instances, the accentuator may act as a chemical catalyst: in others it probably exerts a physical effect, such as the reduction of surface tension. It is unfortunate that another word *accelerator* has been used to describe a class of additives which improve certain neurological metal impregnation techniques by some mechanism that is equally obscure.

Progressive and regressive staining

Histological staining methods fall into two groups. Either the reaction is allowed to progress until the intensity of staining is satisfactory, or the reaction is allowed to go too far and the superabundance of dye is removed slowly and carefully until the desired result has been obtained. The former is known as *progressive* staining and is appropriate when the dye has a specific affinity for a particular tissue component. If, however, the tissue is overstained, with subsequent removal of the excess dye, the method is described as *regressive*. Regressive staining is appropriate when a dye tends to stain too many tissue components but does not become equally firmly attached to them all. It is also appropriate when the affinity of the dye for the tissue component is very strong, so that the removal of excess dye can be carried out in a suitably leisurely manner. The general term for removing the unwanted excess of dye is *differentiation* and the agent that does the removing is known as a *differentiator*. Regressive staining (with differentiation) is practised with many simple dyes and mordanted dyes. There is, of course, no reason why a dye that is used regressively in one staining method should not be used progressively in another.

Counterstains

The first essential of every staining technique is that it shall demonstrate particular components with precision. Often, however, the significance of these components can be understood only when they are considered in relation to the section as a whole. For this purpose it is common practice to use one or more additional stains to show the other components of the tissue. These additional stains are called *counterstains* and should be chosen according to the following rules. They must be of a contrasting colour. They should be pale to avoid masking the specific stain. The counterstaining solution should not itself remove any of the specific stain, nor should the counterstain demand any special treatment (e.g. differentiation) that would do so. Commonly a counterstain is chosen that stains directly, without a mordant, since direct stains are, by and large, very readily differentiated. Occasionally, however, the counterstain is used before the specific stain (e.g. haematoxylin in the Alcian blue method). A method may, of course, use as a counterstain a dye that has a specific use in another method.

CHAPTER 8

Practical Basis of Staining

Dyes and staining solutions. Staining racks and jars. Preliminary treatment of paraffin sections. Finishing paraffin sections. Aqueous mounting media. Labelling slides. Storing slides. Restaining.

Dyes and staining solutions

The solvent for almost every histological stain is either water, or alcohol, or a mixture of the two. Tap water is unsatisfactory; distilled water is always suitable although, for certain methods, this will need to be glass-distilled. In this category are metal impregnation methods and Romanowsky stains. De-ionized water may be used in place of ordinary distilled water, but should not be substituted for glass-distilled water. For alcoholic stains, industrial methylated spirit (74° O.P.) is a satisfactory solvent in almost every instance. On the rare occasions that pure ethanol ('absolute alcohol') is needed in the methods described in the following chapters, that fact is specifically stated.

Staining solutions rarely need to be freshly prepared, although in some cases two or more stock solutions are mixed immediately before use. Since many staining solutions keep for long periods, it is a wise precaution to filter them immediately before use. This is particularly necessary with alcoholic solutions which often throw a sediment because of evaporation. It is not a good plan to filter freshly made solutions, since this will remove any undissolved particles. When a solution is in routine use, and is left in a staining jar, it should be filtered from time to time. Staining solutions and stock solutions should be kept in well-stoppered bottles away from direct sunlight. Most of them may be stored at room temperature without deterioration; when a solution needs to be kept cool, this is specified in the methods that follow. Dye powders should also be stored in subdued light in a cool place. A few substances (e.g. fast red salt B) should be stored at 0–4°C.

All reputable manufacturers of dyes submit them to chemical and chromatographic analysis before they are sold. Often the dyes are also tested for histological use. There may, however, be considerable variations between dyes from different manufacturers and even, on occasion, between two batches from the same manufacturer. It is therefore prudent to compare a new batch of dye with one that is known to give good results before relying on the new batch to stain any important sections. Most of the dyes produced at the present time are considerably purer than they were in the past. A few of the old staining methods, however, probably depended on the presence of impurities in the dyes of that time. All the methods that are mentioned in the following chapters make use of dyes that are currently available. Anyone who is curious enough to follow methods from the old literature should be prepared for a disappointment if current dyes are used.

Although histological staining methods may seem at first sight to be pure chemical processes, they are in fact more closely analogous to cooking recipes. The experienced worker soon learns to make allowances for the method of fixation, for the type of section (paraffin, frozen, nitrocellulose, etc.), and for variations in the tap water from one region to another. Beyond that, there is an indefinable personal skill that comes with familiarity; no one should condemn a new method because it has failed to give good results on the first few attempts.

Staining racks and jars

Even the simplest staining method consists of several steps, making use of one reagent after another. If the section is mounted on a slide, the reagents can be poured on to it successively at suitable intervals. The alternative is to put the reagents into containers (staining jars), and to move the slide from one jar to the next.

Sometimes there is nothing to choose between the two methods, but usually there are good reasons for choosing one or the other. Many staining methods are best carried out by combining the two.

It is essential to use a jar in the following circumstances: a reagent needs a long time to act (e.g. overnight), or is volatile (e.g. an alcoholic staining solution); the temperature is critical and an incubator is used; a reagent is dangerous to handle (e.g. strong acid), or becomes dangerous when dry (e.g. ammoni-

G

acal silver). A jar is preferable, although not essential, when the number of sections is large, or the solution keeps well and is frequently used. When the section is not attached to a slide (e.g. a nitrocellulose section), it must of course be stained by moving it from jar to jar.

On the other hand, it is much better to pour a reagent on to the slides when the reaction needs to be observed carefully; for instance any critical differentiation must be done in this way. Another reason for pouring a reagent on to slides might be that the reagent was expensive and only used occasionally.

The choice of staining jars is largely governed by the types of stain used and the volume of work. For many purposes it is best to use jars that are made specifically for the purpose, but almost any type of vessel can be used. It is essential that slides are kept apart during staining. This is easily achieved by using jars with grooved sides into which slides are slotted vertically. These are obtainable in heavy glass with glass caps and are known as Coplin jars; they have five slots to accommodate standard (76 × 25 mm.) slides and need 50 ml. of reagent. Similar jars made of polyethylene are known as Wilson jars; they again have five slots for standard slides but are less satisfactory than glass jars. They are not properly transparent; the grooves are not so smooth, so that the slides are more difficult to insert; and the jars fall over easily because they are so light. When coverslip preparations rather than slides need to be stained, slotted glass jars known as Columbia jars may be used.

It is possible to obtain larger slotted jars to accommodate a greater number of slides (usually horizontally), but it is almost always more convenient to put a large batch of slides or coverslips into a carrier which can be moved from one jar to the next. With a carrier of this type, any kind of jar may be used. Rectangular glass dishes with loosely fitting lids are sold for the purpose. When, however, a method is in constant use, fairly deep, wide-mouthed, screw-topped jars are preferable, especially for volatile reagents.

Slide or coverslip carriers are obtainable in stainless steel or glass. The stainless steel ones are satisfactory for most purposes; they hold more slides and are more durable. Some methods, however, will not work in the presence of metal: glass carriers are therefore used for metal impregnation techniques and some of the methods for demonstrating metal in tissues (e.g. Perls's method).

When slides are stained by pouring reagents on to them, the slides are laid on racks made from two parallel rods of metal or glass straddling a sink. It is important to leave spaces between adjacent slides, otherwise reagents flow between them by capillary attraction and are lost. Once again, metal rods must be avoided when the object of the method is to demonstrate metal in the tissue.

Preliminary treatment of paraffin sections

Most of the sections in a routine laboratory are cut from tissue embedded in paraffin wax. For this reason, staining methods are usually designed primarily for paraffin sections rather than frozen sections or nitrocellulose sections. In the following chapters, all the staining methods are suitable for paraffin sections except where a specific statement is made to the contrary. When we have found a staining method satisfactory for frozen or nitrocellulose sections as well, we have recorded that information with the particular method. General guidance may also be found in the chapters on nitrocellulose (Chapter 18, p. 264) and frozen sections (Chapter 19, p. 274).

Before a paraffin section can be stained, it is necessary to remove the wax which impregnates the tissue. It may also be necessary to remove deposits that formed during fixation; failure to remove these deposits is a common cause of unwanted granular pigmentation in finished sections. The fixatives that give rise to these deposits are mercuric chloride and formaldehyde. There is a third possible cause of fixation deposit; this is dichromate, which may persist in sections from tissue that was inadequately washed after fixation. This, however, should not occur when the tissue has been properly treated at an earlier stage, whereas mercury deposit and formaldehyde deposit are unavoidable in some circumstances, being particularly likely to form when fixation has been prolonged. Mercuric chloride produces much more deposit in neutral or alkaline fluids than in acid fluids such as Susa. Formaldehyde is particularly likely to cause a deposit in acid mixtures or when the tissue contains much blood. When either of these fixation deposits is anticipated, the sections should be treated suitably before they are stained. In routine laboratories it may be easier to treat every section before it is stained rather than to segregate those in which pigment is to be expected. It is better in the long run to treat too many sections than too few since the treatment has no adverse effect on the great majority of staining methods. One exception, however, is the demonstration of argentaffin cells which may be impaired by attempts to remove mercury deposit or formaldehyde deposit. Secondly, care may be needed with frozen sections, since it is impossible to remove formaldehyde deposit without also extracting lipid from the tissue.

In every laboratory it is necessary to remove paraffin wax from sections. Whether or not formaldehyde deposit and mercury deposit need to be removed will depend on the fixing fluids in routine use. Thus one or other of the following schedules should be used, and a suitable row of jars provided. Whichever schedule is used, the procedure is conveniently described as taking the sections to water. When the phrase 'sections to water' is used in the staining methods that follow, it should be assumed that it includes the removal of fixation deposits if that is necessary.

Taking sections to water

The reagent for removing formaldehyde deposit (Barrett, 1944b) is:

Saturated alcoholic solution of picric acid	85 ml.
Alcohol	15 ml.

The reagents necessary for the removal of mercury deposit are:

A. *Lugol's iodine*

Iodine crystals	1 g.
Potassium iodide	2 g.
Distilled water	100 ml.

Grind the iodine and potassium iodide in a mortar with a small volume of water. Pour off the supernatant, add more water and grind again. Repeat until all is dissolved. Finally add the rest of the water to the solution.

B. 3–5 *per cent aqueous solution of sodium thiosulphate*

METHOD I (Removing wax only)

1. Xylene   2–3 min.
2. Alcohol I   1–2 min.
3. Alcohol II   1–2 min.
4. 50% alcohol   1–2 min.
5. Rinse in tap water

METHOD II (Removing wax and formaldehyde deposits)

1. Xylene   2–3 min.
2. Alcohol I   1–2 min.
3. Alcohol II   1–2 min.
4. Alcoholic picric acid $\frac{1}{2}$–2 hrs.
5. Running tap water until colourless   (10–15 min.)

METHOD III (Removing wax and mercury deposit)

1. Xylene   2–3 min.
2. Alcohol I   1–2 min.
3. Alcohol II   1–2 min.
4. 50% alcohol   1–2 min.
5. Running tap water   1–2 min.
6. Lugol's iodine   2–3 min.
7. Rinse in tap water
8. Sodium thiosulphate until colourless   (1–2 min.)
9. Running tap water   5–10 min.

METHOD IV (Removing wax and both deposits)

1. Xylene   2–3 min.
2. Alcohol I   1–2 min.
3. Alcohol II   1–2 min.
4. Alcoholic picric acid $\frac{1}{2}$–2 hrs.
5. Running tap water until colourless   (10–15 min.)
6. Lugol's iodine   2–3 min.
7. Rinse in tap water
8. Sodium thiosulphate until colourless   (1–2 min.)
9. Running tap water   5–10 min.

Note

Experienced technicians will find it possible to reduce some of these times, especially if the slides are agitated briskly in the reagents. Provided that the sections do not wash off the slides, this will do no harm. There are, however, two stages that should never be cut short: these are the washes in running tap water after picric acid and sodium thiosulphate, since either of these substances is likely to interfere with subsequent staining if not completely removed.

As already stated, sections should never contain dichromate deposit. If, however, they do, this can be removed by treatment with 1 per cent hydrochloric acid in 70 per cent alcohol for 20–30 minutes. It would be convenient to do this between stages 3 and 4 of any of the methods listed above, although any other order for the removal of the various pigments may be used if preferred.

Finishing paraffin sections

Stained sections are usually mounted in a resinous medium which forms a transparent layer of suitable refractive index between the slide and coverslip. Resinous media are dissolved in organic solvents such as xylene and are not miscible with water or alcohol. Almost all dyes used in histological staining methods are dissolved in either water or alcohol, hence the stained sections need to be passed through suitable intermediary reagents after they have been stained and before they can be mounted. This is exactly analogous to the dehydration and clearing of a piece of tissue. When the last stage of a staining method is an aqueous solution, the section is dehydrated in alcohol and cleared in xylene. When a staining method ends with an alcoholic solution, only a rinse in alcohol is needed before the section is cleared in xylene.

Resinous media are usually obtained from commercial suppliers. Often the formula has not been published (e.g. M.A.C., Permount, Polymount, X.A.M.). The constituents of other media, such as Canada balsam and D.P.X., are known, but it is usually more convenient to buy them ready-made. Those who wish to make their own D.P.X. should use the second formula of Kirkpatrick and Lendrum (1941). These authors proposed the abbreviation B.P.S. for this medium to distinguish it from their original D.P.X. (Kirkpatrick and Lendrum, 1939) in which tricresyl phosphate had been used as a plasticizer. Nevertheless, the initials D.P.X. persisted after the formula was altered, and we believe that the second formula (that of B.P.S.) is used for the preparation of at least some of the D.P.X. manufactured commercially. The second formula (Kirkpatrick and Lendrum, 1941) is as follows:

Dibutylphthalate	5 ml.
Xylene	35 ml.
Distrene 80	10 g.

Place the mixture in a closed container in a 56°C incubator until the distrene has dissolved.

In the staining methods that follow, the phrase 'dehydrate, clear, and mount' is used, rather than a repetition of the details of the sequence, which is as follows:

1. 70% alcohol	1–2 min.
2. Alcohol I	1–2 min.
3. Alcohol II	1–2 min.
4. Xylene	at least 2 min.
5. Mount in a resinous medium	

Sections are more often attached to slides than to coverslips. The following instructions apply to slides. (For sections attached to coverslips see Note iv below.) The first step is the removal of excess xylene from the ends and back of the slide. This is best done with a fluff-free cloth. A generous quantity of mounting medium (free from all air bubbles) is then applied to the slide or coverslip; in either case the next step is to lower the side gently on to the coverslip which instantly sticks firmly enough for the slide to be turned right side upwards. With a finger-nail or pencil-point the coverslip may then be pressed down until the whole of its lower surface is covered by mounting medium. If too much of the medium is used, it exudes around the edges of the coverslip and should be left until it has hardened before being removed. When hard, the excess of resinous medium can be lifted by a sharp instrument (e.g. a razor blade) and peeled off in strips.

Notes

(i) After certain staining methods, the section is transferred directly to undiluted alcohol, omitting stage 1. When this is necessary, it is indicated in the staining schedule by the use of the phrase 'clear and mount'.

(ii) Alcohol II must be free from water.

(iii) The xylene must be pure and, above all, must not have been used for the removal of wax from unstained sections since traces of wax are apt to produce crystals in the mounting medium after an interval, thus spoiling the finished preparation (Kirkpatrick and Lendrum, 1941).

(iv) If the section is attached to a coverslip, it is convenient to lay the coverslip, section upwards, on filter paper which will remove the xylene from the other side. Mounting medium may be applied to slide or coverslip, and the procedure completed in the usual way.

(v) If the mounting medium is applied to the section rather than the dry glass, it will spread more freely because the section is still damped with xylene; moreover, it is easier to avoid bubbles in the finished preparation. There is, however, a risk of contaminating the stock of mounting medium by lifting small pieces of section from the slide (or coverslip) when the glass rod is returned to the bottle of medium. These small pieces will reappear on slides mounted subsequently and may be dangerously confusing, especially in cytological laboratories (Graham, 1963). To avoid this possibility, the medium should always be allowed to drop on to the section: it should never be dabbed on.

(vi) The coverslips (or slides) that are used for covering sections must be absolutely clean. Usually it is sufficient to polish them with a fluff-free cloth, but occasionally they are so dirty that it is necessary to soak them in alcohol before polishing.

(vii) When the section is attached to a slide, very viscous mounting media should be avoided, since a thick layer will make it impossible to examine the section with a high power microscope objective that has a small working distance.

Aqueous mounting media

A small number of stains do not lend themselves to mounting in resinous media, because they are dissolved by the dehydrating agent, the clearing agent, or the solvent of the medium. Stains for lipids in frozen sections fall into this category and so do a few stains that are used on paraffin sections (e.g. methyl violet for amyloid). For these stains an aqueous mounting medium must be used. Many aqueous media are available, but they all share two disadvantages when compared with resinous media. First, the medium does not form a strong seal between slide and coverslip, so that the latter is easily dislodged. Secondly, air-pockets are apt to form because of continued evaporation. For these two reasons, a continuous ring of waterproof and rapidly hardening glue is applied around the edge of the coverslip to seal it to the slide. Such glues are known as ringing media, and many types are available. Usually a specially prepared ringing medium is bought from one of the suppliers of histological reagents. Gold size is suitable and so is waterproof glue (e.g. Durofix). In any case, it is easier to apply aqueous media and ringing media if circular coverslips are used rather than rectangular ones. When these media are in constant use, a special turntable will simplify ringing, and will improve the appearance of the finished slides. The best aqueous media are glycerine-jelly and Apáthy's mountant. Glycerine-jelly is easier to prepare but is not suitable for use after every stain (e.g. methyl violet for amyloid). It also needs to be melted before use; this must be done with caution, otherwise air bubbles appear. Apáthy's mountant is fluid at room temperature and may be used after any stain. It is, however, more tedious to prepare.

Apathy's Mountant

This is the original formula (Apáthy, 1892) except for the addition of sodium chloride. The presence of salt was found to improve aqueous media by preventing certain stains (in particular methyl violet) from diffusing out of the tissue into the medium (Highman, 1946).

Gum arabic (gum acacia)	50 g.
Cane sugar	50 g.
Sodium chloride	5 g.
Distilled water	50 ml.
Thymol	a few small crystals

Warm the gum, sugar, salt, and water until all the solids are dissolved (this may take several hours). Whilst still warm, filter through a pad made of several layers of damped muslin. Dissolve the thymol separately by heating it with 1–2 ml. of distilled water and add it to the mixture, which is then ready for use and should be dispensed into several small containers. So long as these are airtight, the medium may be kept indefinitely at room temperature.

Glycerine-jelly

This is the original formula of Kaiser (1880).

Gelatin	10 g.
Distilled water	60 ml.
Glycerol	70 ml.
Phenol	a few crystals

Dissolve the gelatin in the water with gentle heat. Add the glycerol and phenol, mix, filter through damp glass wool or muslin, and dispense into small vessels before cooling. Thymol may be used instead of phenol.

For use, melt in an incubator or water-bath; do not heat over a naked flame as this causes air bubbles to appear.

Labelling slides

Slides have usually been marked with a writing diamond before they were stained. Diamond marks cannot, however, be seen easily when the slides are filed, so that it is almost universal practice to label them again after they have been stained. This may be done by writing on the slide itself with glass-writing ink, or a paper label may be attached and then inscribed. Glass-writing ink has the advantage of permanence; once it has dried it resists water or organic solvents. It is, however, less easy to apply, since it dries too readily on the pen. Moreover, a slide labelled by this method is not easily identified if it is filed vertically in a row. Paper labels are easier to write. They may be obtained already printed with the name of the department. Self-adhesive labels are easier to use than those that need to be moistened.

In any case the label should be applied to the end of the slide opposite to the diamond mark; this arrangement allows the slide to be identified when either end is broken. It is worth considering the use of a variety of colours of ink as an additional aid to identification. A new colour might be used, for example each year; or separate colours for slides of different types (biopsy, necropsy, research, etc.).

Storing slides

The most important feature of any filing system is that slides must be kept in the dark; almost every histological stain will fade on prolonged exposure to light. The second point to be borne in mind is that a file of slides is very heavy; thus a basement should be used for any large collection.

The most compact system is a bank of drawers in which the slides stand vertically in a solid row. This is satisfactory if all the slides are of the same size, but may be confusing when slides of different sizes are in routine use. Before filing slides in drawers of this type, it is essential to verify that the mounting medium is thoroughly dry, otherwise the slides will stick to one another in solid masses.

The alternative for a large collection is to put the slides into cards—which may either be made or bought. These are then filed in standard office filing drawers. Four slides of the usual size (76 × 25 mm.) are comfortably accommodated in a card that fits into a 5 × 3 in. card index filing drawer.

When a small reference collection needs to be consulted often, the slides may be filed flat in drawers, or in trays within boxes. These systems waste too much space to be used for routine storage. A more compact file for a special collection is that in which the slides are fitted into plastic frames, many such frames being suspended in a box. This would be too expensive for the routine storage of a large collection.

Restaining

There are several reasons why it might be necessary to remove the stain from a section and then restain it by the same method or a different one. In some cases the first attempt has been unsuccessful; in others a stain has faded because of age or exposure to light. Sometimes the block is not available so that no new sections can be prepared, or only one section from the block (or only one smear) contains a special feature, and merits examination by more than one staining method.

If the section has been mounted, it will be necessary to soften the mounting medium and remove the coverslip. With a resinous medium this may take time if it has hardened, but xylene will soften even the hardest medium if warmed in an incubator (56-60°C) for a few days. Aqueous media may be softened in warm water after the ringing medium has been scraped away, but care is necessary as the section is liable to be damaged. The section is then returned to water (using the sequence of xylene and alcohol if necessary).

The easiest way to remove most stains is to soak the section in a 1 per cent aqueous solution of potassium permanganate for 5 minutes. After rinsing off surplus permanganate with distilled (not tap) water, the section is treated with a 5 per cent aqueous solution of oxalic acid until the colour has been removed. The oxalic acid is then washed out with several changes of

distilled water. Once again tap water must be avoided since
it may give rise to crystals of calcium oxalate in the section.
After washing, the section is ready for staining. There is no
satisfactory way of decolorizing some preparations (e.g.
Perls's method for ferric iron, and the per-iodic acid Schiff
reaction). However, it is always possible to remove the counterstain from sections stained by these methods; this allows a new
stain to be applied on top of the residue of the old, and is almost
always satisfactory.

After a section has been decolorized, any of the common
histological staining methods may be applied. Some histochemical methods, however, may well fail to work depending on
how the section was treated during its first staining.

CHAPTER 9

Haematoxylin and Eosin

General notes. Eosin. Haematoxylin. Interchangeability of haematoxylin mixtures. Staining machines. Harris's haematoxylin. Ehrlich's haematoxylin. Stock alcoholic solution. Weigert's hæmatoxylin. Heidenhain's haematoxylin. Carazzi's haematoxylin.

MORE sections are stained with haematoxylin and eosin than by any other method and the majority of histological diagnoses can be made without using any other stain. This is because haematoxylin and eosin will show most histological structures, and are particularly suitable for the demonstration of nuclei which are the most important structures in almost every section. Even when not sufficient by themselves, haematoxylin and eosin will usually provide enough information to indicate which other staining methods are likely to be rewarding.

Although every technician stains enormous numbers of sections with haematoxylin and eosin, the results are surprisingly variable and it is not unusual for individual sections or whole batches to be far from perfect. Some of the variations are deliberate, being made to suit the preference of a particular pathologist, and some of the imperfections are due to bad technique at an earlier stage. Many inadequate results, nevertheless, are due to errors in staining, since haematoxylin solutions are inconsistent and demand careful judgement in use. Ideally each section would be stained individually, but in most laboratories the volume of work is so great that it is necessary to use a routine schedule which will be satisfactory for every section. This is particularly important when staining machines are used.

Eosin

Although eosin is the less important half of the haematoxylin and eosin stain, it merits a few notes. Eosin is a synthetic xanthene dye which is usually used as a 0·5 per cent or 1·0 per cent solution in water; this can conveniently be diluted from a 5 per cent stock solution, which also has the advantage of being less susceptible to the growth of moulds. As an alternative the addition of a crystal of thymol or a few drops of formalin will inhibit mould growth, but even when it has become infected, an eosin solution will give satisfactory staining results after filtration.

It would be a mistake to regard eosin as a counterstain whose purpose is to tint everything except the nuclei a uniform pink. Better results are obtained by differentiating the eosin so that different structures are coloured more or less deeply. The degree of differentiation will be a matter of individual taste; when carried to extremes the dye will be almost entirely removed except from red blood corpuscles and eosinophil leucocytes and this may on occasions be useful as a specific staining method for those structures. It should be borne in mind that some fixatives (especially those containing mercuric chloride) render tissue more avid for eosin so that sections are liable to be unpleasantly red after their use unless the differentiation is prolonged. For this reason it is better to segregate sections prepared from tissues fixed in different ways. Very brief eosin staining of osteoid tissue is mentioned elsewhere (p. 291).

Haematoxylin

Haematoxylin is extracted from the heart-wood of the logwood tree (*Haematoxylon campechianum*). Pure haematoxylin is colourless but it can readily be oxidized to the reddish dye haematein which is the active dyestuff in all so-called haematoxylin solutions. This change occurs as soon as the logwood is exposed to air so that pure colourless haematoxylin is never used. Haematein itself is not entirely stable, being rendered colourless by further oxidation. In practice this decay is balanced by the oxidation of at least an equivalent amount of haematoxylin to haematein so that the solution has a useful life of several months or even years. This explains why *haematoxylin* rather than *haematein* is used as the basis of the solution. It is also for this reason that haematoxylin solutions are only useful after the passage of time (*natural ripening*) or the addition of an oxidizing agent (*artificial ripening*). Even a properly ripened solution of haematoxylin needs to be used with a mordant (usually aluminium, iron, or tungsten). This is applied to the section either before the dye or mixed with it.

When first stained with an aluminium (or *alum*) haematoxylin, nuclei are a dark red colour. In order to change this to blue
and to stabilize the dye, the sections must be treated with a weak
alkali. In most regions the tap water is alkaline and may be
used for this process which is referred to as *blueing*.

In almost all nuclear staining schedules, haematoxylin is used
as a regressive stain. There are two exceptions to this rule: first,
it is occasionally expedient to use haematoxylin progressively
for urgent methods; secondly, haematoxylin is sometimes used
as a counterstain and may then follow a stain that would be
removed if the haematoxylin were differentiated. Whenever
possible, progressive staining is to be avoided because it either
leaves the nuclei too pale or colours cytoplasm with the haematoxylin. When haematoxylin is used regressively, the degree of
differentiation can be varied to suit individual tastes but, unfortunately, it is not possible to lay down strict rules about the
time necessary for proper differentiation. The chief reason for
this is variation in the staining power of the haematoxylin
solution, all such solutions being subject to unpredictable re-
newal and decay of the active principle haematein described
above. In practice it is relatively easy to differentiate iron
haematoxylins, since the only problem is to decide when the
section is sufficiently pale, and any doubts can be resolved by
microscopical control. With alum haematoxylins, however,
assessment is more difficult, since the sections turn red in the
differentiating fluid, thus presenting the problem of how to
judge the degree of differentiation in shades of red when the
ultimate results will be blue. It is possible to blue the section in
tap water from time to time, returning it to the differentiating
fluid as often as necessary, but with practice it is soon possible
to recognize the exact shade of bright salmon pink that will give
the correct result. It is well to know what tissue is being stained
because a section that is crowded with nuclei (e.g. lymph node)
will be quite dark, whereas tissue in which nuclei are sparse will
be relatively pale. In every case it is of the utmost importance
to agitate the sections briskly in the differentiating fluid if uniform coloration is to be obtained.

Interchangeability of Haematoxylin mixtures

Many haematoxylin mixtures have been used; these are often

known by the name of the worker who first used them. Some are suitable only for special purposes but others fall into groups and are more or less interchangeable; it would be superfluous to give full details of all of them. The following paragraphs include the names of all the well-known mixtures and are intended to show which of them is likely to be a satisfactory substitute in a method that specifies a mixture not ready to hand.

For routine haematoxylin and eosin staining, the four mixtures in common use are those of Harris (1900), Ehrlich (1886), Cole (1943), and Delafield (Prudden, 1885). Of these, Cole's and Delafield's mixtures have no particular advantages over the others, one or other of which could be substituted for them in any circumstances. Ehrlich's haematoxylin has certain advantages over Harris's, and these are listed in the notes that accompany the method (p. 103). However, Harris's haematoxylin can always be used in place of Ehrlich's even though the results may on occasion be slightly inferior. Harris's is the most widely used haematoxylin of this group, but this is partly because it produces good results when used with stains other than eosin. There can be no serious objection to using Cole's, Delafield's or Ehrlich's haematoxylin in place of Harris's in haematoxylin and eosin methods, but it must be emphasized that these mixtures are not as versatile as Harris's and may not necessarily be satisfactory substitutes in methods other than haematoxylin and eosin. Confusion may arise unless it is remembered that in some methods Harris's haematoxylin is used at half strength, and for some purposes the acetic acid is omitted.

The four mixtures already mentioned are not satisfactory for staining frozen sections or in cases where haematoxylin is being used as a counterstain. They produce very heavy staining results, and in some cases the alcohol content is too high. Good results can, however, be obtained with Carazzi's (1911), or Mayer's haematoxylin, or with Harris's haematoxylin used at half strength. Although Mayer (1903) published his final formula after many modifications and amendments, we have consistently preferred the results that we have obtained with Carazzi's less elaborate mixture which shows no tendency to stain cytoplasm. Half-strength Harris's haematoxylin gives results that are almost as good, but again we prefer Carazzi's mixture which has the additional advantage that it remains stable for a long period. The three mixtures are, however, interchangeable and there is no serious objection to using any of them in place of one of the others.

Weigert's (1904) haematoxylin is sometimes used with eosin (especially for sections of brain) but its chief use is in methods where it is followed by a 'searching' counterstain such as picric acid. For this purpose there is no other satisfactory haematoxylin mixture in common use, although a similar result is obtained with the nuclear staining method that uses celestine blue followed by haematoxylin.

Heidenhain's (1896) haematoxylin is not usually used in combination with eosin, but it has a place in the staining of sections that reject other haematoxylin mixtures. Such sections include those from tissue that was fixed in osmium tetroxide mixtures, or tissue that spent too long in decalcifying fluid, or was stored for a very long time in fixative or in alcohol. Heidenhain's haematoxylin is not exclusively a nuclear stain although, used with orange G, it is a favourite method for the demonstration of mitoses and other fine nuclear detail. Other structures that can be demonstrated include mitochondria, muscle striations, and keratin, depending on the extent to which the stain is differentiated. There is no alternative haematoxylin mixture to Heidenhain's for its particular purposes.

Haematoxylin is used in many staining methods for structures *other than nuclei*. The mixtures used for these methods are usually known by the names of their originators. The methods do not fall within the scope of this chapter and details of the ones in current use will be found in the appropriate later chapters. In order to prevent confusion we have, however, listed the well-known names of such haematoxylin mixtures here. Mallory's phosphotungstic acid haematoxylin is a connective tissue stain of wide application (p. 114). Haematoxylin mixtures that have been used to demonstrate myelin (p. 239) include those of Kultschitzky, Loyez, Spielmeyer, and Weigert. Copper and lead may be demonstrated by Mallory and Parker's haematoxylin. Mayer was responsible for many haematoxylin mixtures in addition to that already mentioned. The one most likely to cause confusion is Mayer's (1896) mucihaematein which has been used for the demonstration of mucin. Yet another

H

use for haematoxylin is as an elastic stain in Verhoeff's method.

Staining machines

At first sight the haematoxylin and eosin methods should be particularly suitable for mechanical staining. In most laboratories the method is used daily for a large number of sections. In practice, however, there are several reasons why it has not proved universally popular and why the results are not always as consistent as might have been expected. In busy laboratories, most of the solutions may need changing frequently since the troughs on most machines contain small volumes compared with those used for hand staining. Moreover the process of changing those on the machine is more laborious and on the whole the machine proves to be wasteful of reagents. Secondly, much of the time taken up by any staining schedule is occupied in loading slides into staining racks and in covering the stained sections with coverslips and labelling them. Hand staining can be done in small batches that follow one another at frequent intervals whereas the machine accepts and delivers considerable numbers at intervals of 40–60 minutes only. This may also be a cause of delay when a single section or a small group require urgent staining. Thirdly, many laboratories use more than one fixative and prefer to vary the times of staining and differentiation to obtain the best results; machines do not lend themselves to such variations.

Nevertheless there are many situations in which staining machines can be used with profit, especially where many sections of the same or similar tissue are prepared. Examples include the preparation of class teaching sections and the work of many specialist diagnostic or research laboratories.

When a haematoxylin and eosin method is carried out by machine, the practical problem is the frequent use of running tap water. Machines may be equipped with this but it is usually preferable to find a substitute for at least some of these washes to obviate the piping necessary for the supply and removal of water and the risk of flooding. In the published methods, running tap water is required after haematoxylin, after differentiation, and after eosin. When the machine is programmed to remove fixation deposits before staining, another washing stage is introduced before the haematoxylin.

Of these washes, that after haematoxylin is the least important, and little or no harm would be done if still tap water were used at this stage. After differentiation, however, proper blueing is essential, and the process rapidly neutralizes the alkali in a trough of still tap water. If running water is not used at this stage, it will be necessary, therefore, either to provide a series of at least three troughs of still tap water, or to use a stronger alkali (such as 1 per cent 0·880 ammonia in tap water). After eosin, adequate washing is necessary for the differentiation of the stain, although some differentiation also occurs in the alcohols used for dehydration. It is, however, undesirable to carry much eosin into these alcohols since any substantial concentration would cause unwanted additional staining of the sections. At this stage at least two troughs of still tap water should therefore be used. When fixation deposits are removed on the machine, it is important to wash the sections well, since both picric acid and sodium thiosulphate inhibit haematoxylin staining. At least two troughs of tap water will therefore be necessary.

A haematoxylin and eosin schedule modified for use with a staining machine has been published by Longnecker (1966).

Harris's haematoxylin and eosin

A popular method for routine use (Harris, 1900). The haematoxylin does not need time to ripen. Results are consistent and the staining schedule is fairly rapid.

REAGENTS

A. *Harris's haematoxylin*

Haematoxylin	1 g.
Alcohol	10 ml.
Potassium alum (aluminium potassium sulphate)	20 g.
Distilled water	200 ml.
Mercuric oxide	0·5 g.
Glacial acetic acid	8 ml.

Dissolve the haematoxylin in the alcohol. Dissolve the alum in the water using heat. Mix the two solutions together; heat to boiling-point; add the mercuric oxide. Cool rapidly by immersing the flask in cold water. When cold, add the acetic acid. The solution is then ready for use and will keep its staining properties for 3–4 months.

B. *1 per cent hydrochloric acid in 70 per cent alcohol*

C. *Eosin*

Eosin (yellowish, water and alcohol soluble)	1 g.
Distilled water	100 ml.
Thymol	1 small crystal

METHOD

1. Sections to water.
2. Harris's haematoxylin 10–15 minutes.
3. Blue in running tap water for at least 5 minutes (see Note i).
4. Differentiate in acid alcohol 10–15 seconds.
5. Blue in running tap water for at least 10 minutes (see Note i).
6. Eosin 5–10 minutes (see Note ii).
7. Running tap water 3–5 minutes.
8. 50% alcohol 2–3 minutes.
9. Dehydrate, clear, and mount.

RESULTS

Nuclei; calcium deposits; bacteria: *blue*.
Mucin; cartilage: *pale blue-grey*.
Red blood corpuscles; eosinophil leucocytes: *red*.
Cytoplasm of other cells: *shades of pink*.

Notes

(i) Running tap water will only blue haematoxylin if it is alkaline (hard water). In regions where the water is neutral or acid (soft water), the stages 3 and 5 above should be replaced by immersion for one-half to one minute in Scott's tap water substitute. (Scott, 1912).

Sodium bicarbonate	3·5 g.
Magnesium sulphate	20 g.
Tap water	1000 ml.
Thymol	1 small crystal

Dissolve the salts separately; then mix.

(ii) In some places the tap water removes eosin from sections unusually rapidly. This can be prevented by the addition of 1 per cent calcium chloride to the eosin. The time needed for staining is then greatly shortened (to about 1 minute). Washing time should also be reduced to about 1 minute.

(iii) If staining machines are used, it may be preferable to avoid the use of running water (p. 98).

(iv) For progressive staining, Harris's haematoxylin should be used for 1–2 minutes.

(v) Since it contains very little alcohol, Harris's haematoxylin is suitable for frozen sections (p. 160).

(vi) Slight fading of the haematoxylin occurs after some years, even if sections are stored in the dark.

Common faults

(i) Groups of tiny dark grey or black granules are due to precipitation of haematoxylin. These lie on top of the section and appear particularly commonly on parts that contain mucus. The only way of avoiding this precipitate is to filter the haematoxylin staining solution about once a week.

(ii) Dull red or brown staining of nuclei is due either to over-ripe haematoxylin or to insufficient blueing after differentiation. This appearance should not be confused with red staining of the nucleolus when all the other nuclear chromatin is blue—a common result with Harris's haematoxylin.

(iii) Nuclei appear as blue rings with colourless centres when the haematoxylin staining time has been too short.

(iv) Uniformly weak staining of the nuclear membrane and chromatin is usually due to over-differentiation.

(v) Sections in which the nuclei are blue and congested without proper chromatin detail have not had sufficient differentiation. In very bad cases the cytoplasm is an unpleasant slaty-blue colour.

Ehrlich's haematoxylin and eosin

Excellent for routine use although requiring more care than Harris's haematoxylin. Many users prefer the results, which are more precise. (Ehrlich, 1886.)

REAGENTS

A. *Ehrlich's haematoxylin*

Haematoxylin	80 g.
Alcohol	2400 ml.
Potassium alum (aluminium potassium sulphate)	240 g.
Distilled water	1200 ml.
Glycerol	1200 ml.
Glacial acetic acid	120 ml.

Dissolve the haematoxylin in the alcohol. Dissolve the alum in the water using heat; whilst warm add the glycerol and allow to cool. Add the haematoxylin solution in small volumes to the alum solution, shaking well between each addition. Add the glacial acetic acid and shake well.

The solution must now be allowed to ripen in clear glass bottles in the light. The bottles should be covered but not stoppered. Ripening will take 6–8 weeks and the solution will then keep its staining properties for many years.

B. *1 per cent hydrochloric acid in 70 per cent alcohol*

C. *Eosin*

Eosin (yellowish, water and alcohol soluble)	1 g.
Distilled water	100 ml.
Thymol	1 small crystal

METHOD

1. Sections to water.
2. Rinse in alcohol.
3. Ehrlich's haematoxylin 45 minutes.
4. Blue in running tap water for at least 5 minutes (see Note i).
5. Differentiate in acid alcohol 15–20 seconds.
6. Blue in running tap water for at least 15 minutes (see Note i).
7. Eosin 5–10 minutes (see Note ii).
8. Running tap water 3–5 minutes.
9. 50% alcohol 2–3 minutes.
10. Dehydrate, clear, and mount.

RESULTS

As for Harris's haematoxylin and eosin above.

Notes

(i) In regions where the tap water is neutral or acid (soft water), Scott's tap water substitute should be used at stages 4 and 6. See Note i to Harris's haematoxylin and eosin above.

(ii) In some places the tap water removes eosin from the sections unusually rapidly. See Note ii to Harris's method above.

(iii) If staining machines are used, it may be preferable to avoid the use of running water (p. 98).

(iv) Ehrlich's haematoxylin has certain advantages over other alum haematoxylin formulae, including Harris's. Fine nuclear chromatin is shown more precisely. The stained sections are even less liable to fading. Ehrlich's haematoxylin will stain some sections that the others will not (e.g. sections from tissue that had been stored too long in fixative or subjected to fierce acid decalcification).

(v) The long period needed for ripening may be regarded as a disadvantage. It certainly means that Ehrlich's haematoxylin is unlikely to be chosen unless its need has been foreseen. Methods for hastening the ripening process are available but are not recommended because they spoil the keeping properties of the stain. In an emergency the stain may be ripened artificially by the addition of sodium or potassium iodate (50 mg. for every gram of haematoxylin) (Lillie, 1965).

(vi) Another disadvantage is the length of time required for staining. This is due to the inhibitory effect of the glycerol which, however, is valuable in preventing evaporation.

(vii) Ehrlich's haematoxylin is unsuitable for frozen sections because of its high alcohol content.

(viii) Ehrlich's haematoxylin will not be used where strict economy is obligatory since the glycerol and the high concentration of haematoxylin make it relatively expensive.

Common faults

Sections stained by Ehrlich's haematoxylin may show any of the faults listed under Harris's haematoxylin above. An additional cause of dull red or brown nuclear staining is the use of unripened stain.

Stock alcoholic haematoxylin solution

A ripened alcoholic solution of haematoxylin which keeps indefinitely. It may be diluted as required and used in many methods.

Haematoxylin	20 g.
Alcohol	100 ml.

Allow to ripen in a clear glass bottle in the light for at least 4 weeks.

Weigert's haematoxylin

An iron haematoxylin which withstands picric acid and is therefore valuable for many special stains. Also good for staining brain sections (Weigert, 1904).

REAGENTS

A. *Weigert's solution A*

Haematoxylin	1 g.
Alcohol	100 ml.

Allow to ripen for 4 weeks before use.

A better alternative is to dilute 5 ml. of stock alcoholic haematoxylin solution (above) with 95 ml. of alcohol. The solution will keep indefinitely.

B. *Weigert's solution B*

30% aqueous solution of ferric chloride	4 ml.
Distilled water	100 ml.
Conc. hydrochloric acid	1 ml.

The solution will keep indefinitely.

C. *Weigert's haematoxylin*

Mix equal volumes of *solution A* and *solution B*, and use within 30 minutes.

D. *1 per cent hydrochloric acid in 70 per cent alcohol*

METHOD

1. Sections to water.
2. Weigert's haematoxylin 15–20 minutes.
3. Running tap water for at least 5 minutes (see Note i).
4. Differentiate in acid alcohol 5–10 seconds.
5. Running tap water for at least 10 minutes (see Note i).
6. Counterstain. Weigert's haematoxylin is particularly suitable for use with the van Gieson counterstain and its modifications (p. 111) or with trichrome stains (pp. 116-122). If an eosin counterstain is required, use the eosin schedule given under Harris's or Ehrlich's haematoxylin and eosin above.

Notes

(i) In regions where the tap water is neutral or acid (soft water), Scott's tap water substitute should be used at stages 3 and 5. (see Note i to Harris's haematoxylin and eosin on page 100.)

(ii) If staining machines are used, it may be preferable to avoid the use of running water (p. 98).

Heidenhain's haematoxylin

Will stain sections that are resistant to other haematoxylin mixtures; capable of producing very precise detail; popular for photography; not exclusively a nuclear stain. (Heidenhain, 1896.)

REAGENTS

A. *Iron alum solution*

Iron alum (ammonium ferric sulphate)	5 g.
Distilled water	100 ml.

The solution will keep indefinitely.

B. *Haematoxylin solution*

Haematoxylin	0·5 g.
Alcohol	10 ml.
Distilled water	90 ml.

Allow to ripen for 4 weeks. A better alternative is to dilute 2·5 ml. of stock alcoholic haematoxylin solution (above) with 7·5 ml. of alcohol and 90 ml. of distilled water. The solution will keep indefinitely.

METHOD

1. Sections to water.
2. Iron alum solution 30 minutes to 24 hours (see Note ii).
3. Rinse in tap water.
4. Heidenhain's haematoxylin solution 30 minutes to 24 hours (see Note ii).
5. Rinse in tap water.
6. Differentiate in iron alum solution 1–30 minutes using careful microscopical control (see Notes iii and iv).
7. Running tap water 5 minutes.
8. Counterstain if required. Suitable counterstains include the van Gieson method and its modifications (p. 111),

trichrome methods (pp. 116–122), a saturated solution of orange G in alcohol for 2–3 minutes, and eosin as used with Harris's or Ehrlich's haematoxylin above.

Notes

(i) The iron alum solution is used as both mordant (stage 2) and differentiator (stage 6).

(ii) Sections should be treated with mordant (stage 2) and haematoxylin solution (stage 4) for about the same length of time. The optimum time varies according to the fixation of the specimen. After most fixing fluids (formalin-saline, mercuric-chloride-formalin, Susa, Bouin's fluid, and Carnoy's fluid), 30 minutes may be sufficient although one hour is better. After fixing fluids that contain dichromate (Helly's fluid and Zenker's fluid) at least three hours will be needed. Sections will need up to 24 hours in each solution when the tissue was fixed in osmium tetroxide or had been stored too long in fixing fluid or alcohol.

(iii) Heidenhain's haematoxylin produces a dark grey or black colour. What structures are stained will depend on the degree of differentiation. Mitochondria are decolorized very quickly and cross-striations of muscles rather more slowly while nuclei are relatively resistant to differentiation. Keratin and red blood corpuscles remain heavily stained and the cytoplasm of other cells remains dull grey.

(iv) Differentiation is slower if the iron alum solution is used at half-strength for stage 6. If by chance a section has been over-differentiated, it should be returned to Heidenhain's haematoxylin for a period equal to the original staining time.

(v) Heidenhain's haematoxylin is resistant to fading provided that the iron alum has been thoroughly removed by washing.

Carazzi's haematoxylin

A pale precise haematoxylin which is very successful as a counterstain. Not intended for use with eosin as a histological stain although smears can be stained satisfactorily. (Carazzi, 1911.)

REAGENTS

A. *Carazzi's haematoxylin*

Haematoxylin	0·5 g.
Glycerol	100 ml.
Potassium alum (aluminium potassium sulphate)	25 g.
Distilled water	400 ml.
Potassium iodate	0·1 g.

Mix the haematoxylin with the glycerol. Dissolve the potassium alum in almost the whole volume of distilled water *without using heat* (this may take many hours). Mix by adding the alum solution in small volumes to the haematoxylin solution, shaking well between each addition. Dissolve the potassium iodate in the rest of the distilled water (say 10 ml.) using very little, if any, heat, and add it to the mixture. Shake well. The solution is then ready for use and will keep its staining properties for 4–6 months.

B. *1 per cent hydrochloric acid in 70 per cent alcohol*

USES

Carazzi's haematoxylin may be used either as a progressive stain or as a regressive stain. For progressive staining (e.g. with Congo red, the per-iodic acid Schiff method, and histochemical techniques for enzymes) the section is counterstained with Carazzi's haematoxylin for 1–2 minutes and then blued in tap water for 5–10 minutes (see Note i). Carazzi's haematoxylin is more often used as a regressive stain (for fat-stained frozen sections, for smears, or in conjunction with such stains as alcian blue and mucicarmine. Sections are then stained for 10 minutes, blued in tap water for 5 minutes, differentiated in acid alcohol for 5–10 seconds, and blued in tap water for 10 minutes (see Note i).

Notes

(i) In regions where the tap water is neutral or acid (soft water), Scott's tap water substitute should be used. See Note i to Harris's haematoxylin and eosin (p. 100).

(ii) Carazzi's haematoxylin is particularly suitable for use as a counterstain because nuclei alone are stained: it does not stain cell cytoplasm or substances such as mucus. In this respect it is better than Mayer's widely recommended haematoxylin (commonly known as Mayer's haemalum).

(iii) Many published special staining methods specify Mayer's haemalum. We have found that Carazzi's haematoxylin will give results that are as good or better. This is equally true when Carazzi's haematoxylin is substituted for Mayer's in methods that specify nuclear staining by celestine blue and haematoxylin.

CHAPTER 10

Connective Tissues

General notes. Collagen: Curtis; van Gieson. Elastic: Weigert; Verhoeff. Phosphotungstic acid haematoxylin. Trichrome stains: Picro-Mallory; Goldner; MSB. Schmorl's picro-thionin. Chloranilic acid.

MANY of the special staining methods used in histological laboratories are not perfectly specific: a single method may be used for one purpose with one tissue and an entirely different purpose with another tissue. For this reason, any classification of staining methods must be arbitrary. In this chapter and the following ones, we have tried to arrange methods according to their commonest or most important uses. When a method has additional uses, a cross-reference has been inserted.

The present chapter is concerned with stains for connective tissues, including fibrous tissue (collagen), elastic tissue, and various types of muscle; stains for fibrin have been added for convenience. Some types of connective tissue are dealt with in more appropriate places; thus, methods for reticulin and basement membranes are to be found in Chapter 16 which is devoted to silver impregnation methods. Mucopolysaccharides (including cartilage and amyloid) are dealt with separately (Chap. 12), and so are lipids (Chap. 13). Some methods that we recommend primarily for another purpose may also be useful for connective tissues. The following list includes the most important connective tissues and related substances, with notes of appropriate methods for their demonstration.

Adipose tissue. Composed largely of triglycerides (neutral fats). Demonstrated in frozen sections by Sudan III and IV (p. 160), oil red O (p. 161), Sudan black (p. 162), or phosphine (p. 163). May be seen in paraffin sections after treatment with osmium tetroxide (p. 164).

Amyloid. An abnormal intercellular deposit of protein and polysaccharide. Demonstrable by several special methods (pp. 152–157).

Basement membranes. Delicate sheets between epithelium and connective tissue. Found immediately beneath epithelial coverings and around glands or tubules. Also present around small blood vessels. Demonstrated by the per-iodic acid Schiff method (p. 141) or by silver impregnation (p. 217).

Bone. Sections of decalcified tissue are usually used. Suitable staining methods include haematoxylin and eosin, Curtis's picro-ponceau (p. 110), and Goldner's trichrome (p. 120). Bone canaliculi are demonstrated by picro-thionin (p. 122).

Bone marrow. Demonstrated by Barrett's bone marrow stain (p. 191), or by Giemsa (p. 182).

Calcium. Found in the skeleton; also found in a wide variety of tissues in abnormal conditions. Demonstrated for most routine purposes by the von Kóssa method (p. 210). For specific staining, the chloranilic acid method (p. 123) should be used.

Cartilage. Demonstrated by the per-iodic acid Schiff method, alcian blue, or toluidine blue.

Collagen. Forms the connective tissue scaffolding of all tissues except brain and spinal cord. Also present in dense masses in tendons, ligaments, etc. Stained specifically by the Curtis and van Gieson methods (p. 110). Counterstained in trichrome methods (see below) but not coloured specifically. Some collagen contains mucopolysaccharide which may be demonstrated by alcian blue (p. 145).

Elastic tissue. Found throughout the connective tissue but particularly plentiful in arteries, veins and skin. Demonstrated by Weigert's method (p. 111), Verhoeff's method (p. 113), or aldehyde fuchsin (p. 201).

Fibrin. Found in blood-clot and inflammatory exudate. (Small arteries and other structures sometimes undergo a degenerative process in which they are converted into a homogeneous material which gives staining reactions identical with those of true fibrin. This is accordingly referred to as 'fibrinoid' degeneration.) Demonstrated by trichrome stains (p. 116) and by phosphotungstic acid haematoxylin (p. 114).

Muscle. Demonstrated by trichrome methods (see below) or by phloxine tartrazine (p. 203). Striated muscle (skeletal and cardiac) repay examination with polarized light. Other methods for muscle striations include phosphotungstic acid haematoxylin (p. 114), Heidenhain's haematoxylin (p. 105), and solochrome cyanin (p. 247.)

Reticulin. Fine fibres around small blood vessels and in many organs such as lymph nodes, spleen, and liver. Demonstrated by silver impregnation methods (pp. 213–216).

Curtis's picro-ponceau

SCOPE

A method for collagen. Suitable for paraffin, nitrocellulose, or frozen sections after any fixing fluid.

REAGENTS

A. *Weigert's haematoxylin* (p. 104)

B. *1 per cent hydrochloric acid in 70 per cent alcohol*

C. *Picro-ponceau mixture*

1% aqueous solution of Ponceau S	10 ml.
Saturated aqueous solution of picric acid	90 ml.
Glacial acetic acid	1–2 ml.

METHOD

1. Sections to water.
2. Weigert's haematoxylin 15–20 minutes.
3. Running tap water at least 5 minutes.
4. Acid alcohol 5–10 seconds.
5. Running tap water at least 10 minutes.
6. Picro-ponceau 2–5 minutes.
7. Rinse briefly in running tap water (see Note i).
8. Dehydrate rapidly, clear, and mount (see Note i).

RESULTS

Collagen: *red*.
Nuclei: *grey*.
Other structures: *yellow*.

Notes

(i) Water removes the red colour, so that the final rinse must be brief. Alcohol removes the yellow colour, so that dehydration should be rapid.

(ii) Weigert's haematoxylin is used because the mordant is iron. Ordinary (aluminium-mordanted) nuclear haematoxylin would be removed by the picric acid.

(iii) This modification of the van Gieson (1889) method was made by Curtis (1905), who substituted ponceau S for the original acid fuchsin. We prefer Curtis's method for routine use because ponceau S gives a much more permanent result than acid fuchsin. It has been said that ponceau S is less satisfactory than acid fuchsin for very young collagen, but we are not convinced that this is so.

van Gieson's picro-fuchsin

This method is almost identical with that of Curtis above. The only difference is at stage 6, where van Gieson's picro-fuchsin is used for 2–5 minutes instead of Curtis's picro-ponceau. All other stages of the method are the same. The results are identical except that acid fuchsin gives a brighter pinkish-red than ponceau which gives a slightly browner red. Fuchsin fades much more rapidly.

van Gieson's picro-fuchsin

1% aqueous acid fuchsin	10 ml.
Saturated aqueous picric acid	100 ml.

Weigert's elastic stain (Hart's modification)

SCOPE

An excellent method for demonstrating elastic fibres, including fine fibres, but has the disadvantage of being slow (overnight). When speed is important, we recommend Verhoeff's method (see below) or aldehyde fuchsin (p. 201). Suitable for paraffin, nitrocellulose or frozen sections after any fixing fluid.

REAGENTS

A. *Weigert's stock solution*

Resorcin-fuchsin	1·5 g.
95% alcohol	200 ml.
Concentrated hydrochloric acid	4 ml.

Boil for 20 minutes in a water-bath. A long-necked flask should be chosen, to reduce evaporation. Cool. The solution will keep for many months.

B. *1 per cent hydrochloric acid in 70 per cent alcohol*

C. *Working solution*

Weigert's stock solution	5–20 ml.
Acid alcohol (solution B)	45–30 ml.
Total	50 ml.

The exact proportion varies with each new batch of stock

solution, and should be discovered by trial and error. An ideal mixture will stain all elastic fibres, including fine ones, but no other tissue component. This working solution will stain dozens of sections without exhaustion. It should be replaced after 2–3 weeks, or sooner if much of it evaporates.

D. *Harris's haematoxylin* (p. 99)

E. *Curtis's picro-ponceau mixture* (p. 110)

METHOD

1. Sections to water.
2. Rinse in alcohol.
3. Elastic stain (working solution) overnight. The container should be closed.
4. Rinse in acid alcohol.
5. Running tap water at least 10 minutes.
6. Harris's haematoxylin 10 minutes.
7. Running tap water at least 5 minutes.
8. Differentiate in acid alcohol 10–15 seconds.
9. Running tap water at least 10 minutes.
10. Curtis's picro-ponceau mixture 2–5 minutes.
11. Rinse rapidly in running tap water.
12. Dehydrate rapidly, clear, and mount.

RESULTS

Elastic fibres: *black*.
Collagen: *red*.
Nuclei: *grey*.
Other structures: *yellow*.

Notes

(i) Weigert (and many later authors) did not add the acid until the dye had been dissolved in alcohol, and the solution cooled. We have obtained more consistent results by adding the acid to the mixture before it is boiled.

(ii) Deterioration of the elastic stain may occur quite suddenly. The working solution must be discarded as soon as it shows any tendency to stain cytoplasm. When this occurs, the dark colour of the elastic stain is often modified by the counterstain so that, for instance, van Gieson's and Curtis's stains produce unpleasant dark greens and reddish-browns.

(iii) A dark bluish-mauve band across the slide (glass as well as section) is a sign that evaporation has occurred.

(iv) Weigert (1898) described the preparation of this stain, which he used at full strength. He did, however, indicate that longer staining with diluted stain was satisfactory. Hart (1908) published the first method to include staining overnight. Carleton and Leach (1938) did not like the results after fixation in Heidenhain's Susa; some later authors have held the same opinion. The results with undiluted Weigert's stain are unsatisfactory, but if Hart's modification is used, Susa gives perfectly satisfactory results.

(v) The elastic stain may be used with a simple counterstain such as neutral red, but we prefer to use haematoxylin and Curtis's stain since these provide a more complete picture of the connective tissue. If required, the method may be combined with alcian blue (p. 145).

If Curtis's mixture is used, protracted washing and dehydration will weaken the red and yellow colours respectively.

(vi) When van Gieson's and Curtis's stains are used on their own, an iron-mordanted haematoxylin is preferred since it will withstand picric acid. When Weigert's elastic stain is added to the schedule, an alum haematoxylin is satisfactory because the ferric chloride in the elastic stain serves as a mordant.

(vii) For those who prefer to prepare their own resorcin-fuchsin, the method is as follows:

Add 200 ml. distilled water to 2 g. basic fuchsin and 4 g. resorcinol and bring to the boil. While boiling, add 25 ml. 30 per cent aqueous ferric chloride with constant stirring. Continue to boil and stir for 5 minutes. A dark precipitate of resorcin-fuchsin forms. When cool, filter, and keep the precipitate (which will amount to 1·5 g.). This should be allowed to dry on the filter paper. Weigert's stock solution is prepared by adding the filter paper with the precipitate to alcohol and hydrochloric acid as above.

Verhoeff's elastic stain

SCOPE

A rapid method for demonstrating elastic, but fails to demonstrate fine fibres. When time permits, Hart's modification of Weigert's stain is preferable. Suitable for paraffin or frozen sections after any routine fixing fluid (Verhoeff, 1908).

REAGENTS

A. *Saturated aqueous solution of mercuric chloride*

I

B. *Verhoeff's elastic stain*

20% alcoholic haematoxylin (p. 103)	5 ml.
Alcohol	15 ml.
10% aqueous ferric chloride	8 ml.
Lugol's iodine (p. 84)	8 ml.

This mixture must be freshly prepared.

C. *2 per cent aqueous ferric chloride*

D. *Curtis's picro-ponceau* (p. 110)

METHOD

1. Sections to water.
2. Mercuric chloride 30 minutes in a closed vessel.
3. Rinse in water.
4. Verhoeff's elastic stain 15–30 minutes.
5. Rinse in tap water.
6. Differentiate in ferric chloride until the elastic fibres stand out sharply.
7. Running tap water 2–3 minutes.
8. Alcohol 5–15 minutes to remove iodine.
9. Running tap water 5 minutes.
10. Picro-ponceau 2–5 minutes.
11. Rinse briefly in water.
12. Dehydrate rapidly, clear, and mount.

RESULTS

Elastic fibres: *black.*
Collagen: *red.*
Nuclei: *grey.*
Other structures: *yellow.*

Phosphotungstic acid haematoxylin

SCOPE

A stain with many uses (see Results below). Suitable for paraffin, frozen and nitrocellulose sections after any routine fixing fluid (see Note v). Of many variants derived from the original method of Mallory (1897–8; 1900–1), this one (Lieb, 1948) has given the best results in routine use but is not our first choice for the nervous system (p. 252).

REAGENTS

A. *0·5 per cent aqueous potassium permanganate.* This should be freshly prepared from a stronger stock solution (not weaker than 1 per cent).

B. *2 per cent aqueous oxalic acid*

C. *4 per cent aqueous iron alum (ferric ammonium sulphate)*

D. *Phosphotungstic acid haematoxylin*

Haematoxylin	0·5 g.
Phosphotungstic acid	10 g.
Distilled water	500 ml.
0·25% aqueous potassium permanganate	25 ml.

Dissolve the haematoxylin in about 50 ml. of water with gentle heat. Dissolve the phosphotungstic acid in the rest of the water with heat. When cool, mix the two solutions and add the permanganate. The solution is ready for use the following day and improves if kept for some weeks.

METHOD

1. Sections to water.
2. Permanganate 5 minutes (see Note i).
3. Rinse in distilled water (see Note ii).
4. Oxalic acid 5 minutes.
5. Rinse in distilled water (see Note ii).
6. Iron alum 1 hour.
7. Rinse in distilled water.
8. Phosphotungstic acid haematoxylin 2–6 hours (see Note iii).
9. Dehydrate, clear, and mount.

RESULTS (see Note vi)

Nuclei; red blood corpuscles; intercellular bridges (prickles) of squamous epithelium; cilia; mitochondria; glial fibres: *blue*.

Fibrin; striations of skeletal and cardiac muscle: *darker blue*
Myelin: *lighter blue*.

Collagen; cartilage and bone matrix; reticulin; elastic fibres: *reddish-brown*.

Cytoplasm: *pale brown to pale pink*.

Notes

(i) Treatment with permanganate must be timed carefully. Too short a time will lead to excessively blue results; prolonged treatment produces sections that are red with little or no blue in them.

(ii) Tap water must be avoided before and after oxalic acid.

(iii) A section should be rinsed in alcohol and examined microscopically after two hours in the stain and every hour thereafter until the result is satisfactory.

(iv) On no account must sections be washed in water after haematoxylin since this destroys the red colours.

(v) This method may be used after any routine fixing fluid. If, however, the fluid contained dichromate, much better results will be obtained with every kind of tissue if Russell's phosphotungstic acid haematoxylin method (p. 252) is used instead.

(vi) Phosphotungstic acid haematoxylin stains a great variety of structures, but is particularly useful for muscle striations, intercellular bridges, fibrin, and cilia. For its use in the nervous system, see page 252.

Trichrome stains

The name trichrome should mean no more than three-coloured. In histological laboratories, however, the meaning has become restricted to a family of staining methods in which several dyes are used for the demonstration of connective tissue and cell cytoplasm. Most of these are variants of the original methods of Mallory and Masson. In recent years, however, entirely new dyes and new methods have been employed to obtain comparable results.

Mallory (1900–1) used acid fuchsin, then phosphomolybdic acid, and finally a mixture of orange G and aniline blue. Masson (1929) used haematoxylin followed by a counterstain of the Mallory type. Among the suggestions made by Masson were the replacement of aniline blue by light green, and the use of a mixture of ponceau and fuchsin in place of simple acid fuchsin. Many other alternatives are possible, including the use of phosphotungstic acid rather than phosphomolybdic acid, and the replacement of the red dye (fuchsin or ponceau-fuchsin) by azocarmine, azophloxine, Biebrich scarlet or erythrosin. A more radical alteration was the use of picric acid as a dye (Lendrum and McFarlane, 1940). New dyes were introduced by Lendrum *et al.* (1962) who devised a method that makes use of Martius yellow, brilliant crystal scarlet, and aniline blue.

Trichrome stains provide a good general picture of connective tissue and cytoplasm; they are commonly used for sections of muscle, bone (especially undecalcified sections), and fibrin (e.g. in thrombi). They would not be the first choice for demonstrating collagen or nuclei. For black and white photography, the best results are obtained with one of the green variants rather than a blue one.

Of the many trichrome methods available, we recommend three which have proved satisfactory in routine use. The picro-Mallory method (McFarlane, 1944) gives the most attractive results and the widest variety of informative colours. It requires more care than the others. The intensity of colour (particularly blue) can be varied to suit individual sections. This method has proved valuable for sections of kidney, in which basement membranes of glomerular capillaries are particularly sharply stained. It is particularly useful for revealing residual tissue architecture in sections of necrotic debris, or in tissue that spent too long in fixing or decalcifying fluid or was fixed in osmium tetroxide. The modification of Masson's method by Goldner (1938) is simpler to use. It provides particularly satisfactory results with sections of brain and bone and is suitable for nitro-cellulose sections. The MSB method (Lendrum *et al.*, 1962) is the simplest for routine use and the most suitable for demonstrating fibrin.

Although trichrome methods may be used after any routine fixing fluid, the most brilliant results are obtained when tissue is fixed in a fluid containing mercuric chloride or picric acid.

Picro-Mallory

SCOPE

Suitable for paraffin sections after any routine fixing fluid except Susa which gives mediocre results. Pieces of tissue must be thin and thoroughly fixed.

REAGENTS

A. *Weigert's haematoxylin* (p. 104)

B. *Picro-orange*

Orange G	0·75 g.
Saturated alcoholic solution of picric acid	300 ml.
20% alcoholic haematoxylin (p. 103)	50 ml.
Alcohol	50 ml.

C. *Red mixture*

Acid fuchsin	2·5 g.
Ponceau 2R	2·5 g.
1% aqueous acetic acid	500 ml.

D. *2 per cent aqueous acetic acid*

E. *Stock differentiator*

Phosphotungstic acid	100 g.
Picric acid	11·6 g.
Alcohol	380 ml.
Distilled water	20 ml.

F. *Red differentiator*

Stock differentiator	160 ml.
20% alcoholic haematoxylin	80 ml.
Alcohol	80 ml.
Distilled water	80 ml.

G. *Blue mixture*

Aniline blue	10 g.
Distilled water	400 ml.
Glacial acetic acid	10 ml.

Add the dye to the boiling distilled water, boil for a few minutes and then add the acetic acid. Cool and filter.

H. *Blue differentiator*

Stock differentiator	80 ml.
Distilled water	320 ml.

All these solutions keep well.

METHOD

1. Sections to water.
2. Weigert's haematoxylin 15–20 minutes.
3. Running tap water 5–10 minutes.
4. Picro-orange 3–5 minutes.
5. Wash in tap water until only the red blood corpuscles remain yellow (see Note i).
6. Red mixture 5–10 minutes.
7. Rinse in weak acetic acid.

8. Red differentiator until only the fibrin and muscle remain red (see Note ii).
9. Rinse in tap water.
10. Blue mixture 5–10 minutes.
11. Rinse in weak acetic acid.
12. Blue differentiator 1–2 minutes.
13. Rinse in weak acetic acid.
14. Dehydrate rapidly, clear and mount.

RESULTS

Muscle: *red.*
Fibrin: *bright red.*
Red blood corpuscles: *yellow.*
Platelets: *blue-grey.*
Nuclei: *grey.*
Nucleoli: *dark red.*
Collagen; basement membranes; reticulin; elastic fibres: *blue.*
Other structures: *shades of pale red, blue and purple.*

Notes

(i) The removal of picro-orange by washing in tap water requires very careful control. If the wash is too brief, fibrin and muscle tend to resist the red mixture and appear orange when the stain is completed. More often the wash is too long, so that some yellow is removed from red blood corpuscles, allowing them to take up red dye and become orange. The correct time for washing in water depends on the hardness of the water used. Soft water takes anything up to 5 minutes: hard water may remove enough picro-orange in 15–30 seconds. Very hard water should be diluted with distilled water.

(ii) Differentiation of the red colour needs careful control; sections must be agitated and should be examined at intervals of ½–1 minute. Differentiation will be complete in 1–5 minutes.

(iii) Many picro-Mallory methods are available. This one was published by McFarlane (1944) and has been slightly modified by the addition of haematoxylin to the picro-orange and red differentiator to reinforce nuclear staining (A. M. Barrett, unpublished).

(iv) If green is preferred to blue, use a 0·2 per cent solution of light green in 2 per cent acetic acid instead of the blue mixture and omit the blue differentiator. When light green is used, the nuclei are slightly more conspicuous, but fine structures such as capillary basement membranes are not as clear.

Goldner's method

SCOPE

Suitable for paraffin or nitrocellulose sections after any routine fixing fluid. This is a slight modification of the method published by Goldner (1938).

REAGENTS

A. *Weigert's haematoxylin* (p. 104)

B. *1 per cent hydrochloric acid in 70 per cent alcohol*

C. *Stock solution of 1 per cent aqueous Ponceau 2R*

D. *Stock solution of 1 per cent aqueous acid fuchsin*

E. *Stock solution of 1 per cent aqueous azophloxine*

F. *Red mixture*

1% Ponceau 2R	6 ml.
1% acid fuchsin	2 ml.
1% azophloxine	1 ml.
2% aqueous acetic acid	9 ml.
Distilled water	72 ml.

G. *0·2 per cent aqueous acetic acid*

H. *Orange mixture*

Orange G	8 g.
Phosphotungstic acid	16 g.
Distilled water	400 ml.

I. *0·2 per cent light green in 0·2 per cent aqueous acetic acid*
All these solutions keep well.

METHOD

1. Sections to water.
2. Weigert's haematoxylin 15–20 minutes.
3. Running tap water 5 minutes.
4. Acid alcohol 5–10 seconds.
5. Running tap water 5–10 minutes.
6. Red mixture 5 minutes.
7. Rinse in weak acetic acid.

8. Orange mixture 5 minutes.
9. Rinse in weak acetic acid.
10. Light green 1–5 minutes (see Note).
11. Weak acetic acid 5 minutes.
12. Dehydrate, clear, and mount.

RESULTS

Muscle; fibrin; keratin: *orange-red*.
Red blood corpuscles: *orange-yellow*.
Nuclei: *blue-black*.
Nucleoli: *purple-red*.
Collagen; basement membranes; reticulin; elastic fibres: *green*.
Other structures: *shades of pale pink, grey and yellow*.

Note

Sections vary considerably in their affinity for light green. For good results, the time in light green should be determined by inspecting the sections microscopically every minute or so.

Martius-Scarlet-Blue (MSB)

SCOPE

Suitable for paraffin sections after any routine fixing fluid. (Lendrum *et al.*, 1962.)

REAGENTS

A. *Weigert's haematoxylin* (p. 104)

B. *1 per cent hydrochloric acid in 70 per cent alcohol*

C. *Yellow mixture*

Martius yellow	0·5 g.
Phosphotungstic acid	2 g.
Water	5 ml.
Alcohol	95 ml.

D. *Red mixture*

Brilliant Crystal Scarlet 6R	1 g.
Glacial acetic acid	2·5 ml.
Distilled water	97·5 ml.

E. *1 per cent aqueous phosphotungstic acid*

F. *Blue mixture*

Aniline blue	0·5 g.
Glacial acetic acid	1 ml.
Distilled water	99 ml.

METHOD

1. Sections to water.
2. Weigert's haematoxylin 15–20 minutes.
3. Running tap water 5 minutes.
4. Acid alcohol 5–10 seconds.
5. Running tap water 5–10 minutes.
6. Rinse in alcohol.
7. Yellow mixture 2 minutes.
8. Rinse in tap water.
9. Red mixture 10 minutes.
10. Rinse in tap water.
11. Phosphotungstic acid 5 minutes.
12. Rinse in tap water.
13. Blue mixture 10 minutes.
14. Rinse in tap water.
15. Dehydrate, clear, and mount.

RESULTS

Fibrin: *bright red.*
Muscle: *red.*
Red blood corpuscles: *yellow.*
Nuclei: *grey.*
Collagen; basement membranes; reticulin; elastic fibres: *blue.*
Other structures: *pale.*

Schmorl's picro-thionin

SCOPE

A method for bone canaliculi. Suitable for frozen or nitro-cellulose sections not less than 15 μ thick. May be used after all routine fixing and decalcifying fluids (Schmorl, 1907).

REAGENTS

A. *Thionin solution*

    Saturated solution of thionin in 50%
        alcohol   1 ml.
    Distilled water   10 ml.

B. *Saturated aqueous solution of picric acid*

METHOD

1. Sections to water.
2. Running tap water for at least 10 minutes.
3. Thionin 5–10 minutes (see Note).
4. Rinse in tap water.
5. Picric acid ½–1 minute.
6. Rinse in tap water.
7. Differentiate in 70% alcohol until no more blue clouds of stain come out of the section (5–10 minutes).
8. Dehydrate, clear, using carbol-xylene (p. 286), and mount.

RESULTS

    Bone canaliculi: *dark brown to black*.
    Nuclei: *reddish-brown*.
    Other structures: *yellow or brownish-yellow*.

Note

    Good results are usually obtained when sections are stained in thionin for 5 minutes. With some batches of dye, however, the time may need to be prolonged. If the results are unsatisfactory after 10 minutes staining, the method should be repeated with a thionin staining solution to which 1–2 drops of strong ammonia have been added.

Chloranilic acid

SCOPE

    A method for calcium, suitable for any type of section or smear. Fixing fluids must not be acid. They and all other reagents must be free from calcium; tap water must not be used in their preparation. This is a precise histochemical method; in practice the von Kóssa method (p. 210) is more suitable for almost all routine purposes. The use of chloranilic acid for histological sections was described by Eisenstein *et al.* (1961) and by Carr *et al.* (1961). The method that we use is that of R. A. Klein (unpublished), and has given good results.

REAGENTS

A. *Saturated solution (about 1 per cent) of chloranilic acid in 96 per cent alcohol*
   Filter before use.

B. *Carazzi's haematoxylin* (p. 106)

C. *1 per cent sodium bicarbonate in distilled water*

METHOD

1. Sections to alcohol.
2. Chloranilic acid 5–15 minutes in a closed vessel (see Note ii).
3. Wash in distilled water.
4. Carazzi's haematoxylin 1 minute.
5. Sodium bicarbonate $\frac{1}{2}$–1 minute.
6. Dehydrate, clear, and mount.

RESULTS

   Calcium: *dark brown crystals.*
   Nuclei: *pale blue.*

Notes

   (i) All reagents, including those used after the chloranilic acid, must be calcium-free.
   (ii) When calcium is plentiful, a dense growth of dark crystals may make high power examination difficult. These crystals are less obtrusive when the staining time is limited to 5 minutes. In extreme cases the chloranilic acid should be diluted with up to three parts of 96 per cent alcohol.
   (iii) Alternative counterstains which may be used include eosin, methylene blue, neutral red, and light green.

CHAPTER 11

Pigments

Classification of pigments. Identification. Characteristics. Ferro-
cyanide and ferricyanide methods: Perls; Tirmann; Schmorl.
Fouchet for bile. Diazo for argentaffin. Rubeanic acid for copper.
Mallory for lead. Chromaffin. Bleaching methods.

Classification of pigments

When a pigment appears in a histological section, three
possible sources must be considered. First, the pigment may
have been produced within the body, in which case it is known
as an *endogenous* pigment. Secondly, the pigment may be a
foreign substance that found its way into the tissue during life;
in this case it is known as an *exogenous* pigment. Thirdly, the
pigment may have appeared in the tissue after removal from the
body; pigments of this third type are classified among the artefacts.

Some pigments are of little or no importance but obviously
none of them can be dismissed as trivial before being identified.
It is therefore necessary for every routine laboratory to employ
a comprehensive range of methods for identifying the common
pigments. As a matter of convenience, this chapter also deals
with some common unpigmented artefacts and also with certain
unpigmented exogenous foreign substances.

Of the endogenous pigments, some are normally present in
certain tissues in the body; they may, however, be of diagnostic
significance when they also occur in tumours derived from those
tissues. Such pigments include melanin, argentaffin pigment,
and chromaffin pigment. Other endogenous pigments are not
strictly normal but are readily produced as a result of illness or
injury. The commonest pigments of this type are bile and
haemosiderin. A very common endogenous pigment is lipofuscin; this is found within the cytoplasm of ageing cells in many
organs and is of no importance once it has been identified.

An exogenous pigment that is found in almost every individual is carbon which accumulates in the lungs from smoke in

the inspired air. Other foreign substances that may be found in
lungs as a result of inhalation include silica dust, asbestos
particles, and iron ore, all of which have been responsible for
industrial diseases. Foreign material may be found in tissues as
a result of direct implantation; examples include tattoo pigment,
surgical sutures, surgical glove powder, and the sequels of
trivial accidents such as splinters beneath the skin and broken
pencil lead in the gum. A rarer cause of exogenous pigment
deposition is ingestion of heavy metals such as lead or copper.
A pigment may also be deposited as a result of infection by
malaria.

Artefacts that must be borne in mind if confusion is to be
avoided include fixation deposits due to formaldehyde, mercuric
chloride and dichromate. Foreign bodies that may be seen in a
stained section or smear include splinters of wood or cork from
a chopping board, talc particles or starch grains from glove
powder, and airborne dust particles such as pollen grains and
fungus spores.

Identification

In many instances, it is possible to make an accurate guess
about the nature of a pigment from its appearance and situation.
When this is so, all that is needed is confirmation by the simplest
available method. In other instances, there are only a small
number of likely possibilities; duplicate sections are then stained
in turn by appropriate methods, beginning with the easiest.

Much time may be saved at the outset by examining the section with a polarizing microscope and (when possible) with a
fluorescence microscope. When polarized light is used, it is
necessary to bear in mind that certain normal tissues are birefringent, notably bone, keratin, and collagen (especially in tendons and ligaments). After making allowances for these, it is
easy to demonstrate suture materials of all kinds, talc and silica
particles, fragments of wood, formaldehyde deposit, malaria
pigments, and certain tattoo pigments by polarized light, although
it may not be possible to identify precisely which of these birefringent objects is present. Fluorescence microscopy is useful
for the rapid identification of argentaffin pigment. It also
usually shows lipofuscin.

Characteristics

Argentaffin pigment. Alternative names include chromo-argentaffin pigment and enterochromaffin pigment. First discovered in the Kultschitzky cells (enterochromaffin cells) of the small intestine. May also be seen in small quantities in many other sites. Present in carcinoid tumours (argentaffinomas). Demonstrated by the Masson-Fontana method (p. 211), the diazo method (p. 135), Schmorl's ferricyanide method (p. 133), or fluorescence microscopy. Fixatives other than formalin must be avoided.

Asbestos bodies. Yellow bodies taking many forms including drumsticks and rouleaux; often partly obscured by carbon. Found in the lungs of individuals exposed to asbestos dust. Demonstrated by Perls's method (p. 131) or by phase contrast microscopy.

Bile. Found in the liver in most patients with jaundice; occasionally in other tissues. Withstands paraffin processing except in rare instances (usually infants) when it is present in the unconjugated form and can only be demonstrated in frozen sections. Demonstrated by Fouchet's method (p. 134).

Carbon. Found in all lungs except those of infants; may also be present in lymph nodes of thorax, neck, and abdomen, and sometimes in the spleen. Has been used as a tattoo pigment. The chief constituent of pencil 'lead'. Demonstrated by its ability to resist treatment with strong acids and bleaching solutions.

Chromaffin pigment. Found in the normal suprarenal medulla and in chromaffin tumours (phaeochromocytomas). Demonstrated reliably by fixing the tissue in a fluid that contains dichromate (p. 138). Occasionally seen in routine paraffin sections. Demonstrated by Schmorl's ferricyanide method (p. 133) or by Giemsa's stain (p. 182).

Copper. Found in the liver and eye in cases of Wilson's disease. Demonstrated by rubeanic acid (p. 136).

Dichromate fixation deposit. A fine granular yellowish-brown deposit which interferes with staining (p. 22). Removed by acid alcohol (p. 86).

Formaldehyde fixation deposit. A brown granular deposit seen especially in tissue that contains much blood (p. 16). Demonstrated by polarized light. Removed by alcoholic picric acid (p. 84).

Glove powder. Formerly talc, which provoked a chronic inflammatory reaction if scattered in an operation wound. Nowadays only starch is used for surgeons' gloves although talc is often supplied with gloves used for other purposes. Found as angular pieces of pale or colourless material in tissues after surgical operations carried out several years ago in the talc era. Found also as contaminant particles that fell onto a section or smear during preparation. Demonstrated by polarized light which shows talc as brilliant angular fragments and starch as bright rounded structures with a darker central area.

Haemosiderin. Golden-brown pigment derived from fragmented red blood corpuscles. Seen at the sites of old haemorrhages, infarcts, etc. Seen in the liver and spleen after massive blood transfusion and also in certain blood diseases. Occurs in the pancreas (and elsewhere) in haemochromatosis. Easily confused with calcium in haematoxylin and eosin sections of brain, where it sometimes occurs in an unusual form encrusting small blood vessels and staining with the haematoxylin. Demonstrated by Perls's method for ferric iron (p. 131) or Tirmann's method (p. 132).

Lead. May be seen in cases of lead poisoning. Demonstrated by Mallory's haematoxylin (p. 137).

Lipofuscins. Also known as brown atrophy pigments or wear-and-tear pigments. Found in the cytoplasm of many types of cells, notably neurones, cardiac muscle fibres, and liver cells. Of variable composition. Demonstrated consistently by aldehyde fuchsin (p. 201) or (in frozen sections) by Sudan black (p. 162). Sometimes demonstrated by one or more of the following methods: Sudan black (paraffin sections); per-iodic acid Schiff (p. 141); Masson-Fontana (p. 211); Schmorl's ferricyanide (p. 133); modified Ziehl-Neelsen (p. 176).

Malaria pigment. Intracellular, but otherwise indistinguishable from formaldehyde fixation deposit (Hueck, 1912).

Melanin. Found in normal skin, eye, brain (substantia nigra) and meninges (especially over the medulla). Present in the majority of melanomas. Demonstrated by the Masson-Fontana method (p. 211), or Schmorl's ferricyanide method (p. 133). Removed by bleaching agents (p. 139).

Melanosis coli. Found, not uncommonly, in glandular epithelial cells and large mononuclear phagocytes in the mucosa of the large intestine. Probably derived from food or drugs: not true melanin. Demonstrated by Perls's method (p. 131), the Masson-Fontana method (p. 211), and the per-iodic acid Schiff method (p. 141).

Mercury fixation deposit. Coarse dark brown or black granules of angular and solid appearance. Removed by iodine (p. 84).

Silica. Tiny colourless spicules in fibrous tissue in lungs and thoracic lymph nodes of individuals exposed to silica dust. Demonstrated by polarized light.

Silver. Dark brown or black pigment which may be found in the tissues of silver workers. Removed by 1–2 hours treatment with Lugol's iodine followed by 5–10 per cent sodium thiosulphate.

Stain deposits. Tiny particles of a similar colour to one of the dyes used; usually darker than the stained structures in the section.

Tattoo pigment. Found in the skin and occasionally in local lymph nodes. Very variable in composition. Easier to see in unstained sections. May be demonstrable by polarized light. Often resists bleaching.

Ferrocyanide and ferricyanide methods

Two rather similar reactions have long been known to chemists. Potassium *ferrocyanide* combines with salts of *ferric* iron to form the insoluble pigment Prussian blue (Berlin blue). Likewise, potassium *ferricyanide* combines with salts of *ferrous* iron to form the insoluble pigment Turnbull's blue. Thus ferrocyanide will demonstrate ferric salts, while ferricyanide will demonstrate ferrous salts. It is unfortunate that the re-agents have confusingly similar names and that in each case the product of the reaction is a deep blue pigment. Nevertheless, the reactions are of great value in histology for demonstrating iron in the tissues and, as will be shown later, for other purposes also.

The ferrocyanide reaction was introduced into histology by Perls (1867), and is usually known by his name. It is much the more useful of the two reactions, because most of the iron in tissues is in the ferric state. Ferrocyanide will not, however, demonstrate ferric iron if it is combined with protein. The purpose of the hydrochloric acid in Perls's reagent is to release ferric iron from such compounds as haemosiderin. Even so, not all bound iron is released by hydrochloric acid, so that many compounds (e.g. haemoglobin) cannot be demonstrated by this method.

The ferricyanide reaction for ferrous iron (Turnbull's blue) was also investigated by Perls, who found that it gave inconsistent results with haemosiderin. In practice, this reaction is rarely used in histology as a test for ferrous iron, because very little iron is present in tissues in the ferrous state. It is, however, possible to use the ferricyanide reaction to demonstrate both kinds of iron (ferric and ferrous) if the tissue is first treated with a reducing agent to transform any ferric iron to ferrous. This technique was first published by Tirmann (1898).

No blue pigment is produced if ferricyanide is mixed with a

K

ferric salt. If, however, a reducing agent is added to the mixture, a blue precipitate forms. This is the basis of the so-called Schmorl's ferricyanide method, in which strong reducing agents in the tissues are coloured blue. The reaction is not specific for any particular tissue component but, in practice, has been found useful for melanin, argentaffin pigment, and most lipofuscins; all these pigments have reducing properties. There seems to be no certainty about which of the reagents undergoes reduction. According to Lillie (1965), the ferric iron in the mixture is reduced to ferrous: this promptly reacts with unaltered ferricyanide to produce Turnbull's blue. Others have suggested that the ferricyanide is reduced to ferrocyanide by the tissue component (melanin, etc.). The ferrocyanide then reacts with unaltered ferric iron to form Prussian blue. This second explanation appears to be more popular. It was proposed by Golodetz and Unna (1909) who first made use of the method, and is also favoured by Adams (1956), Pearse (1960), and Drury and Wallington (1967). Schmorl (1934) did not comment on the chemistry of the reaction; he merely published details of the method and recommended it for lipofuscin. It is of no practical importance to know the exact chemical mechanism of the reaction, since in any case a deep blue pigment is deposited at the site of a reducing substance.

There is evidence that melanin may be reacting in two ways in Schmorl's method. As well as having reducing properties, melanin has an affinity for iron salts. If treated successively with ferrous iron and ferricyanide, the melanin is demonstrated by the deposition of Turnbull's blue (Lillie, 1957). This is an entirely different reaction from that of Schmorl's method; in our experience some lipofuscins behave in a similar way.

Other methods make use of the attachment of iron, followed by its demonstration as a blue pigment. An example is Hale's method for acid mucopolysaccharides (p. 148).

Iron can be demonstrated by methods of other types. Quincke (1880) used ammonium sulphide to produce a precipitate of insoluble iron sulphide. This method has the drawback that other metal sulphides are equally dark in colour and equally insoluble. In practice, Quincke's method is commonly combined with ferricyanide. This is because ammonium sulphide is a reducing agent and much of the iron sulphide is in the ferrous state which enables it to react with ferricyanide to form Turnbull's blue. The combined method was first published in a paper by Tirmann (1898), who stated that it had been developed by his colleague Schmelzer.

Perls for ferric iron

SCOPE

Suitable for paraffin, nitrocellulose and frozen sections and for smears. Acid fixing fluids should be avoided because they tend to remove iron from the tissues. False positive results may be obtained if reagents are prepared with tap water or if metal containers are used.

REAGENTS

A. *Perls's reagent*

Potassium ferrocyanide	1 g.	
Distilled water	25 ml.	
13% aqueous hydrochloric acid	25 ml.	

Must be freshly prepared. Stock solutions of ferrocyanide are unsatisfactory.

B. *1 per cent aqueous neutral red*

METHOD

1. Sections to water (see Note i).
2. Wash well in distilled water.
3. Perls's reagent 20–30 minutes.
4. Wash well in distilled water.
5. Running tap water 5–10 minutes (see Note ii).
6. Neutral red 1–2 minutes.
7. Rinse in tap water.
8. Dehydrate, clear, and mount.

RESULTS

Ferric iron: *blue.*
Nuclei: *red.*
Other structures: *shades of pink.*

Notes

(i) Acids remove some of the iron from the sections. If formaldehyde fixation deposit is present, care is needed in the use of alcoholic picric acid. Usually most if not all of the fixation deposit will be removed within five minutes: treatment for this length of time removes little or no iron.

(ii) All traces of acid ferrocyanide must be washed out of the section before it is counterstained with neutral red. If this is not done, a dark red fine precipitate will form.

(iii) To demonstrate ferrous iron, ferricyanide is used in place of ferrocyanide. In all other respects the method is the same.

Tirmann for ferric and ferrous iron

SCOPE

As for Perls's method above.

REAGENTS

A. *Ammonium sulphide* (concentrated aqueous solution)

B. *Ferricyanide reagent*

Potassium ferricyanide	10 g.
Distilled water	100 ml.
Concentrated hydrochloric acid	1 ml.

Dissolve the ferricyanide in the water with gentle heat. Cool and add the hydrochloric acid. This solution must be freshly prepared.

C. *1 per cent aqueous neutral red*

METHOD

1. Sections to water (see Notes i and ii).
2. Wash well in distilled water.
3. Ammonium sulphide 1–2 hours.
4. Wash well in distilled water.
5. Ferricyanide reagent 15 minutes.
6. Wash well in distilled water.
7. Running tap water 5 minutes.
8. Neutral red 1–2 minutes.
9. Rinse in tap water.
10. Dehydrate, clear, and mount.

RESULTS

Ferric and ferrous iron: *blue.*
Nuclei: *red.*
Other structures: *shades of pink.*

Notes

(i) Ammonium sulphide produces black precipitates with salts of other metals, especially lead, silver, and mercury. For this reason it is better to avoid mercuric chloride fixing fluids; if they have been used, the sections must be treated with particular care by iodine (p. 84).

(ii) Formaldehyde fixation deposit must be removed with caution. See Note i to Perls's method above.

(iii) Ammonium sulphide tends to detach sections from slides. A coating of weak nitrocellulose may be necessary (p. 315).

(iv) If stages 4–7 (inclusive) are replaced by a quick rinse in distilled water, the ferric and ferrous iron will be present in the form of dark green to black ferrous sulphide. This is the reaction of Quincke (1880).

Schmorl's ferricyanide method

SCOPE

Suitable for paraffin, nitrocellulose, or frozen sections. The method will demonstrate melanin and lipofuscin after any routine fixing fluid. For intestinal argentaffin pigment, fixatives other than formalin must be avoided. For chromaffin pigment, a dichromate fixing fluid should be used. This modification of the original method is recommended by Lillie (1954) and is satisfactory.

REAGENTS

A. *Ferric ferricyanide reagent*

1% aqueous ferric chloride	30 ml.
1% aqueous potassium ferricyanide	4 ml.
Distilled water	6 ml.

Both the ferricyanide solution and the final mixture must be freshly prepared.

B. *1 per cent acetic acid*

C. *1 per cent aqueous neutral red*

METHOD

1. Sections to water.
2. Wash well in distilled water.
3. Ferric ferricyanide reagent 10 minutes.
4. Wash with acetic acid.
5. Rinse in distilled water.
6. Neutral red 1-2 minutes.
7. Rinse in water.
8. Dehydrate, clear, and mount.

RESULTS

Melanin; intestinal argentaffin; lipofuscin; chromaffin: *blue*.
Nuclei: *red*.
Other structures: *shades of pink*.

Note

If ionizable ferrous iron is present, it will be coloured by the
ferricyanide to give a false positive result. In fact, any iron that is
present will almost certainly be bound to protein and therefore unaffected by ferricyanide in the absence of acid. If a control is required, a duplicate section should be treated with ferricyanide alone,
instead of the ferric ferricyanide reagent.

Fouchet's method for bile

SCOPE

Suitable for paraffin or frozen sections (see Note ii). May be
used after any routine fixing fluid except Helly's fluid. (Hall,
1960.)

REAGENTS

A. *Fouchet's reagent*

25% aqueous trichloracetic acid	100 ml.
10% aqueous ferric chloride	10 ml.

Mix and filter immediately before use.

B. *van Gieson's picro-fuchsin* (p. 111)

METHOD

1. Sections to water.
2. Fouchet's reagent 5 minutes.

3. Distilled water 2–3 minutes.
4. Running tap water 2–3 minutes.
5. van Gieson's picro-fuchsin 5 minutes.
6. Dehydrate, clear, and mount.

RESULTS

Bile pigment: *olive green.*
Collagen: *red.*
Other structures: *yellow.*

Notes

(i) The green colour depends on the conversion of bilirubin to biliverdin by Fouchet's reagent.

(ii) Ordinary (conjugated) bile pigment is easily demonstrated in paraffin sections. To show unconjugated bile pigment (e.g. in the brain in cases of kernicterus), frozen sections are necessary, because this type of bile pigment is removed by the organic solvents used for routine paraffin processing.

(iii) The van Gieson counterstain appears to stabilize the biliverdin. If simple counterstains, such as neutral red, are substituted, the biliverdin will fade within a few weeks.

Diazo method for intestinal argentaffin granules

SCOPE

Suitable for paraffin sections of formalin fixed material. From the large number of available diazo methods, we recommend the following, which is taken from Pearse (1960).

REAGENTS

A. *0·1 per cent Fast Red salt B in 0·1M veronal acetate buffer at pH 9·2*

Must be prepared immediately before use. The Fast Red B dyestuff is relatively unstable, even in its solid form, and should be stored at 4°C.

B. *Carrazzi's haematoxylin* (p. 106)

METHOD

1. Sections to water.
2. Fast Red solution at room temperature for 30 seconds.
3. Wash thoroughly in running tap water.

4. Carazzi's haematoxylin 1 minute.
5. Running tap water 5–10 minutes.
6. Dehydrate, clear, and mount.

RESULTS

Intestinal argentaffin granules: *brick red.*
Nuclei: *blue.*
Other structures: *pale yellow.*

Rubeanic acid for copper

SCOPE

For consistent results, the tissue must be fixed in rubeanic acid. Results after alcohol or formalin fixation are unreliable but will be positive if a large amount of copper is present. The method cannot be used after routine fixing fluids that are acid or contain mercury or dichromate (Uzman, 1956).

REAGENTS

A. *Rubeanic acid solution*

Rubeanic acid (dithio-oxamide)	0·1 g.
Alcohol	70 ml.
Distilled water	30 ml.

Dissolve the rubeanic acid in the alcohol with gentle heat, then add the water.

B. *Sodium acetate (anhydrous)*   0·2 g.

METHOD

1. Place a thin piece of tissue (2 mm. or less) in the rubeanic acid solution.
2. After 10 minutes add the dry sodium acetate and mix well. Leave for 1–2 days.
3. 70% alcohol 1–2 hours.
4. 70% alcohol overnight.
5. Dehydrate in alcohol, clear, impregnate and embed in paraffin wax.
6. Cut sections, mount on slides, dry, remove wax with xylene, mount in a resinous medium (see Note ii).

RESULTS

Copper: *dark grey to black*.
Other structures: *unstained*.

Notes

(i) Chemical cleanliness is essential. In particular, the bottles, stoppers, and distilled water must be copper-free.

(ii) Neutral red may be used as a counterstain, in which case the dried sections are taken to water, stained in 1 per cent aqueous neutral red for $\frac{1}{2}$–1 minute, rinsed in water, dehydrated, cleared, and mounted.

(iii) When the tissue has been fixed in alcohol or formalin, paraffin sections may be taken to distilled water and stained by using the same reagents. Place in rubeanic acid solution for 15–20 minutes, then add the dry sodium acetate and leave for 24 hours. Transfer to 70 per cent alcohol for 1–2 hours; repeat with fresh 70 per cent alcohol. Leave in undiluted alcohol overnight, clear, and mount in a resinous medium.

Mallory's haematoxylin method for lead

SCOPE

Suitable for paraffin or nitrocellulose sections of alcohol fixed or formalin fixed material.

REAGENT

Mallory's haematoxylin

Haematoxylin	50 mg.
Alcohol	1 ml.
Saturated aqueous solution of calcium	
carbonate (about 0·15%)	100 ml.

Dissolve the haematoxylin in the alcohol and add the freshly filtered carbonate. This reagent must be freshly prepared (see Note i).

METHOD

1. Sections to water.
2. Mallory's haematoxylin at 54°C for 2–3 hours.
3. Running tap water for at least 10 minutes.
4. Dehydrate, clear, and mount.

RESULT

Lead: *bluish-grey to black.*

Notes

(i) The haematoxylin solution must be absolutely fresh. As soon as ripening begins to occur (within an hour or so) the method gives poor results.

(ii) This is the original method (Mallory, 1938). A rather similar method for lead, copper, and iron, was published the following year in a somewhat confusing paper (Mallory and Parker, 1939).

Chromaffin reaction

If a piece of suprarenal (adrenal) gland is placed in a solution containing chromic acid or dichromate for 12–24 hours, the medulla becomes deep brown whereas the cortex is only slightly coloured (Henle, 1865). The cells that darken are not the neurones of the suprarenal medulla, but cells of a special type that are found in a limited number of situations. Because of their affinity for chrome salts, these are known as chromaffin cells (Kohn, 1898); they are also found in sympathetic ganglia and paraganglia. A few cells in the intestine behave in the same way; these are often known as enterochromaffin cells. Of greater practical importance is the fact that chromaffin cells are present in certain tumours that arise in the suprarenal gland (and occasionally in other sites). These tumours have been variously described as chromaffinomas, chromaffin tumours, and phaeochromocytomas.

As already stated, fresh tissue should be fixed in a mixture containing chromic acid or dichromate, although sometimes it may be possible to produce the pigment by secondary dichromate treatment of tissue fixed in the common fixing fluids. Once the pigment has been formed, it will withstand paraffin processing and may be seen in sections without any additional staining. If, however, a more intense colour is required, diluted Giemsa stain should be used as recommended by Schmorl (1918).

Our custom has been to fix thin pieces of fresh tissue in a mixture of one part formalin and nine parts 2·5 per cent aqueous potassium dichromate. Any mixture containing 2–3 per cent dichromate and 10–20 per cent formalin is satisfactory so long as it does not also contain acid or mercuric chloride.

After 18–24 hours, the tissue is transferred to 2·5 per cent aqueous potassium dichromate for a few days. After thorough washing, it is processed and embedded in paraffin in the usual way. Sections may be examined unstained or lightly stained with neutral red. The pigment is stained dark greyish-green by the Giemsa method (p. 182).

Bleaching methods

Methods for the removal of fixation deposits have already been referred to. Many other pigments may be decolorized by bleaching agents, but in practice these are used for only two purposes. The first is the removal of a large amount of pigment obscuring cellular detail. To do this, a bleaching agent must be chosen which does not damage the other structures in the section. The second use of bleaching agents is to provide information about the identity of a particular pigment. Almost all the common pigments are easier to identify by the special staining methods already described; the exception is carbon, which can only be identified by its ability to withstand all bleaching agents.

Many bleaching agents have been used; the following will cover the requirements of a routine laboratory.

Hydrogen peroxide at a strength of about 10 per cent (30 vols) will bleach melanin in about 24–48 hours.

Potassium permanganate (about 0·1 per cent) for 12–24 hours, followed by 1 per cent oxalic acid for 1–2 minutes will bleach melanin.

Carbon resists all organic solvents, oxidizing agents, strong acids, and strong alkalis. In practice the section is taken to water and immersed in concentrated hydrochloric acid, which will remove all the common pigments except carbon and lipofuscin. The tissue is not destroyed even when this treatment is prolonged for several hours. After thorough washing, the section may be dehydrated, cleared, and mounted.

CHAPTER 12

Carbohydrates

General notes. Per-iodic acid Schiff. Alcian blue for mucin. Mucicarmine. Hale's method. Toluidine blue. Best's carmine. Congo red. Methyl violet. Alcian blue for amyloid. Thioflavine.

ALL tissues contain a carbohydrate component, but this is not often great enough to be demonstrated by stains. A wide variety of carbohydrates occur but the most important from a histological point of view are sugars. In animal tissues these are usually six-carbon sugars or hexoses (e.g. glucose and galactose), but five-carbon sugars or pentoses (e.g. ribose) are also present in many animal tissues as well as being common in plants.

Carbohydrates are frequently encountered in the form of polysaccharides; these are large molecules formed by the polymerization of sugar molecules. Glycogen, starch, and cellulose are examples of simple glucose polymers. Many of the carbohydrates of animals and plants are not composed of simple sugar molecules, but of sugars that have been modified in some way. Thus hexosamines (e.g. glucosamine) may form polymers in a similar way to hexoses (e.g. glucose). Similarly hexuronic acids (e.g. glucuronic acid) may become polymerized. Many naturally-occurring polysaccharides are mixed polymers and contain, for instance, hexosamine and hexuronic acid.

Although pure carbohydrates may be found in animals and plants, they are more often combined with protein or fat or both. When carbohydrate is combined with fat, the compound is known as a glycolipid. A compound composed of carbohydrate and protein is known as a mucoprotein, unless the carbohydrate content is low, in which case the name glycoprotein is used.

Depending upon the amount of hexuronic acid present, a polysaccharide may be neutral or acid. A further reason for acidity is the presence of sulphate groups on many polysaccharides.

Although the most obvious site of mucoprotein and polysaccharide in the body is the mucin secreted by epithelial cells, it must be remembered that very similar substances are present in other situations. These include the granules of tissue mast cells and much of the connective tissue (notably cartilage). These so-called connective tissue mucins are not secreted by epithelial cells.

The term mucin is not precise; it is applied to a variety of mucoproteins and polysaccharides (usually mixed). Likewise, the term mucopolysaccharide has little significance beyond indicating that the polysaccharide in question may be found in mucin.

Amyloid is an abnormal substance deposited between cells. When present, it usually affects several organs. The name means 'starch-like' and was applied because an organ infiltrated with amyloid occasionally turns a blue colour when treated with Lugol's iodine; much more often the colour produced is mahogany brown. Amyloid contains protein and polysaccharide in varying proportions. The reactions are inconstant, so that a negative result by any single method is meaningless; at least two (and preferably more) methods should be tried before deciding that amyloid is not present. It has been stated (Culling, 1963) that unstained paraffin sections of amyloid tissue may change their staining reactions with the passage of time. This has not been our experience.

The methods that follow are suitable for the demonstration of mucin, glycogen, and amyloid; they will cover all the requirements of a routine laboratory. Many other methods depend on the presence of carbohydrate but are included in more appropriate chapters. These include the Feulgen method (p. 185), Jones's method for basement membranes (p. 217), and two methods for fungi—Gridley's (p. 179) and Grocott's (p. 219). Conversely, methods intended for other purposes will sometimes demonstrate mucin but not consistently enough to be useful; these include Ehrlich's haematoxylin, Heidenhain's haematoxylin, and many of the silver impregnation methods. Aldehyde fuchsin (p. 201) stains sulphated mucins well, probably by attachment to the sulphate.

The Per-iodic acid Schiff method

SCOPE

Suitable for paraffin or frozen sections after any fixing fluid.

This is the original method (McManus, 1946) except for the Schiff reagent, which is that recommended by Lillie (1951b), and the counterstains.

REAGENTS

A. *0·5 per cent aqueous per-iodic acid*

B. *Schiff's reagent*

Basic fuchsin (see Note i)	1 g.
Sodium metabisulphite	1·9 g.
N/1 hydrochloric acid	15 ml.
Distilled water	85 ml.
Activated charcoal	0·5 g.

Dissolve the basic fuchsin and metabisulphite in the acid and water. Shake frequently during two hours. Add the charcoal and shake well for 1–2 minutes. Filter and store at 0–4°C. The solution should be colourless; when it becomes coloured it must be discarded. In any case, the reagent loses its properties in 6–8 weeks.

C. *Sulphurous acid rinse*

10% aqueous sodium metabisulphite	6 ml.
N/1 hydrochloric acid	5 ml.
Distilled water	to 100 ml.

This solution must be freshly prepared but the constituents may be kept as stock solutions, in which case the metabisulphite is stored at 0–4°C.

D. *Carazzi's haematoxylin* (p. 106)

E. *Saturated solution (0·3 per cent) of tartrazine in cellosolve*

METHOD

1. Sections to water.
2. Per-iodic acid 2 minutes.
3. Running tap water 5 minutes.
4. Rinse in distilled water.
5. Schiff's reagent 15–20 minutes in a Coplin jar.
6. Sulphurous acid rinse 2 minutes.
7. Sulphurous acid rinse 2 minutes.
8. Sulphurous acid rinse 2 minutes.

9. Running tap water 5-10 minutes.
10. Carazzi's haematoxylin 1 minute.
11. Running tap water 5-10 minutes.
12. Rinse in alcohol.
13. Tartrazine $\frac{1}{2}$–1 minute.
14. Rinse in alcohol.
15. Clear, and mount.

RESULTS

Positive result: *magenta* (see Note v).
Nuclei: *greyish-blue*.
Other structures: *yellow*.

Notes

(i) Not every sample of basic fuchsin is satisfactory for this method. Suitable dye is often designated by the suppliers 'for Feulgen' or 'for Schiff'.

(ii) The usual problem with this method is too much non-specific staining. This occurs if the section spends too long in per-iodic acid or is not washed sufficiently after it. Another cause is recolorization of Schiff's reagent by exposure to air if it is not used in a Coplin jar. Omitting or curtailing the sulphurous acid rinses will increase the non-specific staining in our experience. Other authors have claimed satisfactory results when these rinses are entirely omitted, provided that the section is thoroughly washed in water after Schiff's reagent. Possibly their tap water is less alkaline than ours.

(iii) When particularly accurate results are required, a duplicate section should be used as a control, omitting the per-iodic acid. Another useful control is a section known to be positive by the method; one of these should be used to test every new batch of reagent, and from time to time as the batch ages.

(iv) For glycogen, a duplicate section should be treated with amylase (diastase) before being stained. This will remove any glycogen that is present. Saliva will usually work well, although individuals differ in this respect, and in any case the amylase content falls after eating. The alternative is to purchase malt diastase, from which a weak (0·1 per cent) solution is freshly prepared in distilled water. In our experience, malt diastase deteriorates in a month or two.

In practice, the control section is taken to water, washed well in distilled water, and covered with saliva or diastase solution at 37°C for 30 minutes. To prevent drying, the slide should be enclosed in a Petri dish. The control section is then washed well in running tap water, after which it joins the untreated section in per-iodic acid.

(v) So many structures are positive by the per-iodic acid Schiff method, that interpretation is sometimes difficult. In addition to a list of structures for which we have found this method valuable in routine work, we therefore add a list of positive structures that may be encountered by chance, some of which are potentially confusing.

We have deliberately used the method to show the following: mucin (all of which stains except for non-sulphated acid mucopolysaccharides), glycogen, basement membranes, hyaline and fibrinoid degeneration of arteries, diabetic glomerular lesions, hyaline membrane of infants' lungs, certain pituitary cells (see p. 197), fungi and parasites, megakaryocytes, Russell bodies in plasma cells, the glycolipid of Gaucher's disease, the trophoblast layer of the placenta, and the following parts of the eye; corneal collagen, including Bowman's and Descemet's membranes, lens capsule, retinal rods, and vitreous body.

The following are sometimes or always positive. The method might be employed for their demonstration, although usually an alternative is at least equally good. Some of the following are apt to cause confusion. Woven bone, some cartilage, corpora amylacea of brain and prostate, tubular epithelium of infants' kidneys, hyaline casts, cerebrosides, fibrin, melanosis coli pigment, lipofuscin, thyroid colloid, amyloid (weak), mast cell granules, agar, cellulose, nitrocellulose, gelatin, albumin, and glycerol in old museum specimens. For a review of the substances that are positive by this method, see Lillie (1950).

(vi) Schiff's reagent (leuco-basic-fuchsin) may be prepared according to a wide variety of formulae. We have preferred Lillie's mixture because it is easier to prepare than others.

(vii) The theoretical basis of the method depends on two stages: first the production of aldehydes and, secondly, their demonstration. Per-iodic acid produces aldehydes when it acts on any molecule in which adjacent carbon atoms bear hydroxyl groups (Malaprade, 1934). In chemical terms this arrangement may be represented $-CHOH-CHOH-$ and is described as a $1:2$ glycol configuration. This is converted to two aldehyde groups $(-CHO + OHC-)$. The reaction does not occur if either of the hydrogen atoms is substituted by some other radical r to produce $-CrOH-CHOH-$. Since Malaprade's original observations, it has been shown that per-iodic acid produces aldehydes if an amino rather than a hydroxyl group is attached to one of the carbon atoms $(-CHNH_2-CHOH-)$, or if one of the hydroxyl groups has been oxidized $(-CHOH-CO-)$. The reaction is also given by compounds in which an amino group is partly substituted by another radical $(-CHNHr-CHOH-)$.

Once the aldehydes have been formed, they produce a magenta colour by reacting with Schiff's reagent which thus marks the site of glycol groups or their amino equivalents. Plainly the reaction will not be positive if the precursor substance is diffusible, if the aldehydes are diffusible, or if their concentration is too low for a detectable colour to be formed (Hotchkiss, 1948).

The virtue of per-iodic acid is that it does not further oxidize the aldehydes once they have been formed. Many other procedures make use of Schiff's reagent as a sequel to the chemical formation of aldehyde groups by other oxidizing agents. These include chromic acid in the Bauer reaction and in Gridley's method (p. 179), permanganate in the Casella reaction, lead tetra-acetate (Crippa), and sodium bismuthate (Lhotka). Although the results of many of these methods overlap, they are not identical since the oxidizing agents react differently (Lillie, 1951a; 1965). The Feulgen reaction is closely analogous in that hydrochloric acid produces aldehyde groups by hydrolysis, and these are demonstrated by Schiff's reagent. Lipids with aldehyde groups may be shown to be present in cell cytoplasm by the plasmal reaction.

Somewhat similar results are obtained when silver is used instead of Schiff's reagent to mark the aldehydes produced by per-iodic acid (Jones's method, p. 217), or by chromic acid (Grocott's method, p. 219).

Alcian blue for mucin

SCOPE

A stain for acid mucopolysaccharides. Suitable for paraffin or frozen sections after any routine fixing fluid. The original method (Steedman, 1950) has been modified many times; we have used a method derived from Lison (1954). Alcian blue may be combined with many other stains (see Note i).

REAGENTS

A. *Weigert's haematoxylin* (p. 104)

B. *1 per cent hydrochloric acid in 70 per cent alcohol*

C. *Alcian blue solution*

1% aqueous alcian blue	100 ml.
1% aqueous acetic acid	100 ml.
Thymol	a few small crystals

The mixture keeps for several months but must be filtered immediately before use.

D. *Curtis's picro-ponceau mixture* (p. 110)

METHOD

1. Sections to water.
2. Weigert's haematoxylin 20 minutes.
3. Running tap water 5 minutes.
4. Acid alcohol 10–20 seconds.

L

5. Running tap water 5 minutes.
6. Alcian blue solution 10 minutes.
7. Rinse in tap water.
8. Picro-ponceau mixture 1–2 minutes.
9. Rinse briefly in water.
10. Dehydrate rapidly, clear, and mount.

RESULTS

Acid mucopolysaccharides: *bluish-green.*
Nuclei: *dark grey.*
Collagen: *red.*
Other structures: *yellow.*

Notes

(i) The bond between alcian blue and acid mucopolysaccharides is strong and the colour is intense. For these reasons, the method lends itself to a wide variety of counterstains, and may be used in conjunction with many other staining methods.

For a combined alcian blue and per-iodic acid Schiff method, omit Weigert's haematoxylin (stages 2–5 above), prolong the alcian blue staining to two hours, wash well in water, and then use the per-iodic acid Schiff method (p. 141).

For a combination with phosphotungstic acid haematoxylin, omit Weigert's haematoxylin, stain with alcian blue, and then use the phosphotungstic acid haematoxylin method (p. 114).

When combining alcian blue with aldehyde fuchsin, use the aldehyde fuchsin (p. 201) first but omit the counterstain. Transfer the section from stage 9 of the aldehyde fuchsin method to alcian blue staining solution for 10 minutes, rinse, dehydrate, clear and mount.

For a combination with an elastic stain, use Hart's modification of Weigert's method (p. 111) as far as stage 9. Transfer the section to alcian blue staining solution and complete the method as above (stages 6–10).

Other counterstains may be used in place of the picro-ponceau mixture. The mucopolysaccharides stain a brighter blue when the section is counterstained with 1 per cent aqueous chlorantine fast red 5B (15 minutes after 10 minutes mordanting with 1 per cent aqueous phosphomolybdic acid). Useful results are sometimes obtained when alcian blue is combined with phloxine: use the alcian blue method above as far as stage 6 and then transfer the section to stage 5 of the phloxine tartrazine method (p. 203).

(ii) In addition to its use as a routine stain for mucopolysaccharides (mucus, cartilage, etc.), alcian blue has been used in special ways for the demonstration of amyloid (p. 154), and as a pituitary stain (p. 197).

Mucicarmine

SCOPE

Suitable for paraffin, nitrocellulose, and frozen sections, and for smears. This is the modification by Southgate (1927) of the original method of Mayer (1896).

REAGENTS

A. *Carazzi's haematoxylin* (p. 106)

B. *1 per cent hydrochloric acid in 70 per cent alcohol*

C. *Mucicarmine*

Carmine (powder)	1 g.
Aluminium hydroxide	1 g.
50% alcohol	100 ml.
Aluminium chloride (anhydrous)	0·5 g.

Add the carmine and aluminium hydroxide to the alcohol in a long-necked 500 ml. flask. Grind the aluminium chloride in a mortar and add it to the mixture. Mix well, heat rapidly to boiling-point and boil for 2½ minutes; the mixture must be shaken frequently. Cool rapidly under a running tap and filter when cold. This solution keeps for about 3 months.

D. *Saturated solution of tartrazine in cellosolve*

METHOD

1. Sections to water.
2. Carazzi's haematoxylin 10 minutes.
3. Wash in tap water 5 minutes.
4. Acid alcohol 5–10 seconds.
5. Wash in tap water 10 minutes.
6. Mucicarmine 20–30 minutes.
7. Rinse in tap water.
8. Rinse in alcohol.
9. Tartrazine ½–1 minute.
10. Rinse in alcohol.
11. Clear, and mount.

RESULTS

Epithelial mucin: *red.*
Nuclei: *blue.*
Other structures : *yellow.*

Notes

(i) Not every sample of carmine will give good results. When a new batch of carmine is used in this method, a known positive section should be stained.

(ii) It is essential to prepare the mucicarmine according to Southgate's exact instructions.

(iii) Mucicarmine is better than any other stain for distinguishing cryptococci. It also stains the mucin in some gastric carcinomas better than other methods.

Hale's method

SCOPE

Demonstrates acid mucopolysaccharides (Hale, 1946). Suitable for paraffin or frozen sections. Any fixing fluid may be used so long as dichromate and chromic acid are avoided.

REAGENTS

A. *Dialysed iron mixture*

Dialysed iron solution	25 ml.
12·5% aqueous acetic acid	25 ml.

Mix immediately before use.

B. *Perls's reagent* (p. 131)

C. *1 per cent aqueous neutral red*

METHOD

1. Sections to water.
2. Dialysed iron mixture 10 minutes.
3. Wash well several times with distilled water (see Note i).
4. Perls's reagent 10 minutes.
5. Rinse in distilled water.
6. Running tap water 5–10 minutes.
7. Neutral red ½–1 minute.
8. Rinse in tap water.
9. Dehydrate, clear, and mount.

RESULTS

Acid mucopolysaccharides: *blue.*
Nuclei: *red.*
Other structures: *shades of pink.*
(Ferric iron: *blue.*)

Notes

(i) Sections must be washed thoroughly after the dialysed iron mixture, otherwise the whole section becomes blue in Perls's reagent.

(ii) Dialysed iron solution is available from laboratory suppliers. Those wishing to prepare their own should consult the paper by Rinehart and Abul-Haj (1951). The method is tedious.

(iii) If the section contains ionizable ferric iron, this also will be blue. A control section may be treated with Perls's reagent only.

Toluidine blue for mucin

SCOPE

Stains acid mucopolysaccharides metachromatically, especially when these are sulphated. Suitable for paraffin and frozen sections. For ordinary purposes, any routine fixing fluid may be used.

REAGENT

1 per cent aqueous toluidine blue
The solution improves with keeping.

METHOD

1. Sections to water.
2. Toluidine blue 3–4 minutes.
3. Rinse in tap water.
4. Dehydrate in butanol.
5. Clear in xylene, and mount.

RESULTS

Acid mucopolysaccharides: *reddish-purple.*
Nuclei: *blue.*
Other structures: *shades of light blue.*

Notes

(i) Butanol is used for dehydration because the metachromatic colour is removed from some tissue constituents by ethanol. As an alternative to butanol, some workers have used acetone.

(ii) The dye reacts strongly with sulphated polysaccharides, such as mast cells and cartilage, and the bond is relatively resistant to ethanol, so that these structures can often be seen, metachromatically stained, in routine sections counterstained with an appropriate dye (see Note iii below). Non-sulphated acid polysaccharides, on the other hand, stain more weakly, and the dye is susceptible to removal if ethanol is used for dehydration. For a comprehensive review of the metachromatic staining of polysaccharides, see Schubert and Hamerman (1956).

(iii) A number of other stains may be used in place of toluidine blue. A 1 per cent aqueous solution of any of the following dyes may be substituted: thionin, safranin, Bismarck brown, azure A, and azure C. Metachromatic staining may be seen with methylene blue, cresyl violet, and occasionally with neutral red, but we should not use any of these dyes deliberately for this purpose.

(iv) Although human mast cells are comparatively robust and capable of withstanding routine fixing fluids, those in some other species require special methods of fixation, using alcohol or Carnoy's fluid.

Best's carmine

SCOPE

A specific method for glycogen. Suitable for paraffin sections. For a discussion of fixation see Note iv. This is the method published in Best's third paper on the subject (Best, 1906).

REAGENTS

A. *Ehrlich's haematoxylin* (p. 101)

B. *1 per cent hydrochloric acid in 70 per cent alcohol*

C. *Best's carmine, stock solution*

Carmine (powder)	6 g.
Potassium carbonate (anhydrous)	3 g.
Potassium chloride	15 g.
Distilled water	180 ml.
Strong ammonia (0·880)	60 ml.

Add the dye and salts to the water in a long-necked litre flask. Boil carefully for 5 minutes. Cool, and add the ammonia. Filter before use. The mixture keeps for a month or two in a refrigerator.

D. *Best's carmine, working solution*

Stock solution	12 ml.
Strong ammonia (0·880)	18 ml.
Methanol	18 ml.

This mixture must be freshly prepared.

E. *Best's differentiator*

Alcohol	80 ml.
Methanol	40 ml.
Distilled water	100 ml.

METHOD

1. Remove wax with xylene.
2. Rinse twice with alcohol.
3. Ehrlich's haematoxylin 20 minutes.
4. Rinse in 70% alcohol.
5. Acid alcohol 5-10 seconds.
6. Rinse rapidly in water.
7. Best's carmine, working solution 5–10 minutes in a closed vessel.
8. Best's differentiator until the background is clear ($\frac{1}{2}$–5 minutes).
9. Dehydrate, clear, and mount.

RESULTS

Glycogen: *red.*
Nuclei: *blue.*
Other structures: *unstained.*

Notes

(i) This is a temperamental method which cannot be relied upon to give consistent results. On occasions the stock solution requires less dilution with ammonia and methanol; it may even give better results if used undiluted. Differentiation needs careful observation because the glycogen may easily be decolorized.

(ii) Because the method is inconsistent, a known positive section should always be used as a control. Glycogen may be removed from a duplicate section as an additional control if required. This can be done with saliva or diastase (see Note iv on p. 143).

(iii) Aqueous solutions are avoided as far as possible, since they may remove some of the glycogen. For this reason, Ehrlich's haematoxylin is preferred to an aqueous mixture. There is no need to use running tap water to blue the haematoxylin, since blueing occurs in the strongly alkaline carmine solution. Some authors recommend that sections be coated with nitrocellulose (p. 315) as an additional precaution.

(iv) Different authors have expressed conflicting opinions about the fixation of tissue for the preservation of glycogen. These may be classified in three groups. One view is that aqueous fixing fluids must be avoided and that any alcoholic mixture is suitable. The second view is that picric acid should be used, preferably in an alcoholic mixture. The third view is that any routine fixing fluid is satisfactory and that an ordinary formalin solution gives perfectly good results.

When tissue contains an abundance of glycogen, it is certainly true that some of it will be demonstrable in sections, no matter what fixing fluid is used. It is equally true that such tissue imparts a milky opalescence to neutral buffered formalin solution after a few days. Our belief is that picric acid should be used in an alcoholic solution whenever tissue is suspected of containing glycogen in small amounts. A suitable fluid is that of Gendre (1937) which consists of 80 parts of a saturated solution of picric acid in 95 per cent alcohol, 15 parts of formalin, and 5 parts of glacial acetic acid. This should be freshly prepared and will fix thin pieces of tissue in 1–4 hours. After fixation, tissue is washed in 80 per cent alcohol, and may be dehydrated, cleared, impregnated, and embedded in the usual way.

As an additional precaution, we have preferred to mount sections on slides by floating them on 70 per cent alcohol instead of water.

Congo red

SCOPE

A method for amyloid. Suitable for frozen or paraffin sections after any routine fixing fluid. The original method (Bennhold, 1922) was considerably improved by Puchtler, Sweat and Levine (1962). We recommend their method.

REAGENTS

A. *Carazzi's haematoxylin* (p. 106)

B. *1 per cent hydrochloric acid in 70 per cent alcohol*

C. *Stock saturated solution of sodium chloride in 80 per cent alcohol*
   This solution is stable.

D. *Alkaline alcohol*

Stock solution (above)	50 ml.
1% aqueous sodium hydroxide	0·5 ml.

   Filter and use within 15 minutes.

E. *Stock solution of Congo red*
   Saturated solution of Congo red in stock solution C.

   This keeps for several months, but should be allowed to stand for 24 hours before use.

F. *Working solution of Congo red*

Stock solution of Congo red   50 ml.
1% aqueous sodium hydroxide   0·5 ml.

Filter and use within 15 minutes.

METHOD

1. Sections to water.
2. Carazzi's haematoxylin 10 minutes.
3. Running tap water 5 minutes.
4. Acid alcohol 5–10 seconds.
5. Running tap water 2 minutes.
6. Wash well in distilled water.
7. Alkaline alcohol 20 minutes in a closed vessel.
8. Congo red (working solution) 20 minutes in a closed vessel.
9. Dehydrate, clear, and mount.

RESULTS

Amyloid: *orange red and dichroic* (see Note ii).
Nuclei: *blue.*
Other structures: *unstained to yellow.*
(Elastic fibres are often orange red, but are not dichroic.)

Notes

(i) The method works well with paraffin sections but staining is even stronger when frozen sections are used.

(ii) Amyloid is feebly birefringent when unstained. If stained with Congo red it is strongly birefringent (Divry and Florkin, 1927). Furthermore, it is dichroic; that is to say polarized light not only shows it bright against a dark background, but shows it in a colour that differs from the original, namely bright yellow-green. When the Nicol prism or polarizing film is rotated, the amyloid can be seen to change from orange red to a darker brownish red and then suddenly to green which increases in brightness until the background becomes dark. This property is not shared by any of the other tissue components that sometimes stain with Congo red.

Methyl violet

SCOPE

A metachromatic stain for amyloid. Suitable for frozen or paraffin sections, after any routine fixing fluid; formalin gives the best results. An aqueous mounting medium should be used because the dye is removed by alcohol (Cornil, 1875).

REAGENTS

A. *1 per cent aqueous methyl violet*

B. *0·2 per cent aqueous acetic acid*

METHOD

1. Sections to water.
2. Methyl violet 3–5 minutes.
3. Rinse in tap water.
4. Differentiate in acetic acid until cellular detail is apparent and the amyloid stands out in a contrasting colour ($\frac{1}{2}$–2 minutes).
5. Running tap water 5–10 minutes.
6. Mount in Apáthy's medium (p. 89).

RESULTS

Amyloid: *violet-red.*
Nuclei: *dark blue.*
Other structures: *shades of blue.*

Notes

(i) If the mounting medium does not contain salt, methyl violet diffuses into it. For this reason, sodium chloride is incorporated in the Apáthy's medium that we recommend.

(ii) Sections should be examined in white or yellow light without blue filters. In polarized light, the methyl violet stained amyloid may show deep sea-green dichroism if an intense source of light is used.

Alcian blue for amyloid

SCOPE

A method for amyloid. Suitable for frozen or paraffin sections after fixation in any routine fixing fluid. Recently formed amyloid is distinguishable from old deposits. We have used the following method, which is slightly modified from the original (Lendrum, Slidders, and Fraser, 1969).

REAGENTS

A. *Acetic alcohol*

Alcohol	45 ml.
Distilled water	45 ml.
Glacial acetic acid	10 ml.

Prepare fresh each day

B. *Stock solution of alcian blue*
1% alcoholic solution of Alcian blue 8GX

C. *Stock sulphate solution*
1% aqueous solution of sodium sulphate (hydrate)

D. *Alcian blue working solution*

Alcian blue stock solution	45 ml.
Sulphate stock solution	45 ml.
Glacial acetic acid	10 ml.

Mix and allow to ripen for 30 minutes before use. Prepare fresh each day.

E. *Saturated solution (less than 0·5 per cent) of borax (sodium tetraborate) in 80 per cent alcohol*

F. *Weigert's haematoxylin* (p. 104)

G. *Saturated solution of picric acid in 80 per cent alcohol*

H. *Curtis's picro-ponceau mixture* (p. 110)

METHOD

1. Sections to water.
2. Rinse in acetic alcohol.
3. Alcian blue working solution 2 hours in a closed vessel.
4. Rinse in acetic alcohol.
5. Wash in water.
6. Alcoholic borax at least 30 minutes.
7. Wash in water.
8. Weigert's haematoxylin 10–15 minutes.
9. Wash in water.
10. Alcoholic picric acid 1 minute.
11. Rinse in water.
12. Curtis's picro-ponceau 2 minutes.
13. Dehydrate rapidly, clear, and mount.

RESULTS

Recently formed amyloid; mast cell granules; some colloid: *bright green.*

Old amyloid: *pale, dull, blue-green, sometimes brownish.*

Nuclei: *grey.*

Collagen: *red.*

Other structures: *yellow.*

(Mucopolysaccharides stain bluish-green as in the alcian blue method for mucin but less strongly.)

Note

Lendrum *et al.* used celestin blue and haemalum for nuclear staining. We prefer Weigert's haematoxylin because it is a routine stain in many other methods and is simpler to use. It does not, however, give quite such strong results. We use a picro-ponceau counterstain rather than the picro-fuschin mixture of the original method.

Thioflavine T

SCOPE

A fluorescence method for amyloid. Suitable for paraffin or frozen sections after brief fixation in formalin-saline or neutral buffered formalin solution (Vassar and Culling, 1959).

REAGENTS

A. *Carazzi's haematoxylin* (p. 106)

B. *1 per cent aqueous thioflavine T*

C. *1 per cent aqueous acetic acid*

METHOD

1. Sections to water.
2. Haematoxylin 2 minutes.
3. Running tap water 2–3 minutes.
4. Thioflavine 3 minutes.
5. Rinse in water.
6. Acetic acid 20 minutes.
7. Wash well in water.
8. Mount in Apáthy's medium.

RESULTS (with ultra-violet or deep blue light).

Amyloid: *bright yellow*.

Other structures: *dark*.

(Mast cell granules also fluoresce bright yellow.)

(Autofluorescence in other colours may be produced by other tissue components, e.g. elastic fibres.)

Notes

(i) Haematoxylin is used to prevent fluorescence of nuclei.

(ii) Thioflavine T will demonstrate amyloid in cases where other methods have failed.

CHAPTER 13

Lipids

General notes. Fixation and types of sections. Sudan III and IV. Oil red O. Sudan black. Phosphine. Osmium. Cholesterol: Schultz; Polarized light. Baker for phospholipids. Fischler for fatty acids.

THE commonest type of lipid in animal tissue is triglyceride or neutral fat, that is to say an ester composed of three molecules of fatty acid and one molecule of glycerol. Triglycerides are present throughout the tissues, but usually in such small quantities that they cannot be demonstrated by staining methods. In some situations, however, the triglycerides form bulky masses which can be stained and seen; these bulky masses are present in adipose tissue and are fairly common in degenerating cells of the liver and other organs.

Less commonly, triglycerides undergo hydrolysis as a result of disease. When this occurs, free fatty acids may be present in the tissue. These can be demonstrated, for instance, in fat necrosis due to pancreatitis, when pancreatic enzymes escape and attack adjacent tissue.

For transport within the body, and in cell walls, lipid is present in a slightly water-soluble form known as phospholipid. This is composed of two molecules of fatty acid and one molecule each of glycerol, phosphoric acid, and choline. In some phospholipids, ethanolamine or serine takes the place of choline.

By no means all animal lipids are glycerides. The lipids that make up the myelin of the brain are esters of fatty acid with complex alcohols. Some of these brain lipids, known as cerebrosides, also contain other constituents such as sugars and nitrogenous compounds. Similar complex lipids are found outside the brain in rare congenital diseases such as Gaucher's disease and Nieman-Pick's disease.

The sterols are an entirely unrelated family of lipids present in small amounts throughout the body. Sterols are ring compounds, containing three six-membered rings and one five-membered ring; each sterol has a different series of hydroxyl and methyl groups or a different side-chain. The only sterol that is encountered in large enough amounts to be demonstrated histologically is cholesterol.

As a general rule, lipids are insoluble in water but are soluble in organic solvents such as xylene or chloroform. Hence, routine paraffin sections are unsatisfactory for the demonstration of lipids, which are removed by the clearing agent. Either the lipids must be demonstrated by osmium tetroxide before dehydration and clearing, or frozen sections must be used. In a few instances, however, paraffin sections are suitable; thus myelin and some lipofuscins are not entirely dissolved by clearing agents and may be stained in paraffin sections with Sudan black. Another obvious exception to the general rule is phospholipid, which is somewhat soluble in water and must be stabilized (with calcium salts) at an early stage.

Fixation and types of sections

Except for a few special methods like osmium tetroxide, the most suitable fixative for lipids in tissues is formalin. This may be used as formalin-saline or neutral buffered formalin solution, but some subsequent staining methods (e.g. Baker's acid haematein) will not work unless calcium ions are incorporated in the fixing fluid. Since calcium does no harm to any of the tissue components, there is something to be said for using a formalin-calcium mixture whenever it can be foreseen that examination for lipids will be required. A suitable mixture is that published by Baker (1944).

Baker's formalin-calcium

Formalin	10 ml.
Calcium chloride (anhydrous)	1 g.
Distilled water	90 ml.

Keep in a bottle with a small amount of precipitated chalk.

Fixation should be adequate but not unduly prolonged. Between one and seven days will be satisfactory; beyond about eight weeks the lipid is altered so that cutting sections becomes more difficult. For obvious reasons, any fixing fluid that contains a large proportion of organic solvent must be avoided. Mercuric chloride is not entirely satisfactory because it makes frozen sections harder to cut.

As already stated, paraffin sections are suitable for the

demonstration of myelin and some lipofuscins. They are also used when tissue has been treated with osmium tetroxide. For other methods, however, frozen sections are required. These should preferably be cut in a cryostat except when additional mordanting is needed as in Baker's acid haematein method, the Schultz method, and the Fischler method.

Finally the sections will almost always require an aqueous mounting medium. As well as mounting the stained sections, it is useful to mount an unstained section for examination by polarized light.

Sudan III and IV

SCOPE

A method for triglycerides (neutral fats). Frozen sections must be used. Tissue may be unfixed or fixed in any fluid that does not contain a large proportion of an organic solvent. Either formalin-saline, or neutral buffered formalin solution, or Baker's formalin-calcium is preferable, since most other fluids lead to difficulties in cutting frozen sections.

REAGENTS

A. *Sudan staining solution*

Sudan III	1·0 g.
Sudan IV	1·0 g.
70% alcohol	500 ml.

Warm the dyes and alcohol in a long-necked flask over a water-bath at 56°C for 30–60 minutes. Cool. The solution keeps indefinitely in a well-stoppered bottle. Filter before use.

B. *Harris's haematoxylin* (p. 99)

C. 0·5% *aqueous hydrochloric acid*

METHOD

1. Rinse the frozen sections in 70% alcohol.
2. Sudan staining solution 45–60 minutes (see Note i).
3. Rinse in 70% alcohol.
4. Wash in tap water for 3–4 minutes.
5. Harris's haematoxylin 3–4 minutes.
6. Wash in tap water 5 minutes.

7. Differentiate in weak hydrochloric acid 5–10 seconds.
8. Wash in tap water 5–10 minutes.
9. Mount in an aqueous mounting medium.

RESULTS

Triglycerides (neutral fats): *red*.
Nuclei: *blue*.
Other structures: *unstained*.

Notes

(i) A tightly closed vessel must be used to prevent evaporation of the staining solution, otherwise crystals of dye will be deposited on the section.

(ii) This procedure is very similar to the original Sudan III method (Daddi, 1896). Michaelis (1901) introduced Sudan IV (also known as Scharlach R, scarlet red, and Fett ponceau). A mixture of Sudan III and Sudan IV is a stronger stain for fat than either dye on its own (Kay and Whitehead, 1941).

(iii) Although it is possible to remove mercury fixation deposit before the sections are stained, there is no way whereby formaldehyde fixation deposit can be removed without also dissolving the lipid.

Oil red O

SCOPE

Exactly as for Sudan III and IV (above) except that oil red O is particularly suitable for tissue containing lipid in tiny droplets. Lipid dissolves less readily in this staining mixture than in the Sudan mixture (Lillie and Ashburn, 1943).

REAGENTS

A. *Oil red O stock solution*

Oil red O	0·5 g.
Isopropanol	500 ml.

Warm the dye and alcohol in a long-necked flask over a water-bath at 56°C for 30–60 minutes. Cool. The solution keeps indefinitely in a well-stoppered bottle.

B. *Oil red O working solution*

Stock solution	30 ml.
Distilled water	20 ml.

M

Mix well and leave to stand for five minutes. Filter (this may take many minutes). The working solution keeps for several hours.

C. *Harris's haematoxylin* (p. 99)

D. *0·5 per cent aqueous hydrochloric acid*

METHOD

1. Oil red O working solution 5–10 minutes.
2. Wash in water 3–4 minutes.
3. Harris's haematoxylin 3–4 minutes.
4. Wash in tap water 5 minutes.
5. Differentiate in weak hydrochloric acid 5–10 seconds.
6. Wash in tap water 5–10 minutes.
7. Mount in an aqueous mounting medium.

RESULTS

Triglycerides (neutral fats): *deep orange-red.*
Nuclei: *blue.*
Other structures: *unstained.*

Note

It is not possible to remove formaldehyde fixation deposit without also dissolving the lipid. Mercury fixation deposit can, however, be removed in the usual way before sections are stained.

Sudan black

SCOPE

A stain for all kinds of lipid (Lison and Dagnelie, 1935). Usually used with frozen sections, but may be used with paraffin sections for special purposes (e.g. myelin or lipofuscin). If frozen sections are used, fixation should follow the rules given above for Sudan III and IV.

REAGENT

Sudan black

Sudan black B	7·0 g.
70% alcohol	500 ml.

Warm the dye and alcohol in a long-necked flask over a water-bath at 56°C for 30–60 minutes. Cool. The solution keeps indefinitely in a well-stoppered bottle. Filter before use.

METHOD

1. Sections to 70% alcohol.
2. Sudan black 7–10 minutes (see Note i).
3. Rinse in 70% alcohol.
4. Wash in water 3–4 minutes.
5. Mount in an aqueous mounting medium.

RESULTS

Lipids: *black*.
Other structures: *light grey*.

Notes

(i) A tightly closed vessel must be used to prevent evaporation of the staining solution, otherwise crystals of dye will be deposited on the section.

(ii) When frozen sections are used it is not possible to remove formaldehyde fixation deposit without also dissolving the lipid. Mercury fixation deposit can, however, be removed in the usual way before sections are stained.

Phosphine 3R

SCOPE

A fluorescence method for triglycerides (neutral fat). Frozen sections must be used. Tissue should be fixed for a relatively short time (12 hours) in a formalin fixing fluid. Particularly suitable for fine droplets of lipid, because the reagents are aqueous. Preparations are not permanent (Popper, 1941).

REAGENT

0·1 per cent aqueous phosphine 3R

METHOD

1. Rinse frozen sections in distilled water.
2. Phosphine 3 minutes.

3. Rinse in distilled water.
4. Mount in 90% glycerol and examine with the fluorescence microscope.

RESULTS (ultra-violet light)

Triglycerides (neutral fats): *silvery white.*
Other structures: *dark.*
(Coloured autofluorescence may be seen in certain tissues, e.g. elastic fibres.)

Note

According to Volk and Popper (1944), this method demonstrates neutral fats but not fatty acids, soaps, or cholesterol.

Osmium tetroxide

SCOPE

Osmium tetroxide (osmic acid) has long been used for the demonstration of lipid (Schultze and Rudneff, 1865). In the presence of lipid, the osmium tetroxide is reduced to insoluble lower oxides which are deposited in the tissue at the site of the lipid. Since these lower oxides are insoluble in most organic solvents, the tissue can then be processed by the paraffin method so long as the clearing agent is chosen with care. Although it is occasionally desirable to show lipid in paraffin sections, the method is not widely used because it is expensive, fixation is apt to be poor, and the sections obtained are very resistant to counterstains. We have found it useful for the demonstration of tiny fat emboli which are less likely to be dislodged when sections are cut from paraffin blocks rather than frozen tissue.

REAGENT

Flemming's fluid (p. 23)

METHOD

1. Fix thin pieces of fresh tissue (about 1 mm. thick) in Flemming's fluid for 12 hours.
2. Rinse in distilled water.
3. Running tap water 3–4 hours.
4. Dehydrate by successive treatment (about one hour each) with 50, 70, and 90% alcohol and, finally, undiluted alcohol (three times).

5. Clear in chloroform overnight.
6. Impregnate three times with paraffin wax (about 1½ hours each); embed in fresh wax.
7. Cut sections, mount on slides, dry, dewax in chloroform, mount in DPX.

RESULTS

Lipid: *black*.
Other structures: *shades of dull yellow*.

Notes

(i) Avoid xylene and toluene which tend to dissolve the precipitated oxides.

(ii) Few counterstains are worth while. Among the few that can be used are Heidenhain's haematoxylin (p. 105), and the picro-Mallory trichrome method (p. 117).

Schultz for cholesterol

SCOPE

Demonstrates cholesterol and its esters only. Frozen sections (preferably about 20 μ thick) of formalin fixed tissue must be used. Preparations are not permanent. (Schultz, 1924.)

REAGENTS

A. *2·5 per cent aqueous iron alum* (ferric ammonium sulphate)

B. *Acetic-sulphuric mixture*
        Glacial acetic acid 10 ml.
        Concentrated sulphuric acid 10 ml.
Add the sulphuric acid to the acetic acid drop by drop. Use a heat-resistant vessel and keep it cool in ice. The mixture keeps for a few weeks; when discoloured it is useless.

METHOD

1. Rinse frozen sections in distilled water.
2. Iron alum at room temperature for 3 days or at 37°C for 36 hours.
3. Rinse in distilled water.
4. Arrange the section on a slide and remove surplus water.

5. Add one or two drops of acetic-sulphuric mixture to the section and cover carefully with a coverslip. This corrosive mixture must not be allowed to overflow.

6. Examine the section at once.

RESULT

Cholesterol and its esters: *blue or purple or red*; in a few minutes the colour changes to *green*. Within an hour or so, the entire section becomes yellowish-brown. The method can only be regarded as positive if the green colour develops in place of the original blue, purple or red (Lison, 1936).

Polarized light for cholesterol

Subject to certain limitations (see Notes), it is possible to identify cholesterol and cholesterol esters in sections by means of a microscope equipped with polarizing films or Nicol prisms. This is because cholesterol and its esters exist in three different forms at different temperatures (Lison, 1936). At low temperatures (below the melting-point), it forms needle-shaped crystals which are strongly birefringent and very easily seen by polarized light. Above the melting-point but below the clarification-point it forms birefringent liquid crystals. Above the clarification-point it forms droplets that are not birefringent and therefore appear dark in polarized light.

In practice, a mounted unstained frozen section is examined at room temperature. If birefringent needle-shaped crystals are seen, the section is removed from the microscope, warmed, and re-examined. If needle-shaped crystals are still present, it should be warmed more vigorously. Often after warming, the field will be entirely dark, but as the section cools, liquid crystals will appear. These take the form of brightly birefringent spheres each of which has a dark Maltese cross superimposed upon it so that it is divided into four bright quadrants. After an interval of weeks or months at room temperature, these spheres will be re-converted to birefringent needle-shaped crystals. For all practical purposes this sequence of needle-shaped crystals, liquid crystals, dark droplets, seen by polarized light is confirmation of the presence of cholesterol or a cholesterol ester. If, however, the sequence does not occur, it is not safe to conclude that cholesterol is absent.

Notes

(i) An unstained section must be used since the formation of liquid crystals is inhibited by osmium tetroxide and by dyestuffs of the Sudan type.

(ii) The appearances described above are those seen in sections of formalin fixed tissue. Formalin appears to encourage the formation of needle-shaped crystals; if unfixed tissue is examined the cholesterol may be seen initially in the form of liquid crystals, and may only form needle-shaped crystals when refrigerated.

(iii) Cholesterol and its esters are usually present in sections in an impure form. On rare occasions, pure cholesterol may be encountered. Since this does not melt until a temperature of nearly 150°C has been reached, the needle-shaped crystals will persist even if the section is heated to the boiling-point of the aqueous medium.

(iv) Other lipids may exist as birefringent needle-shaped crystals or as birefringent liquid crystals, but the sequence of events described above is confined for all practical purposes to cholesterol and its esters.

Baker for phospholipids

SCOPE

Demonstrates phospholipids (lecithin, cephalin and sphingomyelin). Tissue must be fixed in formalin-calcium; frozen sections must be used (Baker, 1946).

REAGENTS

A. *Formalin-calcium* (p. 159)

B. *Dichromate-calcium*

Potassium dichromate	5 g.
Calcium chloride (anhydrous)	1 g.
Distilled water	100 ml.

The solution is stable.

C. *Acid haematein*

Haematoxylin	0·05 g.
Distilled water	48 ml.
1% aqueous sodium iodate	1 ml.
Glacial acetic acid	1 ml.

Heat the haematoxylin, water, and iodate in a flask until the mixture begins to boil. Cool and add the acetic acid. This solution must be freshly prepared.

D. *Weak borax-ferricyanide*

Potassium ferricyanide	0·25 g.
Borax (sodium tetraborate)	0·25 g.
Distilled water	100 ml.

The solution is stable if kept in a refrigerator.

METHOD

1. Fix thin pieces of tissue in formalin-calcium for 6 hours.
2. Transfer to dichromate-calcium for 18 hours.
3. Fresh dichromate-calcium at 60°C 24 hours.
4. Running tap water overnight (see Note ii).
5. Cut frozen sections 10 μ thick (see Note iii).
6. Treat sections with dichromate-calcium at 60°C for one hour.
7. Wash several times with water.
8. Rinse in distilled water.
9. Acid haematein at 37°C 5 hours.
10. Rinse in distilled water.
11. Weak borax-ferricyanide at 37°C 18 hours.
12. Wash several times with tap water.
13. Rinse in distilled water.
14. Dehydrate, clear, and mount (see Note ii).

RESULTS

Phospholipids (lecithin, cephalin, and sphingomyelin): *dark blue to blue-black*.

Galactolipids: *pale blue*.

Some mucin, nucleoprotein, and some proteins including gelatin: *blue, blue-black, or grey* (see Note i).

Other structures: *pale yellow*.

(Pale dirty blue colours are regarded as negative.)

Notes

(i) For the complete identification of phospholipids, a control block of tissue should be extracted with pyridine which removes all phospholipids and galactolipids, leaving only mucin, nucleoprotein and protein stained by the method. Pyridine extraction is performed as follows:

The control block of tissue is fixed for 20 hours in a mixture containing 50 ml. saturated aqueous picric acid, 10 ml. formalin, 5 ml. glacial acetic acid, and 35 ml. water. It is then treated in turn with: 70 per cent alcohol 1 hour, 50 per cent alcohol 30 minutes, running tap water 30 minutes, pyridine at room temperature 1 hour, fresh pyridine at room temperature 1 hour, pyridine at 60°C 24 hours, and running tap water 2 hours. It is then transferred to dichromate-calcium (stage 2) and treated in the same way as the unextracted tissue.

(ii) Friable specimens may be embedded in gelatin as follows. After dichromate-calcium (stage 3), wash in running tap water 6 hours, impregnate with gelatin and embed in gelatin (p. 285), cut frozen sections and transfer them to dichromate-calcium (stage 6). When gelatin is used, better results are obtained if sections are mounted in an aqueous rather than a resinous mounting medium.

(iii) Sections or gelatin blocks may be stored for a few days in formalin-calcium.

Fischler for fatty acids

SCOPE

Demonstrates fatty acids and soaps. Frozen sections of formalin fixed tissue must be used (Fischler, 1904; Fischler and Gross, 1905).

REAGENTS

A. *Saturated aqueous solution of copper acetate*

B. *Haematoxylin mixture*

Stock 20% alcoholic haematoxylin solution (p. 103)	5 ml.
Alcohol	5 ml.
Distilled water	90 ml.
Saturated aqueous solution of lithium carbonate	2 ml.

This mixture must be freshly prepared.

C. *Weigert's differentiator*

Borax (sodium tetraborate)	2·0 g.
Potassium ferricyanide	2·5 g.
Distilled water	200 ml.

This solution is stable.

METHOD

1. Treat sections with copper acetate at 37°C for 24 hours.
2. Wash thoroughly with distilled water.
3. Haematoxylin 20 minutes.
4. Differentiate in Weigert's differentiator until the red blood corpuscles lose their colour.
5. Wash thoroughly in distilled water.
6. Mount in aqueous mounting medium.

RESULTS

Fatty acids and calcium soaps: *dark blue*.
(Haemosiderin and calcium deposits are also dark blue.)
Other structures: *unstained*.

Notes

(i) The method depends on the formation of copper soaps (salts of copper with fatty acids) which are insoluble. The copper is then stained by haematoxylin, for which it acts as a powerful mordant. Occasionally tissue may contain calcium soaps. These also are insoluble and are demonstrated by the method.

If the tissue is fixed in formalin-calcium, all the fatty acids will be converted to calcium soap.

To distinguish between fatty acids and calcium soaps, a control section is treated with a mixture of equal parts of alcohol and ether. This dissolves fatty acids but not soaps. Used separately, neither alcohol-ether mixture nor weak acid will dissolve the soap, but a solution of hydrochloric acid in alcohol-ether will do so (Lillie, 1948).

(ii) False positive reactions are given by haemosiderin and calcium deposits. The haemosiderin can be identified in a control section stained by Perls's method (p. 131). Calcium deposits may be removed from another control section by dilute hydrochloric acid.

(iii) The haematoxylin mixture and the borax-ferricyanide differentiator are the same as those used by Weigert in his methods for myelin.

(iv) If critical differentiation presents a problem, Weigert's differentiator should be diluted with a large volume of distilled water.

(v) A counterstain such as Sudan III and IV (p. 160) may be used to demonstrate neutral fat.

(vi) If a counterstain is not used, the section may be dehydrated rapidly, cleared, and mounted in a resinous medium.

CHAPTER 14

Micro-organisms and Other Parasites

Bacteria: Gram; Gram-Twort. Acid-fast bacteria: Ziehl-Neelsen; Blue stain for *M. tuberculosis*; Modified Ziehl-Neelsen for *M. leprae*; Fluorescence method for mycobacteria. Fungi: Gridley's method. Inclusion bodies. Miscellaneous parasites: Giemsa.

THE methods detailed in this chapter are used mainly for the demonstration of organisms. There are, however, many types of organisms (especially fungi and miscellaneous parasites) that are well shown by stains not primarily intended for this purpose. These are to be found elsewhere in the book although their uses in the demonstration of organisms are mentioned in the appropriate parts of this chapter.

Bacteria

Apart from acid-fast organisms (see below), bacteria are almost always stained by one or other modification of the Gram (1884) stain. When it is necessary to distinguish Gram-negative bacteria, the Gram-Twort stain gives good results. A stain for all bacteria (not distinguishing Gram-positive from Gram-negative) is Giemsa (p. 182).

Gram's method

SCOPE

Suitable for paraffin or frozen sections after any routine fixing fluid, and for smears fixed dry or wet.

REAGENTS

A. *Lillie's crystal violet*

Crystal violet	5 g.
95% alcohol	50 ml.
Ammonium oxalate	2 g.
Distilled water	200 ml.

Dissolve the dye in the alcohol and the oxalate in the water. Mix. The mixture keeps well but must be filtered before use.

B. *Lugol's iodine* (p. 84)

C. *Acetone*

D. *1 per cent aqueous neutral red*

METHOD

1. Sections to water
2. Lillie's crystal violet 1–2 minutes (see Note i).
3. Rinse in water.
4. Lugol's iodine ½–1 minute.
5. Rinse in water.
6. Differentiate in acetone 10–15 seconds (see Note ii).
7. Running tap water 5–10 minutes.
8. Neutral red ½–1 minute.
9. Rinse in water.
10. Dehydrate, clear, and mount.

RESULTS

Gram-positive organisms: *blue-black*. (Keratin and elastic fibres may also be blue-black.)

Other structures, including Gram-negative organisms: *shades of red*.

Notes

(i) It is particularly important to filter the crystal violet staining mixture before use: stain precipitates are very easily confused with organisms.

(ii) If uneven staining is to be avoided, the slide must be agitated briskly during differentiation.

(iii) This particular modification of the Gram method is due to Lillie (1928). It is simpler than many, and is less likely to over-decolorize the Gram-positive organisms. Lugol's iodine is preferred to the original Gram's iodine mixture because it keeps better.

The Gram-Twort method

SCOPE

As Gram's method above.

REAGENTS

A. *Lillie's crystal violet* (as in Gram's method)

B. *Lugol's iodine* (p. 84—as in Gram's method)

C. *2 per cent acetic acid in alcohol*

D. *Twort's red stock solution*
   0·2 per cent alcoholic neutral red

E. *Twort's green stock solution*
   0·2 per cent alcoholic fast green FCF

F. *Twort's working solution*

Red stock solution	9 ml.
Green stock solution	1 ml.
Distilled water	30 ml.

Mix immediately before use.

METHOD

1. Sections to water.
2. Lillie's crystal violet 3–5 minutes.
3. Rinse in distilled water.
4. Lugol's iodine 3 minutes.
5. Rinse in distilled water.
6. Blot.
7. Differentiate in acetic alcohol until no more colour comes away (the section is now a dirty brown colour).
8. Rinse in distilled water.
9. Twort's working solution 5 minutes.
10. Rinse in distilled water.
11. Differentiate in acetic alcohol until no more red colour comes away (15–30 seconds).
12. Dehydrate, clear, and mount.

RESULTS

Gram-positive organisms: *blue-black.*
(Keratin and elastic fibres may also be blue-black.)
Gram-negative organisms; cell nuclei: *red.*
Other structures: *green.*

Notes

(i) Filter the crystal violet solution immediately before use. Agitate the section during differentiation. (See Notes i and ii to Gram's method above.)

(ii) This combination of Gram's stain with that of Twort (1924) is due to Ollett (1947; 1951), who also modified Twort's mixture by using fast green in place of the original light green.

Acid-fast bacteria

Mycobacteria contain a waxy lipid which makes them difficult to stain. Once a stain penetrates the organisms, however, it is difficult to remove. This latter quality is the basis of the Ziehl-Neelsen stain, which relies on the ability of a mineral acid to decolorize everything except mycobacteria. Although *Mycobacterium tuberculosis* is very resistant to decolorization, other mycobacteria (e.g. *leprae*) are less so and require a modification of the method.

One drawback to the usual Ziehl-Neelsen method is the combination of red and bluish-green colours. As it happens these are the shades that confuse sufferers from the commonest form of colour-blindness. We therefore append an alternative method which makes use of dyes that do not confuse the colour-blind. Those whose vision is normal can use it although they almost always prefer the orthodox Ziehl-Neelsen method.

The Ziehl-Neelsen Method

SCOPE

Suitable for every type of section and smear.

REAGENTS

A. *Carbol fuchsin*

Basic fuchsin	1 g.
Alcohol	10 ml.
5% aqueous phenol	100 ml.

Dissolve the dye in the alcohol and mix with the phenol. The solution keeps well but must be filtered before use.

B. *25 per cent aqueous sulphuric acid*

C. *70 per cent alcohol*

D. *0·25 per cent methylene blue in 1 per cent aqueous acetic acid*

METHOD

1. Sections to water.
2. Carbol fuchsin 7–10 minutes with heat (see Note i).
3. Rinse in water.
4. Sulphuric acid at least 2 minutes.

5. 70% alcohol at least 2 minutes.
6. Sulphuric acid at least 2 minutes (see Note ii).
7. Running tap water at least 5 minutes (see Note iii).
8. Methylene blue ½–1 minute.
9. Rinse in water.
10. Dehydrate, clear, and mount.

RESULTS

Mycobacterium tuberculosis: *red*.
Other structures: *shades of blue*.
(Red blood corpuscles occasionally stain pale pink.)

Notes

(i) Heat is usually applied by means of a flame directly beneath the slide until vapour begins to rise from the stain. The alternative is to use an incubator at about 56°C, in which case the stain must be raised to temperature before the section is placed in it.

(ii) If the section is not fully decolorized at this stage, it is treated alternately with acid and alcohol as often as necessary.

(iii) After decolorization the wash must be thorough. Strong sulphuric acid temporarily converts the dye into a colourless form. A good wash in running tap water restores the colour.

(iv) The counterstain must not be too heavy. Organisms may be hard enough to find even when it is pale.

(v) The credit for this method should really belong to Ehrlich who made the original observation that tubercle bacilli are acid-fast (i.e. once stained they are not decolorized by mineral acid). Ziehl (1882) introduced carbolic acid (phenol) and Neelsen (1883) suggested sulphuric acid rather than nitric.

Blue stain for Mycobacterium tuberculosis

This method is recommended for the colour-blind. The scope, reagents, method, and notes i–iii are identical with the Ziehl-Neelsen method except for the following substitutions.

SUBSTITUTE REAGENTS

A. Prepare *carbol Victoria blue* by using Victoria blue R instead of basic fuchsin. The method of preparation is the same.

D. Replace the acid methylene blue counterstain with *alcoholic Bismarck brown* (p. 194).

SUBSTITUTIONS IN THE METHOD

2. Use carbol Victoria blue instead of carbol fuchsin but in exactly the same way.

8–10. Replace these stages in the Ziehl-Neelsen method as follows:

8. Rinse in alcohol.
9. Bismarck brown 1–2 minutes.
10. Dehydrate, clear, and mount.

RESULTS

Mycobacterium tuberculosis: *blue*.
Other structures: *shades of yellow and brown*.

Modified Ziehl-Neelsen Method for Mycobacterium leprae

SCOPE

Suitable for paraffin sections. Tissue fixed in Susa or in one of the simple formalin mixtures has given good results; our experience is limited to these fluids.

REAGENTS

A. *Carbol fuchsin*
As used in the Ziehl-Neelsen method.

B. *1 per cent hydrochloric acid in 70 per cent alcohol*

C. *Methylene blue as used in the Ziehl-Neelsen method*

METHOD

1. Sections to water.
2. Carbol fuchsin at 56°C for 20–30 minutes (see Note i).
3. Rinse in water.
4. Acid alcohol until the red colour almost but not quite disappears. The entire section should remain faintly pink.
5. Wash in running tap water for 5–10 minutes.
6. Methylene blue ½–1 minute.
7. Rinse in water.
8. Dehydrate, clear, and mount.

RESULTS (see also Note iii)

Mycobacteria (tuberculosis, leprae, and others): *red*.
Red blood corpuscles: *pale pink*.
Other structures: *shades of blue*.

Notes

(i) The carbol fuchsin must be heated to 56°C before the sections are inserted.

(ii) The counterstain must not be too heavy.

(iii) The method also stains the heads of spermatozoa, the clubs of actinomycosis, and some lipofuscins.

(iv) Although this method has given good results with many surgical biopsy specimens, we have not had extensive experience with decrepit bacilli which are said to be very difficult to demonstrate. For these, Wade (1957) recommends his modification of Fite's earlier methods.

(v) A blue stain for *M. leprae* can be achieved if this method is carried out using the substitute reagents described above.

A fluorescence method for mycobacteria

SCOPE

Suitable for all kinds of smears and sections. The preparations lose brilliance and should preferably be examined within about four days. This method is suitable for *M. tuberculosis*; for *M. leprae* see Note iii. (Kuper and May, 1960.)

REAGENTS

A. *Auramine-Rhodamine*

Auramine O	1·5 g.
Rhodamine B	0·75 g.
Glycerol	75 ml.
Phenol crystals liquefied at 50°C	10 ml.
Distilled water	50 ml.

Mix thoroughly and filter before use. The mixture will keep for 2–3 months.

B. *0·5 per cent hydrochloric acid in 70 per cent alcohol*

C. *0·5 per cent aqueous potassium permanganate*

N

METHOD

1. Sections to water.
2. Auramine-rhodamine at 60°C for 10 minutes (see Note i).
3. Running tap water 2 minutes.
4. Acid alcohol 2 minutes.
5. Running tap water 2 minutes.
6. Permanganate solution 2 minutes.
7. Running tap water 2 minutes.
8. Blot dry.
9. Dehydrate rapidly in undiluted alcohol, clear, and mount (see Note ii).

RESULTS (with ultra-violet or deep blue light)

Mycobacterium tuberculosis: *reddish gold.*
Other structures: *dark blue to black.*
Artefacts (when fluorescent): *pale yellow with no tinge of red.*

Notes

(i) The auramine-rhodamine must be heated to 60°C before the sections or smears are inserted.

(ii) Preparations mounted in DPX lose their brilliance within a few days. If 'Fluormount' is used, the deterioration is slower but, even so, it is wise to examine the preparation within four days. 'Fluormount' has the drawback that it does not set nearly so quickly. Bacteriological preparations do not need to be mounted; it is sufficient to dehydrate them rapidly in undiluted alcohol and add the (non-fluorescent) immersion oil directly. Unmounted preparations fade less rapidly.

(iii) For *Mycobacterium leprae*, three modifications of this method are recommended:

(*a*) Stage 1 is replaced by two treatments (of 5 minutes each) with a mixture of two parts of xylene and one part of ground-nut oil. The slide is then blotted dry and transferred to auramine-rhodamine.

(*b*) At stage 4, weak acid is used instead of acid alcohol (0·5 per cent hydrochloric acid in distilled water).

(*c*) After blotting thoroughly (stage 8), alcohol and xylene are avoided, the preparation being either mounted in 'Fluormount' or examined directly with immersion oil.

Fungi

The classification of fungi and similar organisms is beyond the scope of this book, so that the following remarks apply to the so-called 'false fungi' as well as to fungi proper. Those who are faced with the problem of using histological and histochemical methods to identify a particular fungus will obtain useful information from Symmers (1968).

The only staining method for fungi that we have included in this part of the book is that of Gridley (1953). This should not be taken to imply that Gridley's is the only method that we recommend. Grocott's hexamine-silver method for fungi has been put with other silver impregnation methods for convenience (p. 219). There are also other staining methods that may be of immense value in the demonstration and recognition of fungi.

In a haematoxylin and eosin preparation, fungi usually stain sufficiently to arouse suspicion (if not certainly) of their presence. The per-iodic acid Schiff method (p. 141) is useful, since it is available in every laboratory and will stain virtually every fungus. It has the drawback, however, that it often stains too many other things in the section, so that the fungi are obscured. Gram's method (p. 171) stains a part or the whole of most of the common fungi. Mucicarmine (p. 147) has the useful property of staining cryptococci and no other fungi.

Of the special stains for fungi, there is a basic similarity between Grocott's and Gridley's but there are also important differences. Both methods stain dead fungi as well as viable ones, and are sometimes the only methods that will reveal fungi in necrotic tissue. Both are virtually specific for chitin although Grocott's method shows a slight tendency to deposit silver on other structures such as basement membranes. Grocott's gives the more conspicuous result but fails to show any of the internal structure of the fungi whereas Gridley's is more delicate and more detailed.

Gridley's method

SCOPE

Suitable for paraffin sections after any routine fixing fluid.

REAGENTS

A. *Chromic acid*

Chromium trioxide	4 g.
Distilled water	100 ml.

B. *Schiff's reagent* (p. 142)

C. *Sulphurous acid rinse* (p. 142)

D. *Gomori's aldehyde fuchsin* (p. 201)

E. *Saturated solution of tartrazine in cellosolve*

METHOD

1. Sections to water.
2. Chromic acid 60 minutes.
3. Running tap water 5 minutes.
4. Rinse in distilled water.
5. Schiff's reagent in a Coplin jar 15–20 minutes.
6. Sulphurous acid 2 minutes. Repeat this treatment twice more.
7. Running tap water 10–15 minutes.
8. Aldehyde fuchsin in a Coplin jar 20–30 minutes.
9. Rinse in 50% alcohol.
10. Wash well in running tap water.
11. Rinse in alcohol.
12. Tartrazine ½–1 minute.
13. Dehydrate, clear, and mount.

RESULTS

Fungi: *deep rose to purple.*
Elastic and some mucin: *deep blue.*
Other structures: *yellow.*

Inclusion bodies

Viruses and related micro-organisms are too small to be seen individually with the optical microscope. When they are aggregated into masses, however, they may be seen fairly easily. The masses, which are known as inclusion bodies, are found inside cells, either in the nucleus or in the cytoplasm. Depending on the species of virus, the masses are composed predominantly either of deoxyribonucleic acid (DNA) or ribonucleic acid (RNA). They thus show a general tendency to stain in a similar way to nuclei. Many special staining methods for inclusion bodies have been published, but we have not found many of them helpful. On the whole, the most useful results have been obtained with conventional stains for either DNA or RNA according to the type of virus causing the inclusion.

For DNA virus inclusions, good results are obtainable by the Feulgen method (p. 185). For RNA virus inclusions, the pyronin and methyl green stain (p. 187) is recommended provided that it is used with care. A section carefully stained by haematoxylin and eosin will often provide the most information. This is particularly true when Harris's haematoxylin (p. 99) is used, since this mixture tends to stain RNA a reddish colour that stands out clearly against the blue DNA. Laboratories with facilities for fluorescence microscopy should try acridine orange (p. 189) which may give good results. In some cases the phloxine tartrazine method (p. 203) will give a beautiful demonstration. When rickettsial infection is suspected, Giemsa's stain (p. 182) is likely to prove at least as successful as any of the special methods; this stain will also demonstrate virus inclusion bodies in some cases.

Miscellaneous parasites

Histological techniques are rarely the methods of choice for the identification of parasites. It is therefore not surprising that very few specific histological techniques have been developed. Small parasites are more often sought by wet film techniques (e.g. amoebae) or in fixed smears (e.g. malaria). Large parasites are easier to identify when examined in their entirety rather than in sections.

When, however, a parasite is encountered in a section, it may be worth trying the effect of a number of different staining methods. A section stained by haematoxylin and eosin often provides more information than any other, but duplicate sections may sometimes be stained with profit by one or more of the following methods: Giemsa (see below); the per-iodic acid Schiff method (p. 141) or Gridley's stain (p. 179) if much mucus is present; Grocott's method (p. 219); Heidenhain's iron haematoxylin (p. 105); phosphotungstic acid haematoxylin (p. 114).

The following fragments of information may be found useful in specific instances. In chronic lesions many of the larger parasites become impregnated with calcium salts (e.g. schistosoma ova in the bladder; cysticerci). The hooklets of hydatids

(*Taeni echinococcus*) stain a brilliant translucent yellow with picric acid. Amoebae (*Entamoeba histolytica*) usually contain abundant glycogen and may therefore be stained by Best's carmine (p. 150) in addition to the per-iodic acid Schiff method. *Toxoplasma gondii* cysts are stained by the per-iodic acid Schiff method but individual organisms are not. Leishman-Donovan bodies (*L. donovani*) do not stain by Grocott's method or by the per-iodic acid Schiff method and may thus be distinguished from histoplasma. *Pneumocystis carinii* appear practically unstained in haematoxylin and eosin preparations; if their presence is suspected, a smear or section should be stained by Giemsa's method, the per-iodic acid Schiff method, or Grocott's method with prolongation of the time in the silver solution. Malaria parasites may be demonstrated by Giemsa's stain or the Feulgen method (p. 185). Fixing fluids that destroy red blood corpuscles must be avoided. Search for malaria pigment (p. 128) is only possible if a fixing fluid that does not produce formalin fixation deposit has been used; neutral buffered formalin solution or Helly's fluid have been recommended.

Giemsa stain for parasites

SCOPE

Suitable for paraffin sections after any routine fixing fluid. Also suitable for smears which should preferably be fixed in alcoholic mercuric chloride (p. 324) (Giemsa, 1909).

REAGENTS

A. *Weak Giemsa stain*
    Giemsa stock solution (p. 334) 4 ml.
    Buffered distilled water (pH 6·8) 96 ml.

B. *0·5 per cent aqueous acetic acid*

METHOD

 1. Sections to water.
 2. Rinse in distilled water.
 3. Weak Giemsa stain overnight.
 4. Rinse in distilled water.
 5. Weak acetic acid until section is pink (about 1–2 minutes).

6. Wash in tap water.
7. Dehydrate rapidly, clear, and mount.

RESULTS

Many micro-organisms and parasites: *dark blue.*
Nuclei: *blue.*
Other structures: *shades of pink and light blue.*
Chromaffin granules in chrome-fixed tissue: *dark greyish green.*

Notes

(i) Buffered distilled water (pH 6·8) may conveniently be made by using commercially produced buffer tablets.
(ii) Provided that dehydration is rapid, alcohol may be used as after any other staining method.

CHAPTER 15

Intracellular Structures

Nucleic acids: Feulgen; Pyronin and methyl green; Acridine orange. Bone marrow: Barrett's method for marrow; Chromotrope; Bismarck brown. Pituitary: Barrett's method for pituitary; Per-iodic acid Schiff and orange G; Slidders's method. Pancreatic islets: Aldehyde fuchsin; Phloxine tartrazine.

THIS chapter deals with special staining methods for a variety of structures that are found within cells. Nucleoproteins are the chief constituent of the cell nucleus and are sometimes encountered in the cytoplasm as well. Methods for nucleoproteins are important for the recognition of virus inclusion bodies. Many cells are identifiable by the staining reactions of their cytoplasmic granules, and in a few tissues the exact identity of the cells is particularly important. These are tissues in which there is a mixed population of cells that are not easily distinguished in sections stained by haematoxylin and eosin, and include bone marrow, pituitary, and pancreatic islets.

Nucleic acids

Nucleoproteins consist of nucleic acid and protein. They owe their staining qualities to the nucleic acids; these are present in all forms of life, including viruses. In animal tissues two types are present; deoxyribonucleic acid (DNA), which forms most of the nuclear chromatin, and ribonucleic acid (RNA) which is present in both nucleus and cytoplasm. In the nucleus, RNA forms most of the nucleolus, whereas in the cytoplasm it is present in ribosomes. Ribosomes are chiefly concerned with protein synthesis; they are too small to be seen with the optical microscope, so that a stain for RNA will usually appear to stain the cytoplasm diffusely when ribosomes are sufficiently numerous. In a few cells, however, RNA appears to form fairly dense aggregates or granules.

Virus particles contain large quantities of nucleic acid: either DNA or RNA depending on the type of virus. Stains for nucleic acids are therefore valuable for the demonstration of virus inclusion bodies, and may provide limited information about the type of virus present.

The most satisfactory histological method for DNA is the Feulgen reaction; this is specific and does not stain RNA. Conversely, RNA (but not DNA) may be demonstrated by the pyronin and methyl green method. If a fluorescence microscope is available, the acridine orange method may be used; this has the merit of demonstrating DNA and RNA in contrasting colours. Like other fluorescence methods, however, it suffers from the drawback that the stained structures are often difficult to orientate in the section as a whole. A method that stains both DNA and RNA, but does not distinguish one from the other, is gallocyanin chrome alum (p. 233).

In practice, all ordinary requirements will be satisfied by two methods. The Feulgen method is used for DNA inclusion bodies and may also be used for nuclei (e.g. mitoses). The pyronin and methyl green method is used for plasma cells and for RNA inclusion bodies.

Feulgen

SCOPE

A method for DNA; suitable for paraffin sections after any routine fixing fluid except Bouin's fluid. Also suitable for smears fixed chemically or by heat. This method is almost identical with the original (Feulgen and Rossenbeck, 1924).

REAGENTS

A. *N/1 hydrochloric acid*

B. *Schiff's reagent* (p. 142)

C. *Sulphurous acid rinse* (p. 142)

D. *Saturated solution (0·3%) of tartrazine in cellosolve*

METHOD

1. Sections (or smears) to water.
2. Rinse in N/1 hydrochloric acid.
3. N/1 hydrochloric acid at 60°C for 5–10 minutes (see Note i).
4. Rinse in distilled water.
5. Schiff's reagent 1–1½ hours in a Coplin jar.

6. Sulphurous acid rinse 2 minutes.
7. Sulphurous acid rinse 2 minutes.
8. Sulphurous acid rinse 2 minutes.
9. Running tap water 5–10 minutes (see Note ii).
10. Rinse in alcohol.
11. Tartrazine 30–60 seconds (see Note iii).
12. Dehydrate, clear, and mount.

RESULTS

Deoxyribonucleic acid (nuclear chromatin; some inclusion bodies): *magenta* (see Note iv).

Other structures: *yellow*.

Notes

(i) It is essential to raise the temperature of the hydrochloric acid to 60°C before treating the sections; a water-bath is quicker than an incubator. The optimum time in acid varies according to the type of tissue and the method of fixation; for critical work it should be determined by trial and error, but for routine use about 8 minutes is usually satisfactory. Excessive treatment weakens the reaction.

(ii) After sulphurous acid the sections must be washed thoroughly in water or the colour may be weak.

(iii) A green counterstain is often used, but this is more likely to obscure the finest Feulgen-positive structures. If green is preferred, use 1 per cent aqueous light green for 15-30 seconds followed by a rinse in water, in place of stages 10 and 11.

(iv) DNA is the only substance that is Feulgen-positive, so that this method is histochemically specific. It is, however, essential to realize that the terms Feulgen-positive and Schiff-positive are not synonymous. To be Feulgen-positive, a substance must yield aldehyde groups when subjected to mild acid hydrolysis. For precise results a control section should therefore be treated with Schiff's reagent without prior hydrolysis. Only structures that are stained magenta in the test section and unstained in the control may be described as Feulgen-positive. Schiff's reagent is, of course, no more than a marker of aldehyde groups (p. 144), and will show all aldehydes whether liberated by acid hydrolysis or present from the start. Fortunately, pre-existing aldehydes are rare in processed tissue, being virtually confined to elastic fibres, which may therefore appear Schiff positive although not, of course, Feulgen-positive since they are stained equally strongly in the control section. In fresh, unprocessed tissue, aldehydes are plentiful (see below).

(v) Care must be taken when applying this method to frozen sections or to smears that were not fixed in a strong alcoholic fluid. This is because cytoplasm often contains abundant aldehydes which will recolorize Schiff's reagent in test sections and controls. These aldehydes are lipids and are removed during routine processing. They may be removed from frozen sections or from smears by overnight treatment with alcohol.

The demonstration of these aldehyde substances in cytoplasm by Schiff's reagent is the so-called plasmal reaction of Feulgen and Voit (1924), who found that preliminary treatment with mercuric chloride (1 per cent aqueous for 3 minutes followed by thorough washing) gave even stronger results.

(vi) If mineral acids are used for decalcification, the tissue will be unsuitable for the Feulgen method. Formic acid is satisfactory but trichloracetic acid is not.

Pyronin and methyl green

SCOPE

A method for RNA (plasma cells, related 'pyronin-positive' cells, and virus inclusion bodies). Suitable for paraffin sections or smears. May be used after any routine fixing fluid that does not contain dichromate or picric acid. Fixation must not be prolonged (see Note i).

REAGENTS

A. *Stock solution of pyronin*

2 per cent aqueous solution of Pyronin Y extracted ten times with equal volumes of chloroform (the chloroform is always slightly tinted). The solution should be stored over chloroform and may be kept for several weeks.

B. *Stock solution of methyl green*

2 per cent aqueous solution of methyl green extracted at least six times with equal volumes of chloroform; the extraction must continue until the chloroform layer is no longer tinted with methyl violet. The solution should be stored over chloroform and may be kept for several weeks.

C. *Staining mixture*

Pyronin stock solution	12·5 ml.
Methyl green stock solution	7·5 ml.
Distilled water	30 ml.

This solution should be freshly prepared.

D. *n-Butanol*

METHOD

1. Sections to water.
2. Rinse thoroughly in distilled water.
3. Staining mixture 6 minutes in a covered vessel.
4. Blot the section.
5. Butanol 5 minutes.
6. Repeat with fresh butanol.
7. Clear in xylene and mount.

RESULTS

Ribonucleic acid (plasma cell cytoplasm; nucleoli; Nissl granules of neurones; etc.): *red.*

Deoxyribonucleic acid (nuclei): *green or bluish-green.*

Other structures: *colourless to pale pink.*

Notes

(i) For the best results, thin pieces of tissue should be fixed in neutral buffered formalin solution for 18–36 hours. Tissue fixed in this fluid for more than a week gives poor results. In unbuffered formalin-saline the deterioration is quicker. Other fixing fluids are less satisfactory, but fairly good results may be obtained after Carnoy's fluid (2–3 hours), Susa (3–4 hours), and mercuric-chloride-formalin (6–12 hours). Sections of decalcified tissue are unsuitable.

(ii) Different batches of pyronin and methyl green vary in their suitability for this method. We have had good results with dyes manufactured by Merck. In any case, the dyes should be obtained in small packages, since the powders appear to deteriorate after exposure to the atmosphere.

(iii) For complete identification of ribonucleic acid, two control sections should be used. One is incubated at 37°C for one hour with a weak (0·1 per cent) solution of ribonuclease, while the other is incubated with distilled water only. Both are then stained by pyronin and methyl green. Ribonucleic acid is completely destroyed by the enzyme and almost unaffected by the water.

(iv) The use of pyronin and methyl green was first suggested by Pappenheim (1899) who gave few details. More exact instructions were given by Unna (1902). The pyronin and methyl green stain is often known by the names of these two originators. The method we have used is a modification by Kurnick (1955) and has given excellent results.

(v) According to Kurnick (1952), the two basic dyes pyronin and methyl green distinguish the nucleic acids because of different degrees of polymerization; deoxyribonucleic acid being highly polymerized whereas ribonucleic acid is a relatively small polymer.

Acridine Orange

SCOPE

A fluorescence method for nucleic acids, in which DNA is distinguished from RNA. Suitable for frozen sections of unfixed tissue and for smears. For fixation, alcohol, acetic-alcohol (p. 280), alcohol-ether mixture (p. 323), or Carnoy's fluid (p. 20) may be used. This is the method of von Bertalanffy, Masin, and Masin (1956).

REAGENTS

A. *1 per cent aqueous acetic acid*

B. *Stock solution of acridine orange*

Acridine orange	0·1 g.
Distilled water	100 ml.

This keeps well if stored in the dark.

C. *Phosphate buffer*

1/15 M phosphate buffer at pH 6·0.
This should be stored in a refrigerator.

D. *Working solution of acridine orange*

Stock solution of acridine orange	10 ml.
Phosphate buffer	90 ml.

This should be freshly prepared every week.

E. *Calcium chloride solution*

Calcium chloride (anhydrous)	1 g.
Distilled water	100 ml.

METHOD

1. Sections or smears to water.
2. Wash well in distilled water.
3. Rinse with weak acetic acid.
4. Wash well in distilled water.
5. Acridine orange working solution 3 minutes.
6. Wash in phosphate buffer 1 minute.
7. Calcium chloride 30 seconds.
8. Wash in phosphate buffer.
9. Mount in phosphate buffer and examine immediately.

RESULTS (with ultra-violet or deep blue light)

Deoxyribonucleic acid: *green.*
Ribonucleic acid: *orange-red.*

Notes

(i) Preparations should be examined as soon as possible.

(ii) If it is necessary to restain a section by another method, the acridine orange may be removed by washing in 1 per cent acetic acid.

Bone marrow and related cells

The type of staining method chosen will depend on what material is available. For many purposes, the best results are obtained with air-dried smears, for which a stain of the Romanowsky type should be used (pp. 333-335). Histological sections (and smears fixed before drying) may be stained by one or more of the following methods.

A carefully differentiated haematoxylin and eosin section gives a good general view of the marrow. The various types of marrow cells are easier to recognize in sections stained by Barrett's method or the Giemsa method (p. 182). Sometimes all that is required is a method for the identification of a particular type of cell. Unfortunately this is not always possible, and there are many cells for which no specific methods are available. It is, however, comparatively simple to demonstrate eosinophil leucocytes, mast cells, and plasma cells.

Eosinophil leucocytes are conspicuous in sections stained by haematoxylin and eosin if differentiation of the eosin is prolonged. They are stained specifically by chromotrope (see below).

Mast cells and basophil leucocytes can be demonstrated by a number of methods. Of these, perhaps the most reliable is aldehyde fuchsin (p. 201) which does not require skilled differentiation. Traditional methods rely on metachromasia with dyes such as toluidine blue (p. 149) and Bismarck brown (see below); the latter is particularly suitable for distinguishing intact mast cells from ruptured ones, and also permits nuclei to be counterstained in a contrasting colour. Solochrome cyanin (p. 247) is particularly useful for distinguishing mast cells from eosinophil leucocytes, since they are stained different colours; the method does, however, require careful differentiation. Mast cells are also demonstrated by the alcian blue method for amyloid (p. 154). This is complicated but has the merit that differentiation is not critical.

Mast cell granules in human material withstand routine fixing fluids well, so that formalin-saline, neutral buffered formalin solution, Helly's fluid, mercuric-chloride-formalin, and Susa are suitable. In some species, however, the mast cells are destroyed by aqueous fluids; for these it may be necessary to use alcoholic formalin, Carnoy's fluid, or a similar alcoholic reagent.

Plasma cells may be recognizable in haematoxylin and eosin stained sections. For their specific identification, the pyronin and methyl green method (p. 187) must be used.

Megakaryocytes rarely need special stains for their identification. If, however, it is necessary to stain them or their precursors, the periodic acid Schiff method (p. 141) should be used.

Barrett's method for bone marrow

SCOPE

Suitable for paraffin sections, preferably 2–3 μ thick. Helly's fluid gives the best results but other routine fixing fluids may be used. If decalcification is necessary, this should be gentle: Custer's fluid is satisfactory (Barrett, 1944a).

REAGENTS

A. *Carazzi's haematoxylin* (p. 106)

B. *1 per cent hydrochloric acid in 70 per cent alcohol*

C. *Orange mixture*

1% aqueous erythrosin	3 ml.
1% aqueous orange G	9 ml.
Distilled water	6 ml.

D. *Blue mixture*

1% aqueous methylene blue	2 ml.
1% aqueous toluidine blue	1 ml.
Distilled water	17 ml.

Filter before use.

E. *Buffer solution A*

13·6% potassium dihydrogen phosphate	4 ml.
Distilled water	250 ml.

This solution should be kept in a refrigerator.

F. *Buffer solution B*

13·6% potassium dihydrogen phosphate	1 ml.
4% sodium hydroxide	1 ml.
Distilled water	250 ml.

This solution should be kept in a refrigerator.

G. *Working buffer solution* (see Note i)

Buffer solution *A*.	2 parts
Buffer solution *B*.	1–4 parts

This mixture should be freshly prepared as required.

H. *Strong staining mixture*

Orange mixture	0·5 ml.
Working buffer solution	0·5 ml.
Acetone	1·0 ml.

This must be freshly prepared.

I. *Weak staining solution*

Orange mixture	0·1 ml.
Blue mixture	0·1 ml.
Working buffer solution	10 ml.
Distilled water	30 ml.

This must be freshly prepared.

METHOD

1. Sections to water.
2. Carazzi's haematoxylin 10–20 minutes.
3. Running tap water 2–3 minutes.
4. Acid alcohol 5–10 seconds.
5. Running tap water 5–10 minutes.
6. Strong staining mixture 20–30 minutes in a closed vessel (see Note ii).
7. Rinse in distilled water.
8. Weak staining solution overnight in a closed vessel (see Note iii).
9. Dehydrate, clear, and mount (see Note iv).

RESULTS

Eosinophil granules: *orange to scarlet.*

Neutrophil granules: *crimson red.*
Basophil granules: *purple-blue.*
Red blood corpuscles: *pink or orange-pink.*
Nuclei: *grey-blue.*
Other structures: *colourless to blue.*

Notes

(i) The optimum mixture of buffer *A* and buffer *B* varies from one piece of tissue to another. *A* accentuates the red colours and *B* the blue. When the optimum has been discovered for a particular section, the same proportions will give good results with other sections from the same block. For common fixing fluids, the best results are usually obtained as follows: Helly's fluid *A*:*B*::1:2, mercuric-chloride-formalin and Susa *A*:*B*::1:1, formalin-saline and neutral buffered formalin solution *A*:*B*::2:1.

(ii) Stage 6 accentuates the fine granules of neutrophil leucocytes; it may be omitted if these are not important. When included in the method, it may conveniently be performed in a Petri dish with the slide resting on two matchsticks.

(iii) At stage 8, the blue dyes tend to precipitate on new glass. For uniform results, the same Coplin jar should always be used for this mixture. It should be kept filled with distilled water when not in use.

(iv) Impure alcohol and xylene must be avoided. Reagents that have been used for dehydrating and clearing routine batches of sections should not be used.

Chromotrope 2R

SCOPE

A stain for eosinophil leucocytes. Suitable for paraffin sections, frozen sections and smears. Any routine fixing fluid may be used. (Lendrum, 1944.)

REAGENTS

A. *Carazzi's haematoxylin (p. 106)*

B. *1 per cent hydrochloric acid in 70 per cent alcohol*

C. *Carbol-chromotrope*

Phenol	1 g.
Chromotrope 2R	0·5 g.
Distilled water	100 ml.

Warm the phenol crystals until melted. Add the dye and mix

o

well. Dissolve the mixture in the water. The solution keeps for about 3 months.

METHOD

1. Sections to water.
2. Carazzi's haematoxylin 10 minutes.
3. Running tap water 5 minutes.
4. Acid alcohol 5–10 seconds.
5. Running tap water 5–10 minutes.
6. Carbol-chromotrope 30 minutes.
7. Rinse in tap water.
8. Dehydrate, clear, and mount.

RESULTS

Eosinophil granules: *bright red.*
Nuclei: *blue.*
Other structures: *colourless to pale pink.*
(Paneth cells: *rust colour.*)
(Kultschitzky cell granules: *dark brown.*)

Bismarck brown for mast cells

SCOPE

Suitable for paraffin sections after any routine fixing fluid. (Spatz, 1960.)

REAGENTS

A. *Bismarck brown solution*

Bismarck brown	0·5 g.
Alcohol	80 ml.
1% aqueous hydrochloric acid	10 ml.

B. *Carazzi's haematoxylin (p. 106)*

METHOD

1. Sections to 70% alcohol.
2. Bismarck brown at least 30 minutes.
3. Rinse three times quickly with 70% alcohol.
4. Carazzi's haematoxylin 1–2 minutes.
5. Running tap water 5 minutes.
6. Dehydrate, clear, and mount.

RESULTS

Granules of intact mast cells: *yellow-brown*.
Nuclei: *blue*.
Other structures: *colourless to yellow*.
(Other sulphated polysaccharides are also *yellow-brown*).

Pituitary

The pituitary gland or hypophysis is divided into two parts in man; there are additional parts in some other species. The anterior lobe or adenohypophysis is an endocrine gland containing cells of several types: the posterior lobe or neurohypophysis is composed of neural tissue and is connected with the brain by a slender stalk. The posterior lobe is stained by the methods used for other parts of the central nervous system.

When the anterior lobe is stained by combinations of simple acid and basic dyes, the cells fall into three types. About 40 per cent of them contain cytoplasmic granules which stain with acid dyes; these are therefore known as acidophil cells. About 10 per cent contain cytoplasmic granules that stain with basic dyes; these are known as basophil cells. The remaining 50 per cent stain with neither acid nor basic dyes; these are accordingly known as chromophobe cells. By using more elaborate staining methods, however, it has been shown that such a division of the cells of the anterior lobe of the pituitary is an oversimplification. This is not surprising, since there are probably seven separate anterior pituitary hormones, and it is believed that each hormone is formed by a special type of cell. Furthermore, it seems likely that the same cell may present different appearances at different times, being granular (acidophil or basophil) when filled with hormone, and non-granular (chromophobe) when the hormone has recently been secreted.

In due course, no doubt, specific histochemical methods will be developed for each of these cells. At present, however, there is incomplete correlation between the various hormones produced and the results of the many staining methods that have been used; nor is it always possible to correlate one staining method with another. For accounts of the results obtained by a variety of methods, and their relation to the pituitary hormones, the reader may consult Doniach (1960) and Ham (1965).

We have used three methods, each of which has its particular merits. The first is an unpublished modification by A. M. Barrett of Mallory's trichrome method, and gives results of the classical type, showing acidophil, basophil and chromophobe cells. The second is a method derived from Pearse (1950) which makes use of the per-iodic acid Schiff reaction to demonstrate cells containing mucoprotein (basophil and some chromophobe cells). The third method is that of Slidders (1961), and shows two distinct types of basophil cells, as well as giving a clear picture of the acidophil and chromophobe cells.

Barrett's method for pituitary

SCOPE

Suitable for paraffin sections (preferably 2–3 μ thick). May be used after any routine fixing fluid.

REAGENTS

A. *Weigert's haematoxylin* (p. 104)

B. *1 per cent hydrochloric acid in 70 per cent alcohol*

C. *Red mixture* (picro-Mallory; p. 118)

D. *2 per cent aqueous acetic acid*

E. *Blue mixture* (picro-Mallory; p. 118)

F. *Red differentiator* (picro-Mallory; p. 118)

METHOD

1. Sections to water.
2. Weigert's haematoxylin 15–20 minutes.
3. Running tap water 5 minutes.
4. Acid alcohol 5–10 seconds.
5. Running tap water 5–10 minutes.
6. Red mixture 5 minutes.
7. Rinse in weak acetic acid.
8. Blue mixture 3 minutes.
9. Rinse in weak acetic acid.
10. Red differentiator $\frac{1}{2}$–2 minutes (see Note).
11. Rinse in weak acetic acid.
12. Dehydrate rapidly, clear, and mount.

RESULTS

Acidophil granules: *red*.
Basophil granules: *blue*.
Chromophobe cells: *pale blue-grey*.
Nuclei: *dark grey*.
Red blood corpuscles: *orange-red*.

Note

Differentiation should be controlled microscopically and must continue until the acidophil cells are no longer purple but clear red.

Per-iodic acid Schiff and orange G

SCOPE

Suitable for paraffin sections after any routine fixing fluid.

REAGENTS

A-D. As for the per-iodic acid Schiff method (p. 142)

E. *Orange G mixture*

Orange G	2 g.
Phosphotungstic acid	5 g.
Distilled water	100 ml.

Mix well; allow to stand for 24 hours; filter before use.

METHOD

1-11. As in the per-iodic acid Schiff method (p. 142).
12. Orange G 10–20 seconds.
13. Differentiate in running tap water, using microscopical control, until the acidophil cells stand out clearly (15–45 seconds).
14. Dehydrate, clear, and mount.

RESULTS

Basophil granules and granules in some chromophobe cells: *magenta*.
Acidophil granules: *orange*.
Other chromophobe cells: *unstained*.
Nuclei: *dark grey*.
Red blood corpuscles: *yellow*.

Slidders's method

SCOPE

Suitable for paraffin sections (preferably 2–3 μ thick). May be used after any routine fixing fluid.

REAGENTS

A. *Bromine water*

10% aqueous hydrobromic acid	45 ml.
2·5% aqueous potassium permanganate	5 ml.

Mix immediately before use.

B. *Alcian blue mixture*

Alcian blue 8GX	0·1	g.
Concentrated sulphuric acid	1	ml.
Glacial acetic acid	9	ml.
Distilled water	90	ml.

Mix the dye and the sulphuric acid with a glass rod. Cautiously add the acetic acid and mix thoroughly. Add the distilled water; mix; filter before use. This mixture keeps well.

C. *Weigert's haematoxylin (p. 104)*

D. *1 per cent hydrochloric acid in 70 per cent alcohol*

E. *Orange G. mixture*

Orange G	0·5	g.
Phosphotungstic acid	2	g.
Alcohol	95	ml.
Distilled water	5	ml.

Heat the mixture in a water bath; cool; filter before use. This mixture keeps well.

F. *Fuchsin mixture*

Acid fuchsin	0·5	g.
Glacial acetic acid	0·5	ml.
Distilled water	99·5	ml.

This mixture keeps well.

G. *1 per cent aqueous phosphotungstic acid*

H. *Light green mixture*

Light green	1·5 g.
Glacial acetic acid	1·5 ml.
Distilled water	98·5 ml.

This mixture keeps well.

METHOD

1. Sections to water.
2. Rinse in distilled water.
3. Bromine water 5 minutes.
4. Running tap water 2–3 minutes.
5. Rinse in distilled water.
6. Alcian blue ½–1 hour.
7. Running tap water 5 minutes.
8. Weigert's haematoxylin 15–20 minutes.
9. Running tap water 5 minutes.
10. Acid alcohol 5–10 seconds.
11. Running tap water 5–10 minutes.
12. Rinse in alcohol.
13. Orange G 2 minutes.
14. Rinse in distilled water.
15. Fuchsin 2–5 minutes (see Note i).
16. Rinse in distilled water.
17. Phosphotungstic acid 5 minutes.
18. Rinse in distilled water.
19. Light green 1–2 minutes.
20. Rinse in distilled water.
21. Dehydrate, clear, and mount.

RESULTS

S granules of basophil cells: *dark green-blue* $\Big\}$ (see Note ii).
R granules of basophil cells: *magenta red*
Acidophil granules: *orange-yellow.*
Chromophobe cells: *pale grey-green.*
Nuclei: *dark grey.*
Red blood corpuscles: *yellow.*
Connective tissue: *pale green.*

Notes

(i) The acid fuchsin is used as a progressive stain which should be controlled microscopically until the R basophil cells are strongly coloured. If prolonged, the acid fuchsin will stain other structures.

(ii) The division of basophil cells into R and S types is based on their susceptibility to oxidation. These letters were first used by Adams and Swettenham (1958), who used performic acid as the oxidizing agent. They demonstrated that the substance affected by the oxidizing agent (and therefore stained by alcian blue) was a protein rich in cystine. This amino-acid contains sulphur, so that the letter S (for sulphur) was used. Those basophil cells not affected by the oxidizing agent are stained red by the fuchsin. Because of their resistance to oxidation, these cells were called R (for resistant).

Slidders (1961) used bromine water instead of performic acid, in order to cause less damage to the tissue as a whole. He also modified the alcian blue mixture. The method we have quoted is virtually identical with that of Slidders.

Not unexpectedly, the method demonstrates a few other miscellaneous structures, including mast cell granules, keratin, and the neurosecretory substance of the posterior lobe of the pituitary.

Pancreatic islets

Special stains are unlikely to be needed for the exocrine part of the pancreas, although the zymogen granules are well shown by the per-iodic acid Schiff method, and the ducts are lined by an epithelium that is positive to alcian blue.

Methods are, however, occasionally needed for the endocrine cells of the pancreas. These cells are found in the islets of Langerhans, and are of at least two kinds. Beta cells are the most numerous; they are responsible for insulin secretion and are found in insulin-secreting tumours. The remaining cells of the islets have been divided into two types; alpha and delta, although it is possible that the delta cells are no more than immature alpha or beta cells. Islet cell tumours associated with recurrent peptic ulcers are usually of non-beta cell type. For an account of islet cells and tumours, see Evans (1966); for techniques see Pearse (1968).

The important distinction to be made histologically is between beta cells and non-beta cells, and in practice the simple and reliable staining methods are those for beta cells. We have had good results with aldehyde fuchsin and with phloxine tartrazine, both of which demonstrate beta cells specifically.

If a specific method for alpha cells is required, the Gros modification of Bielchowsky's method (p. 237) should be used.

Aldehyde fuchsin

SCOPE

Suitable for paraffin sections after routine fixing fluids except
those containing chrome. Has many uses other than pancreatic
islet cells (see Results). The original method (Gomori, 1950)
was modified by Scott (1952); we have preferred this modification.

REAGENTS

A. *Acidified permanganate*

    1% aqueous potassium permanganate   50 ml.
    Distilled water   50 ml.
    Concentrated sulphuric acid   0·5 ml.

B. *2 per cent aqueous sodium metabisulphite*

C. *Gomori's aldehyde fuchsin*

    Basic fuchsin (see Note i)   1 g.
    70% alcohol   200 ml.
    Concentrated hydrochloric acid 2 ml.
    Paraldehyde (see Note ii)   2 ml.

Dissolve the fuchsin in the alcohol, then add the acid and
paraldehyde. Leave at room temperature for 48–72 hours,
mixing occasionally. During this time the solution becomes
deep purple. Store at 4°C. The solution will keep for 2–3
months.

D. *Löffler's methylene blue*

    1% alcoholic solution of methylene blue 30 ml.
    1% aqueous potassium hydroxide   1 ml.
    Distilled water   90 ml.

This solution keeps well.

METHOD

1. Sections to water.
2. Permanganate 2 minutes.
3. Rinse in distilled water.

4. Sodium metabisulphite until decolorized (1–2 minutes).
5. Running tap water 2 minutes.
6. Rinse in alcohol.
7. Aldehyde fuchsin 2 minutes in a closed vessel.
8. Rinse well three times with 95% alcohol.
9. Wash well in running tap water.
10. Löffler's methylene blue diluted with 9 volumes of distilled water 30–40 seconds.
11. Rinse in tap water.
12. Dehydrate, clear, and mount.

RESULTS

Pancreatic beta cells; pituitary basophil cells; lipofuscin; elastic fibres; sulphated mucopolysaccharides (e.g. mast cells): *purple*.
Other structures: *colourless to pale blue*.

Notes

(i) Not every sample of basic fuchsin is satisfactory for this method. Suitable dye is often designated by the suppliers 'for Feulgen' or 'for Schiff'.

(ii) The paraldehyde must be fresh.

(iii) Other counterstains may be used. Possibilities include orange G (with or without haematoxylin), phloxine followed by light green, trichrome stains, and light green. Halmi (1952), used a special counterstain to demonstrate alpha and delta cells as well as beta cells. This counterstain contains light green 0·2 g.; orange G 1·0 g.; phosphotungstic acid 0·5 g.; glacial acetic acid 1·0 ml.; and distilled water 100 ml. It keeps well. Halmi's method follows the method given above as far as stage 9, but then continues as follows:

10. Weigert's haematoxylin (p. 104) 15–20 minutes.
11. Running tap water 5 minutes.
12. 1% hydrochloric acid in 70% alcohol 5–10 seconds.
13. Running tap water 10 minutes.
14. Rinse in distilled water.
15. Counterstain (as above) 45 seconds.
16. Briefly rinse in 0·2% aqueous acetic acid.
17. Dehydrate, clear, and mount.

Beta cells and other structures stain with the aldehyde fuchsin as before. Alpha cells are *yellow*, delta cells *green*, nuclei *grey*, and collagen *green*.

(iv) For combined staining with aldehyde fuchsin and alcian blue, use alcian blue after stage 9 of this method (see p. 146).

Phloxine tartrazine

SCOPE

Suitable for paraffin sections which should not be thicker than 5μ. Any routine fixing fluid may be used; mercuric-chloride-formalin is particularly suitable. This is very slightly modified from the second published method of Lendrum (1947b) and has several uses (see Results).

REAGENTS

A. *Carazzi's haematoxylin* (p. 106)

B. *1 per cent hydrochloric acid in 70 per cent alcohol*

C. *Phloxine solution*

Phloxine	0·5 g.
Calcium chloride (anhydrous)	0·5 g.
Distilled water	100 ml.

This solution keeps well.

D. *Saturated solution of tartrazine in cellosolve (0·3 per cent)*

METHOD

1. Sections to water.
2. Carazzi's haematoxylin 10 minutes.
3. Running tap water 5 minutes.
4. Acid alcohol 5–10 seconds.
5. Running tap water 5–10 minutes.
6. Phloxine 30 minutes.
7. Rinse in tap water.
8. Rinse in alcohol.
9. Tartrazine until only the red blood corpuscles and pancreatic beta cells remain red (5–15 minutes; see Note i).
10. Rinse in alcohol, clear, and mount.

RESULTS (see Note i)

Pancreatic beta cells; red blood corpuscles; keratin; Paneth cell granules; Russell bodies; fibrin; certain viral inclusion bodies: *red*.

Nuclei: *greyish blue*.

Other structures: *yellow*.

Notes

(i) The tartrazine cellosolve mixture acts both as differentiator and counterstain. The results will depend on the degree of differentiation. Phloxine is readily removed from ordinary cytoplasm and collagen. As differentiation continues, it is removed in turn from muscle, pancreatic beta cells, red blood corpuscles, keratin, fibrin, Paneth cells, and Russell bodies. When phloxine has been removed from all these structures, it will still be present in certain inclusion bodies. Since the results can be varied by altering the time of differentiation, careful microscopical control is necessary.

(ii) Good results are obtained when this method is used after alcian blue (see Note i, p. 146). This combination is suitable for demonstrating Paneth cells in the intestine or inhaled squames in necropsy specimens of lung from stillborn or newborn infants.

(iii) When the method is used for inclusion bodies, sharper nuclear staining may be obtained by using Weigert's haematoxylin which is differentiated in weak (0·2 per cent) aqueous nitric acid.

CHAPTER 16

Silver Impregnations

Theoretical considerations. Practical precautions. Preparation of silver solutions. von Kóssa for calcium salts. Masson-Fontana for melanin and argentaffin pigments. Reticulin: Caldwell and Rannie; James. Gomori for urates. Per-iodic acid silver for basement membranes. Grocott for fungi. Levaditi (Dobell) for spirochaetes; Faine for spirochaetes.

Theoretical considerations

Silver impregnation techniques depend on the chemical reduction of a silver salt so that a deposit of metallic silver is formed. This silver deposit is recognizable in the section as a dark grey or black area. Like any other histological method, silver impregnation is only satisfactory when it is consistent in demonstrating a specific tissue component whilst leaving all other components unaffected. Silver impregnation methods need to be carried out with even more precision than most histological staining methods because a relatively slight alteration in technique may cause the deposit of silver to form on an entirely different tissue component. So long as this tendency can be strictly controlled, it is valuable, and any one of a large number of structures can be demonstrated when a suitable method is chosen and is used with care and judgement. But, on the other hand, any deviation from the correct technique or any carelessness in the preparation or use of reagents is likely to result in unwanted deposits of silver on the wrong tissue components.

In chemical terms, silver impregnation methods may be divided into three kinds. First, the silver salt may react with a tissue component to produce an insoluble silver salt. This can then be reduced to metallic silver. The example of this type of reaction is the von Kóssa method in which silver carbonate and silver phosphate (and occasionally silver urate) are formed. These are then reduced to metallic silver by strong light.

Secondly, the silver salt will be reduced if the tissue contains substances with strong reducing properties. These substances may be present naturally in the tissue, or may have been produced by chemical treatment before the silver salt is applied. Biological substances that have these reducing properties are usually phenolic in character; they include melanin, and the granules in the Kultschitzky cells of the intestinal mucosa and carcinoid tumours. Demonstration of such substances by silver impregnation is often referred to as the *argentaffin reaction*. The practical example of this reaction is the Masson-Fontana method. Preliminary treatment of sections with chromic acid or periodic acid will convert the hydroxyl groups of polysaccharides to aldehyde groups. These aldehyde groups have strong reducing properties and may therefore be demonstrated by a silver impregnation method. Chromic acid is used for this purpose in Grocott's silver method; per-iodic acid is used in the per-iodic acid silver method of Jones which has obvious analogies with the per-iodic acid Schiff reaction.

Thirdly, a deposit of metallic silver may be formed with the help of an added reducing agent. The reducing agent in most methods of this type is formalin, occasionally it is hydroquinone or pyrogallic acid. If the reducing agent merely caused the deposition of metallic silver all over the section, no useful result would be obtained. In practice, however, the silver is deposited on a particular component of the section. The exact component varies from one method to another so that silver impregnation techniques are available for each of the following: reticulin fibres, neurofibrils and axons, glial cells and fibres, and spirochaetes. These tissue components are sometimes described as argyrophil, and this third type of silver impregnation method may be known as the *argyrophil reaction*. The reaction is thought to take place in two stages. To begin with, minute quantities of metallic silver are deposited on a particular structure in the section before any reducing agent has been added. These minute quantities, which are often referred to as 'nuclei', are too small to be detected, even with a high-power microscope. The exact site of deposition of silver nuclei probably depends on the distribution of sulphydryl groups in the tissue. When the reducing agent is added, more metallic silver is formed; this is deposited preferentially upon the existing nuclei, which therefore grow larger and become sufficiently conspicuous to be seen easily with the microscope. Some methods of this type are used solely for the brain, spinal cord, or nerves; practical details of these methods can be found in Chapter 17 which deals with techniques for the nervous system.

Silver impregnation methods are used progressively rather than regressively, although occasionally potassium ferricyanide may be used to remove some of the metallic silver when an excessive amount has been deposited. It is, however, a necessary stage in all silver methods to remove every trace of soluble silver salt from the section after enough deposit has formed. This is done by using sodium thiosulphate and is exactly analogous to the photographic process known as 'fixing'. The process is also referred to as fixing in some histological methods but, for obvious reasons, it is necessary to use the word with care if ambiguity is to be avoided.

When the silver impregnation is complete, there are two additional procedures that may be worth while. The first of these is treatment with a solution of gold chloride. This is known as gold toning and has the effect of removing some of the background discoloration as well as changing the colour of the impregnation from brownish-black to purple-black when metallic gold is deposited in place of the silver. The second optional addition to silver impregnation methods is the use of a counterstain; neutral red is often used; other possibilities include light green, haematoxylin and eosin, and stains of the van Gieson type.

Practical precautions

It will be appreciated that silver impregnation methods require considerable care if good results are to be obtained. They allow far less latitude than the majority of histological methods, in which it is often unnecessary to adhere strictly to the recommended time, temperature, and concentration of solutions. Since silver impregnation methods depend on the deposition of metallic silver, a solution of silver salt is chosen that will readily yield a precipitate. If care is not taken, this precipitate will be deposited on surfaces other than those of the tissue component to be demonstrated. For this reason it is essential to aim at absolute purity and scrupulous cleanliness of all the reagents and glassware that are used. Glass-distilled water must be used at all stages until the excess silver solution has been removed by sodium thiosulphate. The slides should be carefully washed before and after they are treated with silver solution, and this must include the back of the slide as well as the front if contamination is to be avoided. After the first wash, the slide should be handled only by the end that will not be immersed in reagents. Glassware should be thoroughly rinsed several times in glass-distilled water after it has been cleaned by ordinary washing. Less silver will be deposited on the inside of glass vessels if they have been coated with a thin layer of paraffin wax. It is often stated that glassware gives better results when it has previously been used for silver impregnation methods, and has thus become coated with a silver deposit. However, so long as it is completely clean, glass that has not previously been used will give good results. Filter paper is another possible source of impurity since it becomes contaminated by the fingers when it is folded. This can be avoided if a pair of papers are folded together and the outer one (which has been handled) is discarded. It should be obvious that silver impregnation methods need to be carried out in a clean atmosphere; formalin fumes in particular will have disastrous effects.

In some methods, a similar degree of care is needed in timing some of the steps. This is particularly true of gold toning, but applies also to silver impregnation in many of the methods for demonstrating reticulin or axons. When a method calls for a short treatment with the silver salt, this time is usually critical; when the section spends some hours in the silver solution, the time is not usually so important.

When sections are treated for a short and critical time in any reagent, it is obviously essential to ensure proper agitation if a uniform result is to be obtained. This applies especially to silver salts and to the reducing agent when the method includes one.

In a few methods, the section is treated with a warm silver solution. In these methods the temperature is important, and the silver solution must be raised to the correct temperature before the section is placed in it.

No account of practical precautions in the use of silver solutions would be complete without a mention of the hazards involved. Silver nitrate is corrosive, so that both the solid substance and solutions must be handled with care and kept away from clothes and skin. Silver solutions, especially those prepared for impregnation methods, will also produce black discoloration of skin and garments. This may be removed with difficulty from the skin by Lugol's iodine followed by sodium thiosulphate; clothes, however, are likely to be discoloured or bleached by this treatment even if they have not already been rotted by the silver solution.

Another rare but important hazard is explosion. This occurs only with ammoniacal silver solutions that have been kept for many hours or days. It seems to be more likely to occur when the solution is open to the atmosphere and has stood in sunlight (Stewart Smith, 1943; Wallington, 1965). Unwanted ammoniacal silver solutions may be rendered safe by adding an excess of hydrochloric acid or sodium chloride which produce a precipitate of inert silver chloride. If ammoniacal silver solutions are stored, plastic vessels should be used, or glass vessels that have been protected by binding with an abundance of adhesive plaster. Solutions must be kept away from sunlight.

Preparation of silver solutions

Although there are a great variety of silver methods, they almost all make use of one or other of three basic types of silver solution. In the first, ammonia is added to silver nitrate to produce a precipitate of silver hydroxide; this hydroxide is then redissolved by the use of more ammonia. The second type is very similar except that the silver hydroxide precipitate is produced by a different alkali (usually sodium hydroxide); the precipitate is, however, redissolved by ammonia as in the first type. The third type is quite different, making use of hexamine (methenamine) without the addition of any ammonia.

Of these, the first type is the most tedious and requires the greatest judgement. Strong ammonia (0·880) is added drop by drop from a fine Pasteur pipette. It is essential to shake the solution between each drop and to ensure that none of the ammonia falls on the neck of the vessel out of reach of the silver solution. As the ammonia is added, a thick white precipitate forms; beyond a certain point this begins to clear, and at this stage shaking must be particularly thorough. The end point is reached when only a faint milky opalescence persists and the solution smells only weakly of ammonia. Any solution that smells strongly of ammonia is unlikely to be satisfactory.

The second type is simpler in that a measured amount of

P

alkali is added and mixed well to produce a similar precipitate. This is then redissolved by ammonia, which must be added carefully drop by drop with vigorous shaking until the end point described above is reached.

Hexamine silver solutions are simple to prepare. A measured volume of hexamine solution is added to the silver nitrate solution. This yields a white precipitate which redissolves spontaneously when the mixture is shaken well.

Individual methods

The total number of individual silver impregnation techniques and modifications is very large. The following selection has been made to satisfy every likely requirement except for special techniques for the nervous system (Chap. 17).

von Kóssa for calcium salts

Although widely regarded as suitable for the demonstration of calcium, this method in reality demonstrates insoluble phosphates, carbonates, oxalates and urates. For precise histochemical staining of calcium, chloranilic acid (p. 123) should be used. In animal tissues, insoluble phosphates, carbonates and oxalates are virtually always salts of calcium, so that in practice the von Kóssa method is fairly reliable for the demonstration of calcium. Urates, however, may occur in the tissues as insoluble sodium salts, and these also will be positive (see Note iii). The following method, like all those in current use, is an expansion of the original description (von Kóssa, 1901), in which technical details were brief.

REAGENTS

A. *5 per cent silver nitrate* (the concentration need not be exact)
B. *3 per cent aqueous sodium thiosulphate* (the concentration need not be exact)
C. *1 per cent aqueous neutral red* (or other counterstain)

METHOD

1. Sections to water.
2. Wash well in distilled water.
3. Treat with silver nitrate solution in bright light 20–30 minutes (see Note ii).

4. Wash well in distilled water.
5. Sodium thiosulphate 5 minutes.
6. Wash well in running tap water.
7. Neutral red 1 minute.
8. Rinse in tap water.
9. Dehydrate, clear, and mount.

RESULTS

Insoluble calcium salts (also urates): *brown to black*.
Other structures: *shades of pink*.

Notes

(i) The method works after any fixing fluid. However, when the amount of calcium salt in the tissue is small, acid fluids should be avoided because they have a decalcifying action.

(ii) So long as the light is bright, its origin is unimportant. Although bright sunlight or ultra-violet light are often specified, good results are obtained by using an ordinary tungsten filament lamp bulb.

It is, however, important to avoid silver precipitate, which will fall onto the section if the slide is merely flooded with silver nitrate and exposed to light. A glass Coplin jar may be used; better still the slide may be inverted on supports in a Petri dish containing the silver nitrate.

(iii) As already stated, urates will also give positive results which may cause confusion. Urates are readily soluble in alkali and may be removed by treatment for 20 minutes in saturated aqueous lithium carbonate after stage 1 above. The section is then washed well in running tap water before proceeding to stage 2. For the more precise demonstration of urates, see Gomori's hexamine silver method below.

Masson-Fontana for melanin and argentaffin pigments

Masson (1914) demonstrated argentaffin cells and carcinoid tumours of the intestine by using the silver solution of Fontana (1912). The method is more often used for demonstrating melanin.

REAGENTS

A. *Fontana's silver solution*

To 20 ml. of 10 per cent aqueous silver nitrate, add strong (0·880) ammonia until the precipitate dissolves (p. 209).
Add 20 ml. of distilled water and filter before use.

B. *3 per cent aqueous sodium thiosulphate* (the concentration need not be exact)

C. *1 per cent aqueous neutral red* (or other counterstain)

METHOD

1. Sections to water.
2. Wash well in several changes of distilled water for 1 hour.
3. Fontana's silver solution in the dark overnight (see Note ii).
4. Wash well in distilled water.
5. Sodium thiosulphate 5 minutes.
6. Wash well in running tap water.
7. Neutral red 1 minute.
8. Rinse in tap water.
9. Dehydrate, clear, and mount.

RESULTS

Melanin; argentaffin pigment: *black*.

(Lipofuscin and chromaffin pigment are sometimes blackened—see Note iii.)

Other structures: *shades of pink*.

Notes

(i) The method will not work after fixing fluids that contain dichromate. For melanin, any of the other standard fixing fluids gives good results. For argentaffin pigment, fixation in formalin is essential, preferably in a simple formalin-saline mixture.

(ii) For the demonstration of melanin in routine paraffin sections, the silver solution is allowed to act overnight. Argentaffin pigment in paraffin sections is usually demonstrated in an equal time but may take longer; sections should be treated for at least 36 hours before it is decided that a pigment is not argentaffin. For some reason the method is quicker when cryostat sections of fixed tissue are used, 3 hours being long enough for melanin. With frozen sections that are handled loose, the method is quicker still, needing only one hour for melanin.

(iii) Lipofuscin behaves inconstantly in this method, being unaffected in some specimens and blackened in others. Chromaffin pigment is unlikely to survive the type of fixation required by this method. When it does, it will be shown greyish-black.

(iv) An alternative method for melanin and argentaffin pigment is Schmorl's ferricyanide reaction (p. 133). Melanin may also be identified by bleaching reactions (p. 139).

Reticulin

All the silver impregnation methods for reticulin show a basic similarity. Established favourites include the methods of Foot (1924), Gordon and Sweets (1936), and Gomori (1937), all of which yield good results in practised hands. The two methods given below are somewhat more straightforward; the first has given us good results for many years. The second is even simpler; it has not been in use for long, but our experience with it so far has been entirely favourable.

Caldwell and Rannie for reticulin

This method, published by Lendrum (1947a), is consistent in use. Sections are not likely to become detached during treatment. Subsequent counterstaining is easy.

REAGENTS

A. *0·25 per cent potassium permanganate in 0·3 per cent sulphuric acid*

B. *1 per cent aqueous oxalic acid*

C. *2·5 per cent aqueous iron alum (ferric ammonium sulphate)* dissolved without heat

D. *Ammoniacal silver solution*
To 10 ml. of 20% aqueous silver nitrate, add 0·4 ml. of 40% aqueous sodium hydroxide; then add strong (0·880) ammonia until the precipitate dissolves (see p. 209). Make up to 50 ml. with distilled water. Filter. Results are better if the solution is stored overnight before use.

E. *10 per cent aqueous formalin*

F. *0·2 per cent aqueous gold chloride*

G. *5 per cent aqueous sodium thiosulphate*

H. *1 per cent aqueous neutral red* (or other counterstain)

METHOD

1. Sections to water.
2. Acidified permanganate 10 minutes.
3. Oxalic acid 5 minutes.

4. Wash in distilled water.
5. Iron alum 20 minutes (see Note ii).
6. Wash in running tap water 10 minutes (see Note iii).
7. Wash well in distilled water.
8. Ammoniacal silver 3 to 60 seconds (see Note iv).
9. Wash well in distilled water.
10. Formalin solution 1 minute.
11. Wash in tap water.
12. Gold chloride 2 minutes.
13. Wash in tap water.
14. Sodium thiosulphate 3 minutes.
15. Running tap water 5 minutes.
16. Neutral red 1 minute.
17. Rinse in tap water.
18. Dehydrate, clear, and mount.

RESULTS

Reticulin fibres: *black*.
Other structures: *shades of pink*.

Notes

(i) Fixation in formalin-saline solutions gives the best results but the method will work after any of the standard fixing fluids.

(ii) The time in iron alum may be lengthened to as much as 24 hours without ill effects.

(iii) After iron alum, the wash in running tap water must be thorough, otherwise silver will be precipitated at random. On the other hand, too long a wash will reduce the intensity of the reticulin impregnation.

(iv) Within 24 hours of preparation, the ammoniacal silver gives results in about 3 seconds. As the solution ages, the time must be increased.

(v) Gold toning (stages 12 and 13) may be omitted; the collagen will then appear brownish-yellow.

James's method for reticulin

This method gives attractive and consistent results. The times are easily memorized. Sections are less likely to detach during treatment than is the case with most reticulin methods (James, 1967).

REAGENTS

A. *Acidified permanganate*
    0·3% aqueous potassium permanganate
    0·3% sulphuric acid

Mix equal parts immediately before use.

B. *5 per cent aqueous oxalic acid*

C. *5 per cent aqueous silver nitrate*

D. *Ammoniacal silver solution*
    To 20 ml. of 10 per cent aqueous silver nitrate, add strong (0·880) ammonia until the precipitate dissolves (see p. 209). Add one drop of 10 per cent aqueous silver nitrate and 20 ml. of distilled water. Filter; the solution is ready for use; store in the dark.

E. *5 per cent aqueous formalin*

F. *5 per cent aqueous sodium thiosulphate*

METHOD
    1. Sections to water.
    2. Acidified permanganate 5 minutes.
    3. Rinse three times in distilled water.
    4. Oxalic acid 5 minutes.
    5. Rinse three times in distilled water.
    6. Silver nitrate 5 minutes.
    7. Rinse three times in distilled water.
    8. Ammoniacal silver 5 minutes.
    9. Rinse three times in distilled water.
    10. Formalin solution 5 minutes.
    11. Rinse three times in distilled water.
    12. Sodium thiosulphate 5 minutes.
    13. Wash well in running tap water.
    14. Dehydrate, clear, and mount.

RESULTS
    Reticulin fibres: *black*.
    Collagen: *yellow to brown*.

Notes

(i) Fixation in formalin-saline solutions gives good results. Our experience with other fixing fluids is limited, but the method is satisfactory after Heidenhain's Susa.

(ii) The method does not include gold toning. If this is preferred it should be introduced between stages 11 and 12, using 0·2 per cent aqueous gold chloride solution for 2 minutes, followed by a thorough wash in running tap water.

(iii) The method does not include a counterstain. If one is required, it will work better when the sections have been toned with gold chloride.

Gomori's method for urates

A simple method for uric acid and urates (Gomori, 1951). Tissue must be fixed suitably.

REAGENTS

A. *Gomori's silver-methenamine solution* (*stock solution*)

To 100 ml. of 3 per cent aqueous hexamethylenetetramine (sold as 'methenamine' or 'hexamine'), add 5 ml. of 5 per cent aqueous silver nitrate solution. Shake immediately and continue shaking until the white precipitate redissolves. Store in a refrigerator at 4°C. The solution will keep for months.

B. *Stock buffer solution*

Boric acid	1·6 g.
Sodium tetraborate (borax)	1·3 g.
Distilled water to	200 ml.

Store in a refrigerator at 4°C.

C. *Working solution*

Gomori's stock solution	25 ml.
Stock buffer solution	5 ml.
Distilled water	20 ml.

This solution should be freshly prepared.

D. *2 per cent aqueous sodium thiosulphate*

METHOD

1. Xylene (to remove wax) 2 minutes.
2. Alcohol 2 minutes.

3. Working solution of buffered silver 1–2 hours at 45°C in the dark (see Note ii).
4. Rinse in distilled water.
5. Sodium thiosulphate 1 minute.
6. Running tap water 5 minutes.
7. Dehydrate, clear, and mount.

RESULTS

Uric acid and urates: *black*.
(Melanin and some calcium salts—see Note iii): *black*.

Notes

(i) Uric acid and urates are soluble in aqueous fluids. Alcohol is the fixative of choice.

(ii) The silver solution will not give satisfactory results unless it is warmed to 45°C. When the solution is used in a heavy glass Coplin jar, it will need longer than two hours in the incubator before the section is placed in it. A water-bath is quicker.

(iii) Small amounts of calcium salts are unlikely to give false positive results because they are dissolved by the silver solution. If an additional precaution is required, the section should be treated with 0·5 per cent alcoholic hydrochloric acid for two minutes to remove all traces of calcium salts before treatment with the silver solution.

(iv) Sections may be counterstained if this is required.

(v) The silver-methenamine (or hexamine-silver) reagent used in this method, and also in the next two to be described, was first published by Gomori (1946) when he used it to demonstrate polysaccharides.

Per-iodic acid silver method

A method for basement membranes, particularly suitable for those of glomerular capillaries in the kidney (Jones, 1957). Sections must be thin.

REAGENTS

A. *0·5 per cent aqueous per-iodic acid*

B. *Silver solution*

Gomori's silver-methenamine solution
(see 'A' in previous method)   50 ml.
5% borax (sodium tetraborate)   6 ml.

This solution should be freshly prepared.

C. *0·2 per cent aqueous gold chloride*

D. *3 per cent aqueous sodium thiosulphate*

METHOD

1. Sections to water.
2. Rinse in distilled water.
3. Per-iodic acid 15 minutes.
4. Wash well in distilled water.
5. Silver solution 1½–3 hours at 50°C in the dark (see Note iii).
6. Wash in distilled water.
7. Gold chloride 2 minutes.
8. Wash in distilled water.
9. Sodium thiosulphate 2 minutes.
10. Running tap water 5 minutes.
11. If required, counterstain with Harris's or Ehrlich's haematoxylin and eosin (see Note iv).
12. Dehydrate, clear, and mount.

RESULT

Basement membranes: *black*.

Notes

(i) Results are satisfactory after fixation in any of the following: formalin-saline, neutral buffered formalin solution, mercuric-chloride-formalin, Susa, Bouin's fluid, and Carnoy's fluid. Fluids that contain osmium tetroxide or a dichromate are unsuitable.

(ii) Thin sections (1–3 μ) must be used.

(iii) The silver solution will not give satisfactory results unless it is warmed to 50°C. When the solution is used in a heavy glass Coplin jar, it will need longer than two hours in the incubator before the section is placed in it. A water-bath is quicker.

After 1½ hours in the silver solution, the section should be rinsed in distilled water and inspected microscopically. If necessary, it is then rinsed again in distilled water and returned to the silver solution. This inspection should be repeated every half-hour until the result is satisfactory. After 3 hours, however, no further impregnation will occur, and the section should be removed.

(iv) Counterstaining with haematoxylin and eosin gives good results. Most other dyes are inhibited by the long treatment with silver solution.

Grocott's method for fungi

A specific method for fungi; particularly suitable for photography. May be used on sections or smears (Grocott, 1955).

REAGENTS

A. *5 per cent aqueous chromic acid* (chromium trioxide)

B. *1 per cent aqueous sodium bisulphite*

C. *Silver solution*

>
> | Gomori's silver-methenamine | |
> |---|---|
> | solution (see 'A' in Gomori's method | |
> | p. 216) | 25 ml. |
> | Distilled water | 25 ml. |
> | 5% aqueous sodium tetraborate (borax) | 2 ml. |

This solution should be freshly prepared.

D. *0·1 per cent aqueous gold chloride*

E. *2 per cent aqueous sodium thiosulphate*

METHOD

1. Sections to water.
2. Rinse in distilled water.
3. Chromic acid 1 hour.
4. Wash in tap water.
5. Sodium bisulphite 1 minute.
6. Running tap water 5 minutes.
7. Rinse three times in distilled water.
8. Silver solution 30 to 60 minutes at 50°C in the dark (see Note iii).
9. Rinse three times in distilled water.
10. Gold chloride 3 minutes.
11. Rinse in distilled water.
12. Sodium thiosulphate 2 minutes.
13. Running tap water 5 minutes.
14. Counterstain as required (see Note iv).
15. Dehydrate, clear, and mount.

RESULTS

Fungal cell walls: *black*.
Inner parts of fungi; some mucin: *dull purple-red*.

Notes

(i) Results are satisfactory when tissue has been fixed in fluids containing formalin or mercury, and when smears have been fixed in alcohol. We have not used the method after other fixing fluids.

(ii) The method gives good results with sections of the usual thickness (5 μ). For fine detail, thinner sections will be preferred.

(iii) The silver solution will not give satisfactory results unless it is warmed to 50°C. When the solution is used in a heavy glass Coplin jar, it will need longer than two hours in the incubator before the slide is placed in it. A water-bath is quicker.

(iv) Grocott suggested safranin or haematoxylin and eosin counterstains; we have usually used light green.

(v) This method is basically similar to that of Gridley (p. 179). Chromic acid acts on chitin to produce aldehyde groups which are then demonstrated by either Schiff's reagent (Gridley) or methenamine-silver (Grocott).

Levaditi's method for spirochaetes (Dobell's modification)

In this method a piece of tissue is treated before it is embedded in wax. The method is equally suitable for treponema and leptospira. It is particularly useful when a large number of sections is required (e.g. for class use). If paraffin blocks or unstained paraffin sections are the only material available, the method of Faine should be used (see below).

REAGENTS

A. *0·2–0·5 per cent aqueous silver nitrate*

B. *0·5–1·0 per cent hydroquinone in 50 per cent alcohol*

METHOD

1. Thin pieces (1–2 mm.) of thoroughly fixed tissue must be used. The only reliable fixing fluids are formalin-saline and neutral buffered formalin solution.
2. Undiluted alcohol 24 hours.
3. 90% alcohol 24 hours.
4. 70% alcohol 24 hours.
5. 50% alcohol 24 hours.
6. Distilled water 24 hours (change several times).
7. Silver nitrate 24 hours at 37°C in the dark.
8. Distilled water 12–18 hours (change several times).
9. Alcoholic hydroquinone 12–24 hours.

10. Process the tissue by a routine paraffin method.
11. Cut sections at the usual thickness, mount them on slides, remove wax, mount in a resinous medium. A counterstain is not necessary.

RESULTS

Spirochaetes (treponema and leptospira): *black*.
(Other bacteria and fungi may also be demonstrated.)
Other structures: *pale yellow to light brown*.

Notes

(i) Attempts to hasten the method will result in non-specific deposition of silver if any trace of formalin or alcohol persists when the tissue is treated with silver nitrate.

(ii) This differs from the original method (Levaditi, 1905) in which the silver nitrate was reduced by a mixture of pyrogallic acid and formalin. There are many other minor differences. We have not been able to discover whether this modification was ever published by Dobell. It may well have been an unpublished personal communication to Carleton, who included it in the second edition of his book (Carleton and Leach, 1938).

Faine's method for spirochaetes

The advantage of this method (Faine, 1965) is that ordinary paraffin sections are used. The tissue requires no preliminary treatment before sections are cut. If pieces of tissue are available, and time permits, the Levaditi method is easier, especially when a large number of sections is required.

REAGENTS

A. *Stock solution of acetic acid M/5*

B. *Stock solution of sodium acetate M/5*

C. *Working solution of acetate buffer pH 3·6, M/125*

Acetic acid M/5	18·5 ml.
Sodium acetate M/5	1·5 ml.
Deionized or double-glass-distilled water	480 ml.

D. *Working silver solution*
   1 per cent solution of silver nitrate in acetate buffer C.
   The pH must be adjusted to 3·6 at 56°C (see Note iii).

E. *Stock solution of 2 per cent silver nitrate in acetate buffer C*
   The pH must be adjusted to 3·6 at 37°C (see Note iii).

F. *Stock solution of 5 per cent gelatin (see Note ii) in acetate buffer C*
   Dissolve at 56°C. Cool to 37°C and adjust the pH at that temperature to 3·6 (see Note iii).

G. *Stock solution of 3 per cent hydroquinone in acetate buffer C*
   Keep in a cold room. This reagent must be used within 3 or 4 days of preparation.

H. *Developer (working solution)*

   Gelatin solution F at 37°C   60 ml.
   2% silver nitrate E at 37°C   12 ml.

   Add the silver nitrate with constant stirring. Keep in the dark. Immediately before use add:

   Hydroquinone solution G   4 ml.

J. *5 per cent aqueous solution of sodium thiosulphate*

METHOD
1. Sections to water.
2. Wash in acetate buffer C for 2 minutes.
3. Working silver solution D for 30 minutes at 56°C in the dark (see Notes iv and v).
4. Developer H for 10 minutes at 37°C in the dark (see Notes iv and v).
5. Wash twice with acetate buffer C at 37°C in the dark.
6. Sodium thiosulphate J for 5 minutes.
7. Running tap water.
8. Dehydrate, clear, and mount.

RESULTS
   Spirochaetes (treponema and leptospira): *black*.
   Other structures: *pale yellow to light brown*.

Notes

(i) The method is reliable after fixation in formalin-saline or neutral buffered formalin solution. Other fixing fluids give variable results.

(ii) The gelatin must be free from sulphite which is sometimes added as a preservative. Faine used gelatin no. 02-158 from Baltimore Biological Laboratory, Inc., 1640 Gorsuch Avenue, Baltimore, Maryland, USA. We have used Davis Gelatine (caterers' grade), obtained from Davis Gelatine, Ltd., Warwick, England with satisfactory results, although Faine found that 'Bacteriological Gelatine' from Davis Gelatine (Australia) Pty. Ltd., needed preliminary treatment to remove sulphite. This was done by adding 3 ml. of 100 vol. hydrogen peroxide to a solution of 5 g. gelatin in 92 ml. deionized water. The mixture was boiled for 5 minutes and cooled. Four ml. of strong (M/5) acetate buffer were then added to give a final concentration of M/125.

(iii) The pH is critical at stages 3 and 4 of the method. It is insufficient to add the correct amount of buffer: adjustments must be made when the solutions have reached their working temperatures.

(iv) The solutions must be at the correct temperatures before slides are placed in them. A water-bath is better than an incubator, but Coplin jars must be immersed in the bath up to their necks.

(v) A dark room is preferable, but satisfactory results can be obtained by placing the water-bath inside a large black plastic bag.

(vi) If the developer is too hot or sections are left in it too long, the results will be unsatisfactory because of non-specific deposition of silver. This can be removed by the cautious use of 1 per cent aqueous potassium ferricyanide.

CHAPTER 17

Techniques for the Nervous System

Structure of the nervous system. Fixation. Processing and section cutting. General notes on staining. Nissl methods. Methods for axons. Methods for normal myelin. The Marchi method for degenerating myelin. Methods for neuroglia. Brain smears.

HISTOLOGICAL methods for the nervous system employ the same principles as methods used for other tissues: they differ, however, in a multitude of details. The same basic techniques are used: specimens are fixed; tissue is processed so that sections can be cut from wax or nitrocellulose blocks; frozen sections are prepared; finally a variety of dyes and metallic impregnations are used for revealing histological structure. But the individual dyeing and metallic impregnation methods are often peculiar to the nervous system and of no use for sections of any other tissue. Some of these methods demand sections of a particular kind, such as frozen sections, or nitrocellulose sections, or sections from tissue fixed in a special fluid.

Structure of the nervous system

In order to appreciate why methods for the nervous system are different from those used for other tissues, it is necessary to have some knowledge of how the nervous system differs from other parts of the body.

The most important units in the nervous system are the nerve cells or neurones. Each neurone consists of a cell body and a number of fine filamentous processes. The nucleus is in the cell body, which often also contains conspicuous cytoplasmic granules of ribonucleic acid known as Nissl granules. In a typical neurone, one of the filamentous processes is comparatively long; this is known as the axon, the shorter processes being known as dendrites. By and large the nervous system is divided into regions where nerve cell bodies are numerous, and other regions that contains axons but no cell bodies. In the central nervous system (brain and spinal cord), the cell bodies are found in the grey matter, whereas the white matter contains abundant axons but no cell bodies. In the peripheral nervous system, the cell bodies are collected together in the ganglia; they are not found in the nerve trunks.

Most axons are myelinated. If the axon is thought of as an electric wire, the myelin can be regarded as its insulation. Myelin is a complex lipid; it is responsible for the whiteness of the white matter of the brain and spinal cord, and is also present around many of the axons in peripheral nerves.

Many ordinary techniques for staining nuclei and cytoplasm will show nerve cell bodies and Nissl granules. They will not, however, distinguish axons or myelin. Moreover, techniques for demonstrating axons are not suitable for myelin. Thus, the full examination of the normal nerve cell and its myelin sheath may call for three separate histological techniques applied to three separate sections. If the tissue is abnormal, the situation may become even more complicated, since degenerating myelin is demonstrated by techniques that are completely different from those used for normal myelin. Finally, it may be necessary to show evidence of complete myelin degeneration in the form of neutral lipids. Unlike normal or degenerating myelin, these lipids are stained by such dyes as Sudan III and IV.

In addition to neurones, the brain and spinal cord contain a number of supporting cells known as neuroglia or glia. These play no direct part in the transmission of nervous impulses: their functions are structural support, nutrition, and repair. Although analogous to the fibrocytes, fibroblasts, and histiocytes of the rest of the body, the neuroglial cells are quite different in appearance, and require special methods to demonstrate them histologically.

There are three distinct kinds of neuroglial cells: astrocytes, oligodendrocytes, and microglial cells. Each type has a cell body and a number of fine processes. In this they show a resemblance to neurones, but it must be emphasised that neuroglia and neurones are utterly different in function. Staining methods, likewise, are entirely different. It is, of course, true that any nuclear stain such as haematoxylin and eosin will reveal the nuclei of neuroglial cells as well as those of neurones; but the special histological techniques for axons or myelin will not show the processes of neuroglial cells. Conversely, techniques for neuroglial processes will not demonstrate axons, dendrites, or myelin.

Q

As an additional complication, each type of neuroglial cell needs a separate technique for its demonstration. These techniques are tedious and temperamental, and so it is fortunate that they are not very often needed in routine laboratories. The only common requirement is a stain for the processes of astrocytes when these have formed a dense tangled mat in response to brain damage. Luckily these tangles of processes can be stained by phosphotungstic acid haematoxylin, although that method does not show the bodies of the cells; nor will it stain the astrocyte processes in normal brain.

The nervous system contains neurones, myelin, and neuroglia, whereas other organs of the body do not. On the other hand, there are some structures in the nervous system that are similar to those found elsewhere in the body. The blood-vessels in the nervous system are just like those encountered elsewhere; collagen is present in the meninges and in the connective tissue of peripheral nerves. Micro-organisms, pigments, and deposits of tumour in the nervous system are similar to those in other organs. Thus, the great majority of staining methods that are used for other organs will occasionally be needed for sections from the nervous system.

Fixation

Although the principles of fixation, as applied to the brain, are exactly the same as those for any other tissue, two points require emphasis. First, the brain and spinal cord are so delicate that it is impossible to examine them unfixed without damaging their structure, especially if the tissue has been further softened by an infarct or tumour. Therefore, since it is often necessary to fix large pieces or whole brains, a fluid must be chosen that penetrates well without overfixing the outer layers; in practice the only suitable fixing fluid is a formalin solution. Secondly, some histological methods for the nervous system were originally designed for use after a special fixing fluid. Some of these methods have been modified, so that they can be used after conventional fluids. In Weigert's original myelin method, for instance, tissue was fixed in a fluid containing dichromate; modifications in current use incorporate a dichromate solution as a separate stage after the tissue has been fixed in a formalin mixture. Nevertheless, special fixing fluids are still essential for a few methods, notably those of Cajal and Rio-Hortega for the demonstration of glial cells. For these methods, formalin-ammonium-bromide (Cajal, 1916) must be used.

Formalin-ammonium-bromide (FAB)

Formalin	15 ml.
Ammonium bromide	2 g.
Distilled water	85 ml.

For almost every other purpose, brains may be fixed in one of the formalin mixtures that is in general use. Formalin-saline (p. 15) and neutral buffered formalin solution (p. 17) are satisfactory; these fluids are even more effective when the concentration of formalin is increased to 15 per cent. For museum specimens Kaiserling I (p. 340) may be preferred.

When it is important to preserve Nissl substance, small pieces should be fixed in fairly strong alcohol (95 per cent) or in Carnoy's fluid (p. 20). For rapid diagnostic work it may be convenient to use Heidenhain's Susa (p. 18) or Bouin's fluid (p. 20) but these restrict the number of staining methods that can subsequently be used. As described later, alcohol is used for fixing brain smears.

Entire brains should be fixed as soon as possible after removal, before they lose their natural shape. They may be perfused, but more often they are suspended in a large volume of fixing fluid (about 10 litres). The basilar artery is a convenient point of suspension and is strong enough to support an adult brain in the fluid. The basilar artery of an infant's brain, however, is too delicate so that infants' brains cannot be suspended; they are instead laid in a suitably shaped nest of cotton-wool in a sufficient volume of fluid. After a week or two a brain may be cut into slices which will keep their shape, but fixation for three or four weeks is preferable. The process is hastened, to some extent, if the ventricles are drained and filled with fixing fluid. This is done after fixation has continued for about three days; the brain is removed from the fluid and slits are made in the corpus callosum. The brain is then tilted every way until the cerebro-spinal fluid has run out. Before it is resuspended, the brain is submerged and again tilted every way until the ventricles are filled with fixing fluid; very gentle pressure will assist in expelling the air bubbles.

If a brain needs to be cut before it has been fixed, the thick slices may be fixed in a fairly deep flat tray. The bottom of the tray is covered with a layer of cotton-wool, and this in turn is covered with lint to provide a flat surface. The lint should be placed with its fluffy side upwards, since the woven side will pattern the surface of the tissue, and may thus make it unsuitable for use as a museum specimen. The lint must be damped with fixing fluid before the slices are laid on it, otherwise fluff will adhere to the brain and may be difficult to remove later. When the slices have been arranged on the lint, the tray is filled with fixing fluid, care being taken not to pour the fluid directly onto the soft slices.

When blocks of tissue are taken from an entire brain or from a thick slice, it is wise to return these blocks to fixing fluid for a day or more (depending on thickness) before starting to dehydrate them.

Processing and section cutting

It is possible to apply some of the special neurological techniques to any type of section, but many of them demand sections of a particular kind. Thus, some require paraffin sections, others nitrocellulose sections, and others frozen sections. In some instances, frozen sections must be handled free and not attached to slides. Whichever type of section is used, the basic techniques for their preparation are just the same as those used for other tissues. The following notes refer only to the special problems presented by pieces of brain and spinal cord. For general information the relevant chapters should be consulted: routine processing (p. 26); wax embedding (p. 35); cutting ordinary wax sections (p. 61); wax sections from large pieces (p. 302); nitrocellulose techniques (p. 264); and frozen sections (p. 274).

Dehydration must be slow and thorough. Brain and spinal cord are dense tissues so that penetration is slow; on no account should dehydrating times be curtailed. It is better to use a large series of dehydrating alcohols of gradually increasing concentration; an abrupt change to concentrated alcohol will produce shrinkage and distortion.

Clearing, likewise, must be thorough. Some of the lipids in brain and spinal cord are removed by the clearing agent; if these persist in the tissue they will make it difficult to cut sections from the wax block. A gentle clearing agent should be used: rapidly acting ones (xylene; benzene; toluene) should be avoided, since these cause excessive shrinkage and distortion.

Wax impregnation must be performed without overheating the tissue, since heat is apt to give rise to fragmentation by a multitude of hair-line cracks. Cooling may also give rise to difficulties; pieces of brain in ordinary histological wax seem to be particularly susceptible to cracking when they are cooled. For this reason special waxes may be used with profit since these resist cracking when cooled with ice. Proprietary waxes such as Fibrowax are suitable, or ordinary histological paraffin wax may be modified by the addition of beeswax or dental impression wax. (p. 37)

Cutting wax sections calls for a very sharp, well-stropped knife, since any imperfection in the edge will leave a particularly conspicuous line across a section of brain or spinal cord. Sections should be cut as slowly as possible in order to avoid creases, since these are more difficult to remove from sections of brain than from sections of other tissues.

It is often desirable to have sections of two different thicknesses: some of about 5 μ for routine staining methods, and some thicker ones for Nissl or myelin stains. The thickness of the latter should not exceed 10–12 μ otherwise the sections will be likely to wash off the slides during staining.

Mounting wax sections onto slides requires special care in the avoidance of air bubbles because these cause more damage to brain and spinal cord than to most other tissues. An adhesive should be used, preferably smeared on the slide rather than added to the mounting water. Hot mounting water must be avoided; on no account should it be as hot as the melting-point of the wax; ideally it should be about 6°C below this point. Hotter water will cause fragmentation of the section by fine cracks.

Sections must be dried without undue heat; it is particularly important not to exceed the melting-point of the wax while any trace of water remains, since this is another cause of fragmentation of sections. On the other hand, the drying temperature must be at least 37°C, otherwise the sections will fail to adhere to the slides during staining. Drying must be thorough: whenever possible the sections should be left to dry in an incubator overnight.

Frozen sections of brain may be difficult to prepare if the tissue is too cold; sections are then apt to be shattered by fine cracks parallel to the knife edge. Sections are better if the tissue is only just below freezing point; in practice it is easier to freeze it hard to secure the block to the block-holder, and then to warm the surface of the tissue to a suitable temperature by finger pressure.

General notes on staining

Sections of neurological material are stained in just the same way as those of other tissues, using the techniques listed in Chapter 8 (p. 80). Frozen sections are handled in the way described in Chapter 19 (p. 274), and nitrocellulose sections as described in Chapter 18 (p. 264). Many neurological staining methods are long and obviously call for the use of staining jars, as also do the methods that make use of alcoholic reagents or of heat.

As already mentioned, sections of neurological material may be stained by any of the methods that are used for other tissues. Details of these methods can be found in the relevant chapters. For haematoxylin and eosin, many neuropathologists prefer Weigert's haematoxylin to the more usual mixtures. Of the trichrome stains, we have had pleasing results from Goldner's modification of Masson's method (p. 120). Bile may present a special problem in cases of kernicterus, since, in this disease, it dissolves in organic solvents. Fouchet's method is satisfactory if frozen sections are used (p. 134).

Nissl methods

Nissl granules are clumps of cytoplasmic ribonucleic acid. The clumping depends to a large extent on the type of fixation. Nissl (1885) drew attention to the fact that basic aniline dyes would demonstrate these granules after fixation in alcohol. He later (Nissl, 1894) gave the details of a method that made use of methylene blue. Since then, many other so-called Nissl stains have been introduced, including some that are not simple basic aniline dyes.

Fixation is important. The best results are obtained after tissue has been fixed in strong alcohol (80–95 per cent alcohol) or in Carnoy's fluid. Formalin gives uncertain results, especially when fixation has been prolonged.

Sections of any type (paraffin, nitrocellulose, or frozen) may be used for any of the methods that follow, except for gallocyanin chrome alum, which will not stain nitrocellulose sections. When paraffin sections are used, these give better results if they are thicker than usual (10–12 μ).

Combinations of Nissl stains with myelin stains are common; for this purpose either neutral red or cresyl fast violet is usually used for the Nissl granules. See the myelin methods given later in this chapter.

The following methods should satisfy the requirements of a routine laboratory. Each has its merits and drawbacks.

Toluidine blue is a dye that is available in almost every laboratory. The staining method is simple, but skill is needed for precise differentiation. The same remarks apply to the alternative dyes listed with this method.

Cresyl fast violet gives a stronger colour and the staining method is quicker. It needs very careful timing. Success depends to a great extent on whether the particular batch of dye used is satisfactory.

Gallocyanin chrome alum is a progressive stain. Since differentiation is unnecessary, this is a good method when sections are numerous. Staining is slow. The dye solution will keep for only a limited time.

Other methods that will stain Nissl granules, although rarely used for this purpose, include acridine orange (p. 189), and the pyronin and methyl green method (p. 187).

Toluidine blue
(or other simple basic dye–see Note i)

REAGENTS

A. *0·5–1·0 per cent aqueous solution of toluidine blue*
The solution improves with time and may be kept for years.

B. *Gothard's differentiator* (Gothard, 1898)

Creosote	50 ml.
Cajeput oil	40 ml.
Xylene	50 ml.
Alcohol	160 ml.

METHOD

1. Sections to water.
2. Toluidine blue for not less than 30 minutes (see Note ii).
3. Wash in running tap water.
4. Rinse in alcohol.
5. Differentiate, using microscopical control, in Gothard's differentiator until the background is colourless (see Note iii).
6. Rinse twice with alcohol.
7. Clear and mount.

RESULTS

Nissl granules: *blue.*
Nuclei: *light blue.*
Background: *unstained.*

Notes

(i) Any of the following dyes (in 0·5–1·0 per cent aqueous solution) may be substituted for toluidine blue: methylene blue, neutral red, safranin, thionin.

(ii) Results can be obtained by staining for 30 minutes. If time permits, the sections should be stained for longer. Overnight staining gives good results.

(iii) Gothard's differentiator dissolves nitrocellulose and is therefore unsuitable for nitrocellulose sections of loose or friable tissue. For these sections, stages 4 and 5 should be replaced by differentiation in 50–70 per cent alcohol. Paraffin or frozen sections can equally well be differentiated by alcohol but the results will not be as sharp as those given by Gothard's differentiator.

Cresyl fast violet

REAGENTS

A. *Stock solution of 1 per cent aqueous cresyl fast violet* (see Note i)

This keeps well.

B. *Working solution of cresyl fast violet*

Stock solution	6 ml.
Distilled water	54 ml.
10% acetic acid	0·5 ml.

Prepare as required; this solution deteriorates after a few days.

METHOD

1. Sections to water.
2. Cresyl fast violet (working solution) at 56°C. Paraffin sections need 6 minutes; nitrocellulose sections 3 minutes; frozen sections 1–2 minutes.
3. Differentiate in 95 per cent alcohol (see Note ii).
4. Rinse twice in alcohol.
5. Clear and mount.

RESULTS

Nissl granules: *violet.*
Nuclei: *pale violet.*
Background: *colourless.*

Notes

(i) Not all samples of cresyl fast violet are satisfactory. We have had good results with cresyl violet (Merck) and with cresyl fast violet acetate (G. T. Gurr).

(ii) If sections are overstained, the differentiation can be hastened by adding a few drops of cajeput oil to the 95 per cent alcohol.

Gallocyanin chrome alum

According to Einarson (1932), who originated the method, it can be used after most of the standard fixing fluids except Heidenhain's Susa. In our experience, however, alcoholic fluids give the best results and prolonged formalin fixation is unsatisfactory. The method cannot be used with nitrocellulose sections.

REAGENT

Gallocyanin chrome alum

> Chrome alum (chromium potassium sulphate) 10 g.
> Distilled water   200 ml.
> Gallocyanin   0·3 g.

Dissolve the chrome alum in the water, using gentle heat. Add the gallocyanin and mix well. Gradually heat the mixture to boiling point, and boil for 15–25 minutes, shaking frequently. Allow to cool; filter. The solution will keep for 1–2 months.

METHOD

1. Sections to water.
2. Gallocyanin chrome alum overnight.
3. Rinse in distilled water.
4. Dehydrate, clear, and mount.

RESULTS

> Nissl granules; nuclei: *dark blue-black.*
> Background: *colourless.*

Methods for axons

Axons are demonstrated by the use of silver salts. The principles and practical management are similar to those in other silver methods such as that for reticulin (Chap. 16). The methods in current use stem from the work of Bielschowsky, although he was not the first to use silver for this purpose. Bielschowsky published many papers on the subject and modified his method many times. We have used the method recommended in the first and second editions of Carleton's book (Carleton, 1926; Carleton and Leach, 1938). This is based on the schedule in one of Bielschowsky's earlier papers (Bielschowsky, 1904) but makes use of a silver mixture that he introduced later (Bielschowsky, 1909). The method shows not only axons, but also neurofibrils within the cell bodies; these are superbly illustrated in the earlier paper mentioned above.

The chief drawbacks to the Bielschowsky method are the time required and the need for frozen sections. The method was substantially modified by Gros, with great reduction of the time needed. The Gros modification may be used for nitrocellulose sections as well as for frozen sections; it gives moderately good results with paraffin sections. As in the original method, neurofibrils are demonstrated. We have found no published account by Gros herself; the method that we give below is that recommended by Carleton (Carleton and Leach, 1938; Carleton and Drury, 1957). This gives good results and is essentially the same as the earliest report of the method that we have seen (Romeis, 1924).

For use with paraffin sections, we have had the most consistently successful results from the Glees-Marsland modification (Marsland *et al.*, 1954). This method does not always demonstrate neurofibrils but it can be combined easily with a myelin stain such as luxol fast blue; this is far more difficult when frozen sections are used.

The Bielschowsky method

SCOPE

Tissue must be fixed in formalin-saline or neutral buffered formalin solution. Fixation must be thorough but the time is not critical; results can be obtained with tissue that has spent many years in formalin solutions. The method will only work with frozen sections.

REAGENTS

A. *2 per cent aqueous silver nitrate*

B. *Bielschowsky's silver solution*

20% aqueous silver nitrate	5 ml.
40% aqueous sodium hydroxide	6 drops
A brown precipitate forms.	

Strong ammonia (0·880) is added drop by drop with constant agitation until the precipitate is just dissolved. About 5 ml. will be needed.

Distilled water   to 25 ml.

This solution must be freshly prepared and filtered before use.

C. *10 per cent formalin*

This must not be acid: it may be neutralized with magnesium carbonate or (in most regions) made up with tap water.

D. *0·2 per cent aqueous gold chloride*

E. *5 per cent aqueous sodium thiosulphate*

METHOD

1. Well-fixed thin pieces are washed several times with distilled water for at least one hour.
2. Cut frozen sections (about 20 μ thick for axons or 10 μ thick for neurofibrils) and place them in distilled water for at least one hour.
3. Silver nitrate solution in the dark 48 hours. Sections must be flat without overlap.
4. Rinse rapidly in distilled water.
5. Bielschowsky's silver solution for the optimum time. Remove the first section after 3 minutes (see Note).
6. Rinse rapidly in distilled water.
7. Formalin solution 10 minutes. The section must be well agitated when introduced into this solution.
8. Wash in distilled water for at least 15 minutes.
9. Gold chloride solution until sections are pale grey.
10. Rinse in distilled water.
11. Sodium thiosulphate 1 minute.
12. Running tap water 5 minutes.
13. Dehydrate, clear, and mount, using carbol-xylene (p. 286).

RESULTS

Axons; dendrites; neurofibrils: *black.*
Other structures: *grey to light brown.*

Note

Each time the method is used, it will be necessary to discover the optimum time for treatment with Bielschowsky's silver solution. This may be anything from 3 to 10 minutes. The first section is removed after 3 minutes, rinsed and treated with formalin (stages 6 and 7). It is then examined in distilled water under a microscope. If the impregnation is insufficient, the next section is left for an extra minute and the process is repeated until the axons are intensely black. Once the optimum time has been found, it is possible to treat a batch of sections.

The Gros modification

SCOPE

Tissue must be fixed in formalin-saline or neutral buffered formalin solution. The method is suitable for frozen or nitrocellulose sections; it is less satisfactory for paraffin sections because non-specific precipitation usually occurs. This modification is quicker than the original Bielschowsky method; the impregnation is progressive and is controlled microscopically.

REAGENTS

A. *20 per cent aqueous silver nitrate*

B. *20 per cent formalin*
This must not be acid: it may be neutralized with magnesium carbonate or (in most regions) made up with tap water.

C. *Gros's silver solution.*

> 20% silver nitrate   10 ml.

Add strong ammonia (0·880) ammonia drop by drop with constant agitation. A brown precipitate forms. Continue adding ammonia until this just redissolves. Then add 11 more drops. This solution must be freshly prepared and filtered before use.

D. *10 per cent aqueous ammonia*

E. *Distilled water made acid by the addition of a few drops of glacial acetic acid*

F. *0·2 per cent aqueous gold chloride*

G. *5 per cent aqueous sodium thiosulphate*

METHOD

1. Sections to distilled water.
2. Silver nitrate solution in the dark for 1 hour. Sections must be flat without overlap.
3. Treat with 20 per cent formalin. This must be changed several times in the course of about 10 minutes until the solution no longer appears cloudy.
4. Transfer to Gros's silver solution in a shallow vessel under a low-power microscope. Examine until the axons are black on a colourless background (see Note).

5. Transfer to ammonia water to stop the impregnation. Leave for at least five minutes.
6. Wash in acidified distilled water.
7. Gold chloride until the section is bluish-grey.
8. Wash in distilled water.
9. Sodium thiosulphate 5 minutes.
10. Wash well in water.
11. Dehydrate, clear, and mount, using carbol-xylene for frozen or nitrocellulose sections (p. 286).

RESULTS

Axons; dendrites; neurofibrils: *black*.
Other structures: *bluish grey*.

Note

The reaction may be very rapid. If necessary it can be slowed down by rinsing the section briefly in distilled water after treatment with formalin (stage 3). Another way of slowing the reaction is to add a larger excess of ammonia to Gros's silver solution (e.g. 15–20 drops).

The Glees-Marsland modification

SCOPE

Tissue must be fixed in formalin-saline or neutral buffered formalin solution. The method is suitable for paraffin sections of about 6–8 μ thickness. The sections should be mounted on albuminized slides. (Marsland *et al.*, 1954.)

REAGENTS

A. *20 per cent aqueous silver nitrate*

B. *10 per cent aqueous formalin*

This must not be acid: it may be neutralized with magnesium carbonate or (in most regions) made up with tap water.

C. *Glees's silver solution*

| 20% aqueous silver nitrate | 30 ml. |
| Alcohol | 20 ml. |

Add strong ammonia (0·880) drop by drop with constant agitation. A precipitate forms. Continue to add ammonia until this just redissolves. Then add 5 more drops.

D. *0·2 per cent aqueous gold chloride*

E. *5 per cent aqueous sodium thiosulphate*

METHOD

1. Sections to distilled water.
2. Silver nitrate solution at 37°C until sections are amber-coloured (about 25–30 minutes).
3. Rinse in distilled water.
4. Rinse twice quickly (10 seconds) with the formalin solution.
5. Wash off the formalin with Glees's silver solution, flood the slide with this solution, and leave for 30 seconds.
6. Pour off the silver solution and immediately flood the slide with the formalin solution and leave it for one minute.
7. Examine microscopically. If the impregnation is insufficient repeat the treatment with Glees's silver solution (stage 5) followed by formalin (stage 6).
8. When the impregnation is satisfactory, rinse in distilled water.
9. Gold chloride 10 minutes. This stage is optional.
10. Wash in distilled water.
11. Sodium thiosulphate 5 minutes.
12. Wash well in water.
13. Dehydrate, clear, and mount.

RESULTS

Axons and dendrites: *black*.

Other structures: *light grey* (if gold was used).

or: *light yellowish-brown* (if gold was not used).

Methods for normal myelin

As already mentioned, stains that show normal myelin are not satisfactory for degenerating myelin, nor will they show the products of myelin degeneration. Degenerating myelin is demonstrated by methods of the Marchi type, which are discussed later in this chapter. Products of myelin degeneration are usually demonstrated by lipid stains such as Sudan III and IV (p. 160).

The usual purpose of staining normal myelin is to reveal areas where it has undergone complete destruction and is absent; these areas are said to be demyelinated.

Myelin is composed of complex lipids; these are not entirely soluble in ordinary fat solvents, so that parts of the myelin sheaths withstand routine dehydrating and clearing agents. It is for this reason that myelin can be stained in paraffin or nitrocellulose sections when suitable dyes are chosen.

The earliest methods used haematoxylin and depended upon the mordant properties of chromium (and often copper as well). The tissue was mordanted with a chromium salt before being embedded in nitrocellulose or wax. This technique is still in use and is usually known as the Weigert-Pal method. For the various contributions of Weigert, Pal, and Kultschitzky, see the historical note on page 244.

It was later discovered that myelin could be stained with haematoxylin when iron was used as the mordant. In this type of method, the mordant is applied to the section rather than to the piece of tissue. This means that sections from existing nitrocellulose or paraffin blocks can be used: special blocks are unnecessary. Many iron haematoxylin methods have been published for sections of various types (paraffin, nitrocellulose, or frozen). Of these, the Loyez method is among the best for nitrocellulose sections and can easily be adapted for use with paraffin sections.

Recent methods have made use of dyes other than haematoxylin. These dyes, which do not require mordants, include luxol fast blue (or methasol fast blue) and solochrome cyanin.

Fixation in formalin-saline or neutral buffered formalin solution is satisfactory for any of the following methods including that of Weigert-Pal.

Sections of any type (paraffin, nitrocellulose or frozen) may be stained by one or other of the myelin methods. In practice, paraffin or nitrocellulose sections are most commonly used; paraffin sections give better results when they are 10–12 μ thick.

Combinations of myelin stains with nuclear or Nissl stains are common. The combined demonstration of myelin and axons is possible, provided that one of the paler myelin methods is used.

The Weigert-Pal method gives the strongest colour and is particularly suitable for low-power examination of large sections. It is, however, a long and tedious method, and does not combine well with counterstains. Moreover, it is a block impregnation method, requiring a special block of tissue; this makes it impossible to examine small lesions for any tissue components other than myelin. Paraffin and frozen sections are not entirely satisfactory, since they are very brittle: the best results with the Weigert-Pal method are obtained if the tissue is embedded in nitrocellulose.

The Loyez method is simple and satisfactory for nitrocellulose sections. It can also be used for paraffin sections but these tend to wash off the slides during staining. The solutions are easy to prepare and the colour is strong.

Luxol fast blue (or methasol fast blue) gives satisfactory results with paraffin sections. Nitrocellulose or frozen sections can be used, but are less suitable. When neutral red is used as counterstain, the colour is strong; counterstaining with cresyl fast violet gives a more delicate result. In either case the counterstain is more informative than that in most of the other myelin methods. No mordant is required and the reagents are easy to prepare.

Solochrome cyanin is by far the quickest method. It may be used with paraffin sections or with frozen sections (of fixed or unfixed tissue). Sections of 10–12 μ thickness are less likely to wash off the slides than those stained by any of the other myelin methods. Sections can readily be counterstained with neutral red to show Nissl granules. Myelin is stained less intensely by solochrome cyanin than by many of the other stains.

Weigert-Pal

SCOPE

In this method, pieces of tissue are mordanted before cutting sections; the method is not applicable to individual sections of material fixed in ordinary fluids. Originally nitrocellulose was used as the embedding medium and this gives the best results. It is, however, possible to embed the mordanted tissue in paraffin, although the sections may give trouble by washing off the slides during staining, especially when they are large.

R

REAGENTS

A. *Weigert's primary mordant*

Potassium dichromate	5 g.
Chromium fluoride (fluorochrome)	2·5 g.
Distilled water	100 ml.
Acetic acid	1 ml.

Dissolve the salts in the water, using heat. Allow to cool and then add the acetic acid, mix, and filter. This solution must be freshly prepared.

B. *Copper acetate*

Saturated aqueous solution of copper acetate	100 ml.
Distilled water	100 ml.

C. *Kultschitzky's haematoxylin*

Stock 20% alcoholic haematoxylin solution (p. 103)	5 ml.
2% aqueous acetic acid	95 ml.

This mixture must be freshly prepared

D. *0·5 per cent aqueous solution of sodium carbonate*

E. *0·1 per cent aqueous solution of potassium permanganate*
This solution will not keep. It may conveniently be prepared from a 1 per cent stock solution which is stable.

F. *Pal's solution*

Oxalic acid	1 g.
Potassium sulphite	1 g.
Distilled water	100 ml.

Dissolve the salts without using heat. The solution is stable.

METHOD

1. Weigert's primary mordant at 37°C for 5 days. Pieces should be well fixed and no more than 0·3 cm. thick for paraffin embedding (or 0·5 cm. thick for nitrocellulose).

2. Transfer to alcohol without washing. Replace the alcohol several times in the course of 30 minutes (see Note i).

3. Continue the dehydration in alcohol, clear, and embed in paraffin or nitrocellulose. Cut sections (10–12 μ in paraffin: 20–30 μ in nitrocellulose).

4. Sections to water.
5. Copper acetate 30 minutes.
6. Wash repeatedly in distilled water for 5 minutes.
7. Kultschitzky's haematoxylin at 37°C overnight (see Note ii).
8. Wash thoroughly in running tap water.
9. Blue in sodium carbonate.
10. Rinse in distilled water.
11. Differentiate:
    (a) in potassium permanganate until the stain begins to fade from the grey matter in the section (about 30 seconds);
    (b) in Pal's solution for 30 seconds.
    Repeat (a) and (b) alternately until the grey matter is colourless.
12. Wash repeatedly in distilled water for 10 minutes.
13. Wash in running tap water.
14. Blue in sodium carbonate.
15. Counterstain with 1% aqueous neutral red if required.
16. Rinse in tap water.
17. Dehydrate, clear, and mount (see Note iii).

Results

Myelin sheaths; red blood corpuscles: *bluish black*.
Nuclei; Nissl granules: *red* (if counterstained).
Other structures: *colourless to light grey*.

Notes

(i) After 5 days, the mordanting fluid will be turbid. Debris is removed from the tissue by gentle shaking in alcohol. The alcohol is renewed until it is free from particles. At this stage the white matter in the tissue will be dull greenish brown.

(ii) When paraffin sections show a tendency to wash off the slides during staining, they should be coated with thin nitrocellulose (p. 315).

(iii) Nitrocellulose sections are usually cleared in carbol-xylene (p. 273). In the Weigert-Pal method it may be useful to use carbol-xylene for paraffin sections also.

(iv) This variant of the Weigert-Pal method is virtually identical with that recommended by Russell (1939). We have found it to give consistently good results.

Historical Note

Haematoxylin was introduced as a myelin stain by Weigert (1884a; 1884b). He found it far superior to the methods that he had previously used. Initially the mordant was chromium, which was present in the fixing fluid, but later copper was used as an additional mordant (Weigert, 1885). Weigert used borax-ferricyanide to differentiate the stain.

Pal (1886) introduced the permanganate-oxalic-sulphite differentiator that is still in use. He found that it removed more haematoxylin from the background, allowing counterstains to be used. Pal used the same weakly alkaline haematoxylin solution as Weigert.

Kultschitzky (1889) used an acid haematoxylin to stain myelin in a method that was otherwise fairly closely related to that of Weigert.

The names of Weigert, Pal, and Kultschitzky have since been linked in various combinations depending on the use that is made of the contributions of the three original inventors. Thus methods have been named after Weigert, Kultschitzky, Weigert-Pal, Kultschitzky-Pal, and Weigert-Pal-Kultschitzky.

All these methods were originally described before formalin was in use as a histological fixative. In those days it was common practice to use fluids containing chrome salts for fixing every kind of tissue. Thus, Weigert, Pal, and Kultschitzky designed their methods for tissue fixed in chrome salts. It is, however, equally satisfactory to fix the tissue in a formalin mixture and then transfer it to a chrome mordant. This enables the methods to be used for routine material.

Loyez

SCOPE

This method was originally designed for nitrocellulose sections (Loyez, 1910) and gives excellent results. It may also be used for paraffin or frozen sections.

REAGENTS

A. *4 per cent aqueous iron alum (ferric ammonium sulphate)*

B. *Haematoxylin mixture*

> Stock 20% alcoholic haematoxylin solution (p. 103) 5 ml.
> Alcohol   5 ml.
> Distilled water   90 ml.
> Saturated aqueous solution of lithium carbonate   2 ml.

This mixture must be freshly prepared.

C. *Weigert's differentiator*

Borax (sodium tetraborate)	2 g.
Potassium ferricyanide	2·5 g.
Distilled water	200 ml.

METHOD

1. Sections to water.
2. Iron alum overnight.
3. Rinse rapidly in distilled water.
4. Haematoxylin mixture at 37°C overnight (see Note i).
5. Wash well in tap water.
6. Differentiate in iron alum until the grey matter is nearly colourless (see Notes ii and iii).
7. Continue differentiation in Weigert's differentiator until the grey matter is colourless.
8. Wash in distilled water.
9. Wash well in tap water.
10. Dehydrate, clear, and mount.

RESULTS

Myelin sheaths; red blood corpuscles: *black*.
Nuclear chromatin: *black* (inconsistent).
Other structures: *colourless to yellow*.

Notes

(i) Staining at 37°C overnight gives the best results. Fairly good results are obtained at room temperature overnight. When time is limited, sections may be stained at 56°C and examined from time to time; they are removed when dark enough (1–2 hours).

(ii) By careful reduction of the staining time, it may be possible to avoid the need for differentiation.

(iii) As an alternative to stages 6 and 7, acid alcohol may be used for differentiation (1 per cent hydrochloric acid in 70 per cent alcohol). This leaves the myelin blue rather than black, and also fails to decolorize the grey matter completely.

Luxol fast blue
(or methasol fast blue)

SCOPE

This method is particularly suitable for paraffin sections but may also be used for frozen or nitrocellulose sections.

REAGENTS

A. *Luxol fast blue*

Luxol fast blue M.B.S. (or methasol fast blue 2G)	0·5 g.
Alcohol	475 ml.
Distilled water	25 ml.
10% acetic acid	2·5 ml.

The solution will keep for years in a well-stoppered bottle; it should be filtered before use.

B. *0·05 per cent aqueous lithium carbonate*

C. *Working solution of cresyl fast violet* (p. 233) or *1 per cent aqueous neutral red*

METHOD

1. Sections to alcohol (see Note i).
2. Luxol fast blue (or methasol fast blue) at room temperature overnight (or at 56°C for 4–5 hours).
3. Rinse in alcohol to remove excess of stain.
4. Wash in distilled water.
5. Lithium carbonate 5–10 seconds.
6. Rinse several times with 70 per cent alcohol until the grey matter in the section is colourless (see Note ii).
7. Wash in running tap water.
8. Counterstain with:
   Either cresyl fast violet at 56°C for 6 minutes *or* neutral red at room temperature for 10–15 minutes.
9. Rinse in tap water.
10. Dehydrate, clear, and mount.

RESULTS

Using cresyl fast violet:
   Myelin sheaths: *greenish blue.*
   Nuclei; Nissl granules: *violet.*

Using neutral red:
   Myelin sheaths: *dark blue.*
   Nuclei; Nissl granules: *red.*

Notes

(i) Paraffin sections are dewaxed in xylene and then transferred to alcohol. Frozen sections are rinsed in 70 per cent alcohol and then transferred to undiluted alcohol. Nitrocellulose sections (which are already in 70 per cent alcohol) are rinsed in 90 per cent alcohol and then placed directly in the staining mixture.

If fixation deposits are present, it will be necessary to remove these first (p. 84).

(ii) If 70 per cent alcohol fails to decolorize the grey matter, the sections are returned to lithium carbonate (stage 5) for 5–10 seconds and then rinsed again in 70 per cent alcohol (stage 6). Occasionally these two stages may need to be repeated yet again.

(iii) The original method used Luxol fast blue in conjunction with cresyl fast violet (Klüver and Barrera, 1953). The very similar dye Methasol fast blue was used in conjunction with neutral red by Pearse (1955). In our experience, either dye may be used with either counterstain; the results obtained depend entirely on which counterstain is chosen.

Solochrome cyanin

SCOPE

A simple and rapid method suitable for paraffin sections and for frozen sections of fixed or unfixed tissue (Page, 1965).

REAGENTS

A. *Solochrome cyanin solution*

Solochrome cyanin RS	0·2 g.
Concentrated sulphuric acid	0·5 ml.
Distilled water	90 ml.
4% aqueous iron alum (ferric ammonium sulphate)	10 ml.

Place the dye in a 250 ml. flask and add the sulphuric acid. Effervescence occurs. Stir the creamy mixture with a glass rod until all the dye is dissolved. Add the distilled water and then the iron alum. Mix well; filter. The solution keeps well.

B. *10 per cent aqueous iron alum* (ferric ammonium sulphate)

C. *1 per cent aqueous neutral red*

METHOD

1. Sections to water.
2. Solochrome cyanin solution 10 minutes.
3. Wash well in running tap water until blue.
4. Differentiate in 10% iron alum according to the results required (see below).
5. Wash in running tap water for several minutes.

6. Neutral red 1 minute.
7. Rinse in tap water.
8. Dehydrate, clear, and mount.

RESULTS

This method has applications other than the demonstration of myelin sheaths; results will depend on the duration of differentiation.

The dye is firmly bound to myelin sheaths so that they remain coloured when differentiation is continued until the rest of the tissue (including the nuclei) is decolorized. This will occur in about 5 minutes. Nuclei will then take up the red counterstain.

The method is also useful for demonstrating a few other structures to which the dye is less firmly bound. These include the striations of skeletal and cardiac muscle, the intercellular bridges ('prickles') of squamous epithelium, and the granules of eosinophil leucocytes (which contrast strikingly with tissue mast cells when stained by this method).

The dye becomes attached moderately firmly to eosinophil granules, less firmly to intercellular bridges, and only relatively weakly to muscle striations. When the method is used for the demonstration of any of these structures, differentiation must be correspondingly reduced and should be controlled microscopically. With these reduced times of differentiation the nuclei will not be decolorized and will remain blue.

Thus, two sets of results may be tabulated, as follows:

For the demonstration of myelin:

Myelin sheaths: *grey-blue.*
Nuclei; Nissl granules: *red.*
Other structures: *shades of pink.*

For other purposes:

Nuclei; muscle striations; intercellular bridges: *dark blue.*
Granules of eosinophil leucocytes: *light blue.*
Granules of mast cells: *bright red.*
Other structures: *pale grey-blue or light pink.*

The Marchi method for degenerating myelin

When an axon dies, its myelin sheath degenerates. An axon will die if it is separated from the cell body, or if the cell body itself dies. A method that demonstrates degenerating myelin sheaths will therefore show which axons are dead. This information may be of great value in discovering the course of axons throughout the nervous system, since the destruction of a cell body is followed by degeneration of myelin along the entire course of the axon, however complex that course may be. Alternatively, the finding of degenerating myelin in an identifiable position in the central nervous system or in a peripheral nerve may make it possible to discover the site of a lesion some distance away.

Stains for normal myelin may sometimes reveal the abnormality: at an early stage of degeneration the myelin sheath will be misshapen and stain darkly; at a late stage the complete loss of staining will be obvious if the affected area is large. When, however, only a few sheaths are affected, they will be very likely to escape notice unless a method is used that demonstrates degenerating myelin specifically.

Normal myelin is a complex lipid. Like almost all lipids it can be demonstrated with osmium tetroxide. Preliminary treatment with dichromate, however, prevents the reaction. Degenerating myelin contains many unsaturated fatty acids and these too can be demonstrated with osmium tetroxide. In this case, however, the reaction is not prevented by dichromate to an appreciable extent. If, therefore, a piece of tissue is treated with dichromate, the normal myelin is oxidized and becomes unreactive while the degenerating myelin remains reactive to osmium tetroxide. The combination of potassium dichromate and osmium tetroxide was first used by Marchi (Marchi and Algeri, 1885), and methods of this type are still known by his name. Since that date, many modifications have been made, including the replacement of potassium dichromate by other oxidizing agents such as sodium iodate (Busch, 1898) or potassium chlorate (Swank and Davenport, 1935).

Methods of the Marchi type do not give useful results before a significant quantity of unsaturated fatty acid has been formed, so that they are not satisfactory immediately after degeneration has begun. Furthermore, these methods become less satisfactory beyond a certain time because the unsaturated fatty acids are absorbed in the later stages of degeneration. This drawback was appreciated by Marchi and Algeri (1886); they obtained good results one month after injury. Most users of this type of method have found the useful time limits to be 10–60 days. Smith (1951), however, has obtained results as long as 400 days after injury.

In the original method, tissue was fixed in Müller's fluid. Modern practice is to use a formalin-saline mixture for a relatively short time. As a general rule, results are unsatisfactory if formalin fixation is prolonged beyond 72 hours. In skilled hands, however, results have been obtained with tissue that has spent months or even years in a formalin mixture (Smith, *et al.* 1956).

Methods of the Marchi type need a separate piece of tissue; after it has been treated with dichromate and osmium tetroxide, the tissue is not suitable for any other staining method; nor can the Marchi method be combined with other stains.

The method given below is that recommended by Lillie (1948); it does not differ greatly from the original (Marchi and Algeri, 1885; 1886). We have found it satisfactory.

The Marchi Method

REAGENTS

A. *2·5 per cent aqueous potassium dichromate*
   This solution keeps well.

B. *Osmium-dichromate mixture*

2·5% aqueous potassium dichromate	20 ml.
1·0% aqueous osmium tetroxide	10 ml.

These should be mixed immediately before use. The osmium stock solution may be kept in chemically clean, dark glass bottles with a close fitting non-metal cap; the keeping properties are improved by the addition of one drop of saturated aqueous mercuric chloride to every 10 ml. of the solution.

METHOD

1. Fix very thin pieces (1·5–2·0 mm.) in formalin-saline or neutral buffered formalin solution.
2. Potassium dichromate solution for 7–9 days. During this time the fluid should be changed every 2–3 days and should be shaken occasionally to ensure that both sides of the piece of tissue have access to the solution.

3. Dichromate-osmium mixture for 14 days at room temperature in the dark. The fluid should be shaken occasionally and should be changed once after 7 days.
4. Rinse several times with distilled water.
5. Wash in running tap water for 24 hours.
6. Dehydrate in acetone for 30–45 minutes. Repeat with fresh acetone three more times (see Note iv).
7. Clear in petroleum ether (technical grade) for 30 minutes. Repeat once with fresh petroleum ether (see Note iv).
8. Impregnate with paraffin wax for 30 minutes; repeat twice with fresh wax and embed.
9. Cut sections 10–12 μ thick and mount them on slides.
10. Remove the wax with chloroform and mount in a resinous medium (see Note iv).

RESULTS

Degenerating myelin: *black*.
Other structures: *yellow to brown*.

Notes

(i) A common source of artefacts in this method is careless handling of tissue. Spinal cord in particular is liable to kinking, squeezing, and stretching during removal. Manipulation must be very gentle.

(ii) We believe that prolonged fixation gives rise to artefacts, although this has not been the experience of some other users of the method (Smith, 1956).

(iii) Experimental animals should not be killed with ether, since this may give rise to artefacts.

(iv) The black deposit at the site of degenerating myelin consists of lower oxides of osmium. These are slightly soluble in alcohol and some other organic solvents. For this reason the tissue is dehydrated in acetone and cleared in petroleum ether since these do not dissolve the lower oxides. The sections are dewaxed in chloroform rather than xylene for the same reason. The solvents of resinous media, however, dissolve too little of the oxides to make any appreciable difference.

Organic solvents are avoided if frozen sections are cut; moreover these have been recommended by Smith (1956) because artefacts are fewer. In practice, however, frozen sections are often hard to produce because the tissue is very brittle after treatment with dichromate.

Methods for neuroglia

As already mentioned, techniques for the complete demonstration of neuroglial cells are tedious and temperamental; they are rarely used except in special laboratories. In practice it is possible to identify oligodendrocytes in haematoxylin and eosin sections. Microglial cells are phagocytic; they are easily recognized in many sections of abnormal brain by their content of pigment or lipid, which can if necessary be demonstrated by Perls's method or by such stains as Sudan III on frozen sections.

Astrocytes are perhaps the most important of the three types of cells. Astrocytes have numerous well-developed processes which are particularly conspicuous in abnormal brains (e.g. following injury) where they form dense tangles. Fortunately these tangles are demonstrable without undue difficulty by phosphotungstic acid haematoxylin or by the Holzer method.

Fixation of tissue for the phosphotungstic acid haematoxylin stain or for Holzer's method is not critical. Formalin-saline and neutral buffered formalin solution give good results. On the other hand it is extremely important to use the right fixing fluid (formalin-ammonium-bromide) for Cajal's and Rio-Hortega's methods, and tissue must be fixed for the correct length of time for each method. Details are included with the methods.

Sections of any type may be used for phosphotungstic acid haematoxylin and Holzer's method. For Cajal's and Rio-Hortega's methods, frozen sections are essential and these must be handled free, not attached to slides.

Phosphotungstic acid haematoxylin for neuroglial fibres

SCOPE

A consistent and reliable method for paraffin and frozen sections; suitable for nitrocellulose sections if modified (see Note vi). Works well after most fixing fluids including formalin-saline, neutral buffered formalin solution, mercuric-chloride-formalin, Susa, and Helly's fluid. Not a specific method; the merit that most other structures are stained in contrasting colours largely outweighs the drawback that myelin sheaths are stained a similar colour to neuroglial fibres.

Of many variants derived from the original method of Mallory (1897–8; 1900–1), this one is particularly suitable for neuroglial fibres (Russell, 1939) but is not our first preference for structures outside the nervous system (p. 114).

REAGENTS

A. *Acid dichromate solution*

> 2·5% aqueous potassium dichromate   95 ml.
> Glacial acetic acid   5 ml.

B. *Lugol's iodine* (p. 84)

C. *0·25 per cent potassium permanganate*
This should be freshly prepared from a stronger stock solution (not weaker than 1·0 per cent).

D. *5 per cent aqueous oxalic acid*

E. *Phosphotungstic acid haematoxylin solution* (p. 115)

METHOD

1. Sections to water.
2. Acid dichromate solution overnight or longer (see Note i).
3. Running tap water 5–15 minutes.
4. Lugol's iodine 15 minutes.
5. Decolorize in alcohol (about one hour).
6. Rinse in distilled water.
7. Potassium permanganate 5 minutes (see Note ii).
8. Rinse in distilled water (see Note iii).
9. Oxalic acid 5 minutes.
10. Rinse in distilled water (see Note iii).
11. Running tap water at least 5 minutes.
12. Haematoxylin solution overnight or longer.
13. 95% alcohol (see Note iv).
14. Complete dehydration, clear, and mount.

RESULTS

Neuroglial fibres; red blood corpuscles: *dark blue.*
Myelin sheaths: *blue.*
Collagen: *reddish brown.*
Cytoplasm: *pale brown to pale pink.*
(For structures outside the nervous system, see p. 115.)

Notes

(i) Treatment with dichromate may be omitted if tissue was fixed in Helly's fluid.

(ii) Treatment with permanganate must be timed carefully. Too short a time will lead to excessively blue results; prolonged treatment produces sections that are red with little or no blue in them.

(iii) Tap water must be avoided before and after oxalic acid.

(iv) On no account must sections be washed in water after haematoxylin since this destroys the red colours. Usually a brief rinse in 95 per cent alcohol is sufficient before the sections are transferred to undiluted alcohol. If sections are very blue (e.g. after staining for a whole weekend), they may be differentiated to some extent by prolonging treatment with 95 per cent alcohol for up to 5 minutes.

(v) In this method the dichromate acts as a mordant. Permanganate appears to act by removing chromium selectively from some of the tissue elements. The action of iodine is not fully understood, but this probably acts as an additional mordant.

(vi) For nitrocellulose sections, acid dichromate is not used at stage 2. Instead the sections are treated with a saturated aqueous solution of mercuric chloride for 20–30 minutes. The rest of the method is unchanged.

Holzer's method

SCOPE

Suitable for paraffin or frozen sections after fixation in formalin-saline or neutral buffered formalin solution. A quicker method than phosphotungstic acid haematoxylin but more difficult to perform. Specific for proliferated neuroglial fibres in abnormal brains or spinal cords; the lack of background staining may make orientation of the sections difficult. We have obtained satisfactory results with the following method which is slightly modified from the original (Holzer, 1921).

REAGENTS

A. *Phosphomolybdic acid solution*

0·5% aqueous phosphomolybdic acid	10 ml.
Alcohol	20 ml.

Must be freshly prepared.

B. *Alcohol-chloroform mixture*

Alcohol	2 ml.
Chloroform	8 ml.

Must be freshly prepared.

C. *Crystal violet*

Crystal violet	0·5 g.
Alcohol	2·0 ml.
Chloroform	8·0 ml.

Must be freshly prepared and filtered.

D. *10 per cent aqueous potassium bromide*

E. *Aniline-chloroform mixture*

Aniline oil	6 ml.
Chloroform	9 ml.
25% ammonia	1 drop

Must be freshly prepared.

METHOD

1. Section to water.
2. Blot the section.
3. Phosphomolybdic acid solution 2–3 minutes.
4. Blot the section.
5. Alcohol-chloroform mixture.
6. Before the section is dry, flood with staining solution and leave for 30 seconds.
7. Without draining the slide, rinse several times with potassium bromide solution until the green scum disappears and the section appears to be uniformly covered with the solution.
8. Blot the section.
9. Add aniline-chloroform mixture and agitate the slide until only the neuroglial fibres remain coloured.
10. Blot the section.
11. Rinse several times with xylene.
12. Mount.

RESULTS

Neuroglial fibres: *violet*.

Note

Once the procedure is started, it must be completed without delay.

Cajal's method for astrocytes

SCOPE

Tissue should be fixed in formalin-ammonium-bromide for the correct time (see Note i). Frozen sections must be used and must be handled free, not attached to slides. The method is reliable provided that it is carried out with great care. Glass-distilled water must be used; all glassware must be chemically clean; the gold chloride and mercuric chloride must be of analytical quality.

The method below is that recommended by Russell (1939). It differs only in minor details from the original (Cajal, 1913; 1916) and has given us excellent results.

REAGENTS

A. *Formalin-ammonium-bromide* (p. 227)

B. *1 per cent formalin in distilled water*

C. *Cajal's gold solution*

Mercuric chloride	0·5 g.
Distilled water	50 ml.
1% aqueous gold chloride (see Note ii)	10 ml.

Dissolve the mercuric chloride in the water using very gentle heat. Overheating at this stage will ruin the solution; no part of the flask must become uncomfortably hot to the hand. While still warm, add the gold chloride; mix well; allow to cool; filter before use. The stock solution of gold chloride keeps well in a dark bottle but the mercuric chloride solution and the mixture must be freshly prepared.

D. *5 per cent aqueous sodium thiosulphate*

METHOD

1. Fix thin pieces (3 mm.) in formalin-ammonium-bromide for 48–72 hours (see Note i).
2. Cut frozen sections, 15–20 μ thick, and place them in 1% formalin where they should not remain for more than 30–60 minutes.

3. Carry the sections as quickly as possible through two dishes of distilled water.
4. Place the sections flat without creases in Cajal's gold solution in a shallow vessel (e.g. a Petri dish). There must be no more than 10–12 sections in 60 ml. of the solution and they must not overlap. Cover to exclude dust and leave in subdued light at room temperature (see Note v).
5. After about 3 hours examine a section under the microscope from time to time (see Notes iii and iv). When the astrocytes appear dark, remove all the sections and rinse them in distilled water.
6. Sodium thiosulphate 5 minutes.
7. Wash thoroughly in tap water.
8. Dehydrate, clear, and mount, using carbol-xylene (p. 286).

Results

Astrocyte processes and cell bodies: *black and dark brown.*
Capillary walls: *grey.*
Nuclei of other cells: *grey to brown.*
Other structures: *pink to brownish-red.*

Notes

(i) Duration of fixation may be varied according to the results required. Protoplasmic astrocytes are demonstrated when tissue is fixed for not more than 48–72 hours. Fibrillary astrocytes are demonstrated when tissue is fixed for not less than 48–72 hours. Therefore both types can be demonstrated in the same preparation when the tissue is fixed for 48–72 hours.

(ii) Cajal and Russell both specified brown gold chloride rather than yellow gold chloride. It seems doubtful, however, whether all chemical manufacturers label these reagents consistently. We have had satisfactory results using yellow gold chloride (chloro-auric acid $HAuCl_4XH_2O$ supplied by Messrs Hopkin and Williams).

(iii) Impregnation will be complete in 3–4 hours when the room temperature is 18–21°C (65–70°F). In a cooler room the time will need to be increased, whereas in a warmer room (24–25°C) it will be greatly reduced. In both cases, however, there is an increased risk of non-specific precipitation.

The rate of impregnation depends also on the lighting. The times mentioned above apply when the staining vessel is away from direct sunlight and is covered by two sheets of paper folded to make a well-fitting cap. More light will accelerate the impregnation: complete

S

darkness will inhibit it; in either case the risk of non-specific precipitation is increased.

(iv) Beginners (and others who find it difficult to determine whether impregnation is complete by examining a wet section) may prefer to dehydrate, clear, and mount a section quickly, so that they can examine it more carefully. For this reason, we have found it helpful to start with more sections than are required, so that some of them can be used for this purpose and discarded.

(v) Our experience has been limited to specimens of human brain, with which we have obtained good results at room temperature. When the method is used for specimens from other species, it may be necessary to use higher temperatures to obtain satisfactory results. From his experience of Cajal's method with various species, Rio-Hortega (1917) made the following suggestions: cerebrum of dog, cat, or rabbit, 30–35°C; cerebellum of these species, 35–40°C; olfactory bulb of these species, 40–45°C; pineal from large animals (including man), 40°C. Yet another suggestion made by Rio-Hortega in the same note was the use of a saturated solution (about 10 per cent) of mercuric chloride in place of the dilute solution (0·5 g. in 50 ml. in Reagent C above); he used this modified reagent at 35–40°C for 30 to 60 minutes to demonstrate the neuroglia of animals.

Rio-Hortega's method for oligodendrocytes

SCOPE

Tissue should be fixed in formalin-ammonium-bromide for 12–48 hours (12–24 hours in warm climates). Frozen sections must be used and must be handled free, not attached to slides. Glass-distilled water must be used; glassware must be chemically clean; the silver nitrate and sodium carbonate should be of analytical quality.

We have used the following method, which is that recommended by Carleton and Drury (1957); the identical method is given in earlier editions of Carleton's book, and an almost identical method in the fourth edition. It differs only in detail from the original (Rio-Hortega, 1921).

REAGENTS

A. *Formalin-ammonium-bromide* (p. 227)

B. *Distilled water to which a few drops of strong ammonia have been added*

C. *Rio-Hortega's silver solution for oligodendrocytes*

10% aqueous silver nitrate	5 ml.
5% aqueous sodium carbonate (anhydrous)	20 ml.
Strong ammonia (0·880) added drop by drop with agitation until the precipitate just dissolves.	
Distilled water	to 45 ml.

After filtration, the solution is ready for use. Like any other ammoniacal silver solution, it should not be stored.

D. *1 per cent formalin solution*

E. *0·2 per cent aqueous gold chloride*

F. *5 per cent aqueous sodium thiosulphate*

METHOD

1. Fix thin pieces in formalin-ammonium-bromide for 12–48 hours.
2. Transfer to warm formalin-ammonium-bromide (45–50°C) and leave for 10 minutes.
3. Wash several times with distilled water during 2–3 hours.
4. Cut frozen sections, 15–20 μ thick, and place them in ammonia water.
5. Carry the sections as quickly as possible through two dishes of distilled water.
6. Place the sections in Rio-Hortega's silver solution for oligodendrocytes. The solution must be agitated; this can be done by blowing on the surface. Treatment should continue for the optimum time (between one and five minutes; see Note ii).
7. Rinse in distilled water for 15 seconds.
8. Formalin solution for about 1 minute with agitation.
9. Rinse in distilled water.
10. Gold chloride until sections are light grey to the naked eye (10–15 minutes).
11. Sodium thiosulphate for 1 minute.
12. Wash well in water.
13. Dehydrate, clear, and mount using carbol-xylene (p. 286).

RESULTS

Oligodendrocytes and processes: *black*.
Microglial cells are sometimes black also.
Other structures: *pale grey*.

Notes

(i) The key to success with this method is agitation of the sections in the silver solution and the formalin solution. Neglect of this detail will lead to uneven results.

(ii) Each time the method is used, it will be necessary to discover the optimum time for treatment with the silver solution. This may be anything from one minute to five minutes. The first section is removed after one minute, rinsed, treated with formalin, and rinsed again (stages 7, 8, and 9). The wet section is then examined with the microscope. If the impregnation is insufficient, the next section is left in the silver solution for an extra minute and the process is repeated until the oligodendrocytes are intensely black. Once the optimum time has been found, it is possible to treat a batch of sections.

Rio-Hortega's method for microglia

SCOPE

Tissue should be fixed for 2–3 days in formalin-ammonium-bromide. Frozen sections must be used and must be handled free, not attached to slides. Glass-distilled water must be used; glassware must be chemically clean; the silver nitrate and sodium carbonate should be of analytical quality.

Rio-Hortega published many silver carbonate methods for a variety of purposes. The variant given below is virtually identical with that designed specifically for microglia (Rio-Hortega, 1919). It was also favoured by Carleton, who included it in the first three editions of his book (Carleton, 1926; Carleton and Leach, 1938; Carleton and Drury, 1957). We have rarely needed to demonstrate microglia and have little practical experience with this method.

REAGENTS

A. *Formalin-ammonium-bromide* (p. 227)

B. *Distilled water to which a few drops of strong ammonia have been added*

C. *Rio-Hortega's silver solution for microglia*

10% aqueous silver nitrate	5 ml.
5% aqueous sodium carbonate (anhydrous)	25 ml.
Strong ammonia (0·880) added drop by drop with agitation until the precipitate just dissolves.	
Distilled water	to 75 ml.

After filtration, the solution is ready for use. Like any other ammoniacal silver solution, it should not be stored.

D. *5 per cent formalin solution*

E. *0·2 per cent aqueous gold chloride*

F. *5 per cent aqueous sodium thiosulphate*

METHOD

1. Fix thin pieces in formalin-ammonium-bromide for 2–4 days.
2. Transfer to warm formalin-ammonium-bromide (50–55°C) and leave for 10 minutes.
3. Cut frozen sections, about 20 μ thick.
4. Rinse rapidly in ammonia water.
5. Rinse rapidly in distilled water.
6. Place the sections in Rio-Hortega's silver solution for microglia. This must be agitated frequently. Treatment should continue for 10–15 minutes at room temperature.
7. Rinse very quickly in distilled water.
8. Formalin solution for about 1 minute with agitation.
9. Rinse in distilled water.
10. Gold chloride 10–15 minutes.
11. Sodium thiosulphate 1 minute.
12. Wash well in water.
13. Dehydrate, clear, and mount, using carbol-xylene (p. 286).

RESULTS

Microglial cells and processes: *black.*
Oligodendrocytes are sometimes black also.
Other structures: *pale grey.*

Note

As in the previous method, the sections must be agitated when in the silver solution and the formalin solution if even results are to be obtained.

Brain smears

Brain smears are made when a histological diagnosis is needed during the course of a neurosurgical operation. Frequently the only specimens obtainable are tiny fragments of soft and gelatinous material. Such specimens are difficult to handle by frozen section techniques, even when a cryostat is available.

Tissue is smeared before being fixed in any way and the smears are dropped at once into fixing fluid before they begin to dry. Smears are made by compressing the tissue between two glass slides and then gently sliding them apart. In order to avoid unnecessary damage to cells, too much force must not be used in making the smears although tough tumours may need considerable compression before the smears are thin enough.

Fixation by alcohol is simple and satisfactory. In theory a mercuric-alcohol mixture would be better; in practice it confers no advantages, possibly because it does not dissolve any lipid whereas alcohol does.

When a result is required as soon as possible, a simple stain such as toluidine blue is used. If rather more time is available, haematoxylin and eosin (p. 326) may be preferred although Russell, who first used brain smears for diagnosis, recommended eosin and methyl blue (Russell *et al.*, 1937).

Toluidine blue for brain smears

REAGENT

1·0 per cent aqueous toluidine blue

METHOD

1. Fix smears in alcohol for not less than two minutes.
2. Rinse in water.
3. Toluidine blue 2 minutes.
4. Rinse well in water.
5. Differentiate in 70% alcohol.
6. Dehydrate, clear, and mount.

RESULTS

Nuclei: *blue or greenish blue.*
Capillary walls: *lighter blue.*
Red blood corpuscles: *dull green.*
Other structures: *pale blue to colourless.*

Notes

(i) Dehydration and clearing need particular care when parts of the smear are thick.

(ii) Mast cells are not uncommon in some intracranial tumours. The granules of these cells are stained metachromatically by toluidine blue and appear purple.

CHAPTER 18

Nitrocellulose Technique

General notes. Processing. Cutting sections.
Staining. Finishing off.

CELLULOSE NITRATE or nitrocellulose has been used as an embedding medium for many years. The original method made use of celloidin (or collodion); more recently another form has been used as an alternative: this is known as low viscosity nitrocellulose (LVNC). Whichever is preferred, the principle is the same. It consists of impregnating the tissue with progressively stronger solutions of nitrocellulose, which is then allowed to harden by the evaporation of its solvent.

During the many years that nitrocellulose techniques have been in use, they have been modified in points of detail and, as usual, most workers prefer the variant that they have become accustomed to. Some readers, however, may not be confident of their ability with nitrocellulose. For these readers we give a detailed account of the method which we have found satisfactory for routine use, and which has proved easy to follow by newcomers to nitrocellulose techniques. For a traditional (celloidin) method, the reader is recommended to Anderson (1929), or to earlier editions of Carleton's book (Carleton, 1926; Carleton and Leach, 1938; Carleton and Drury, 1957). Much information about the celloidin technique and its modifications will be found in the various editions of *The Microtomist's Vade-mecum* (Lee, 1885, 1890, 1893, 1896, 1900, 1905, 1913; Gatenby *et al.*, 1921, 1928, 1937, 1950).

Whichever nitrocellulose method is chosen, the results will be similar and will show certain advantages and disadvantages when compared with paraffin wax. The most important advantage to be gained by using nitrocellulose is freedom from shrinkage and fragmentation of the tissue. It is therefore the ideal method for tissues which are particularly susceptible to damage of this kind, notably brain which suffers more than most kinds of tissue from the heating that is inevitable when paraffin wax is used. Heat is also detrimental to organs that are partly composed of tough tissue and partly of delicate tissue. Such organs (e.g. eyes) benefit considerably when embedded in nitrocellulose. The other great merit of nitrocellulose is the firm support that it gives to the tissue. For this reason it is often used when high-quality sections are required from decalcified bone or similar dense tissue.

The disadvantages of nitrocellulose are the slowness of the method, the fire-hazards of the reagents used, the difficulty of cutting sections (and especially serial sections) from the blocks, and the relative thickness (10 μ or greater) of the sections produced. Moreover, the sections are tedious to stain since each one must be handled individually.

Celloidin and LVNC are not obtainable as pure substances since they are unstable when dry and are apt to explode. Each may be obtained in the form of fine woolly particles damped by a fluid such as methylated spirit or butanol. Alternatively LVNC may be obtained as a strong solution in alcohol-ether mixture.

Processing

The principle of processing by nitrocellulose methods is analagous to paraffin processing. The tissue must first be thoroughly fixed (preferably in formalin-saline or neutral buffered formalin solution). It is then dehydrated by increasing concentrations of alcohol; this will often need to be done slowly since large and relatively thick pieces of tissue are often selected. From undiluted alcohol the tissue is transferred to a mixture of equal parts of alcohol and ether, and then to a series of solutions of increasing strength of nitrocellulose in alcohol and ether. When it reaches a sufficiently strong solution, it is orientated suitably and the nitrocellulose is allowed to harden.

Low viscosity nitrocellulose schedule

REAGENTS (see Note i)

A. *Alcohol-ether mixture*

Alcohol (methylated spirit 74° O.P.)	100 ml.
Ether (diethyl ether, technical grade)	100 ml.

B. *Thin LVNC*

Thick LVNC (see below)	200 ml.
Alcohol	100 ml.
Ether	100 ml.

Mix thoroughly.

C. *Thick LVNC*

Low viscosity nitrocellulose (damped)	400 g.
Celloidin (damped) (see Note iii)	20 g.
Alcohol	1000 ml.
Ether	1000 ml.

Pour the alcohol on to the LVNC and celloidin; allow to soak for at least 3 hours; add the ether and mix by repeated inversion during several days. Since the degree of damping is inconstant, it may be necessary to adjust this solution, making it thinner by adding alcohol and ether or thicker by adding LVNC. The consistency required is rather thicker than cold treacle but not too thick to pour.

D. *Chloroform* (*technical grade*)

E. *Chloroform and cedarwood oil mixture I*

Chloroform	200 ml.
Cedarwood oil (clearing quality)	100 ml.

F. *Chloroform and cedar wood oil mixture II*

Chloroform	150 ml.
Cedarwood oil	150 ml.

G. *Chloroform and cedarwood oil mixture III*

Chloroform	100 ml.
Cedarwood oil	200 ml.

H. *Cedarwood oil*

METHOD

1. After thorough fixation, the tissue is dehydrated by treating it with increasing concentrations of alcohol. It is better to use many short steps than to jump from low to high concentrations. It is essential also to dehydrate the tissue thoroughly; thick pieces of brain may need as long

as 24 hours at each stage. The concentrations of alcohol are: 50, 70, 80, 90 per cent, and finally three treatments with undiluted alcohol.

2. Alcohol-ether mixture 1–2 days.
3. Thin LVNC (in tightly closed vessel) 1–2 weeks.
4. Thick LVNC (in tightly closed vessel) 1–2 weeks.
5. Embed in fresh thick LVNC. This should be done in a flat-bottomed glass vessel (see Note iv), using sufficient LVNC to form a layer 2–3 cm. thick. The vessel must be sealed or placed in a larger sealed container; in either case, a satisfactory seal would be a well-greased plate of glass.
6. When all air bubbles have risen and burst (usually within about 24 hours), the solvent is allowed to evaporate (see Note i). This must be done very gradually at first; the seal is moved slightly to leave a small aperture for an hour or two, and then replaced until the next day. During several days the time is lengthened progressively until, after about 7–10 days, the seal is left off entirely. Attempts to hasten evaporation cause bubbles to form (see Note v). If the LVNC shrinks too much, more may be added (see Note vi).
7. Evaporation has gone far enough when the LVNC no longer clings to a probe (e.g. a finger nail) although it is still easily dinted by one. It is then removed from the embedding vessel, trimmed to a suitable size (see Note vii) and transferred to chloroform for 1–2 days to harden.
8. The hardened block is transferred successively to mixtures of chloroform and cedarwood oil (E, F, and G above) for 3 days each, and finally to pure cedarwood oil, in which the block may be stored indefinitely both before sections are cut and afterwards.

Notes

(i) Both ether and nitrocellulose are extremely inflammable (nitrocellulose is also explosive if allowed to become dry). At every stage, these reagents must be kept away from naked flames; this is particularly important during the evaporation of the solvent when good ventilation is essential.

(ii) When LVNC is purchased as a strong solution in alcohol-ether, it is often not thick enough for use. In this case it should be allowed to evaporate at room temperature until it thickens to a suitable consistency.

(iii) The small proportion of celloidin in the mixture gives flexibility to the LVNC, which is otherwise apt to produce a rather brittle block. A similar effect can be obtained by the addition of 1 per cent of tricresyl phosphate (Chesterman and Leach, 1949) or 0·5 per cent of castor oil (Moore, 1951) instead of celloidin. These additives are often referred to as plasticizers.

(iv) For obvious reasons the vessel used for embedding should have a flat bottom. Glass is better than metal because it allows bubbles to be seen even when they are trapped below the tissue. Paper or cardboard are poor, because they become drawn in and deformed when the LVNC shrinks. Vessels of rectangular shape are preferable; if circular ones are used the centre of the block is particularly liable to become too thin as it dries, while the edges are correspondingly thicker. The vessel should be of a considerably greater area than the specimen of tissue, since the LVNC sometimes shrinks back from the sides during evaporation, and in any case the edges are likely to be damaged when the block is removed from the embedding vessel.

(v) If bubbles appear in the LVNC block during evaporation, the vessel should be sealed until they rise and burst. Superficial bubbles can be removed with ether vapour—either by pouring the heavy vapour (but no fluid) into the embedding vessel from a bottle of ether, or by putting an open container of ether into the same vessel as the LVNC block and closing the lid.

(vi) When the level of LVNC in the embedding vessel falls too much, it is perfectly satisfactory to add more of the thick solution provided that the vessel is closed for several hours to allow the old and new solutions to mix and the bubbles to escape.

(vii) When evaporated blocks are trimmed, the waste pieces should not be incinerated, nor allowed to fall into the hands of refuse collectors; they should be dissolved in alcohol and ether and used again. When, however, the LVNC has been saturated with cedarwood oil, we dispose of it by adding it in small amounts to a large incinerator where it burns with a bright flare.

Cutting sections

The first problem is to attach the LVNC block rigidly to the block-holder. Like most steps in the LVNC technique, this is somewhat laborious. First the block must be made completely flat on the surface that is to be attached; this is best achieved by rubbing it on fairly coarse sandpaper on a flat surface. The block is then placed in a shallow vessel and supported on two pieces of thin stick or wire. Sufficient alcohol-ether mixture is poured into the vessel to wet the flattened surface and a millimetre or so of the side of the block. It should be left here until the surface becomes tacky; this will take at least 15 minutes ~~but is unlikely to need as long as 30 minutes.~~

Meanwhile the block-holder should be prepared. This must be at least as large as the block, it should have generous criss-cross grooves on its surface to increase adhesion, and it must be firm and incompressible. Very hard wood may be used but resin-bonded compressed textile blocks (e.g. 'Carp') are preferable. The block-holder must first be moistened with alcohol. When the block becomes tacky, the top surface of the block-holder is liberally coated with thick LVNC solution and the block is pressed firmly on to it. It is held in this position with a weight for 5 minutes or so; the block-holder with attached block is then put into chloroform to harden the newly-applied LVNC. The hardening process takes 30–60 minutes but should not be prolonged unnecessarily since chloroform tends to remove cedarwood oil from the block, making subsequent section cutting difficult. Indeed it is a wise precaution to put the block once again into cedarwood oil for 30 minutes or so before sections are cut.

Microtomes used for cutting LVNC sections must have an arrangement for fixing the knife with a considerable angle of slant (Chap. 5, p. 53). This means that a sledge microtome is nearly always used. Traditionally a sledge microtome with moving knife is preferred because the angle of slant can be very large. In practice, however, microtomists who are more accustomed to using a sledge microtome with moving block can obtain perfectly good results with this type of instrument provided that the knife is slanted. Although a plano-concave knife is recommended for cutting LVNC blocks, good sections can be cut with a properly sharpened wedge knife. If the block is oblong, it is fixed on to the microtome so that the short side is to the front, because a long stroke is easy to manage whereas a shorter stroke on a broad front is more difficult. After the block has been orientated, it is cut until all surplus LVNC has been removed from its face exposing the tissue, but on no account should the edges of the LVNC be trimmed since this is likely to loosen it from the block-holder.

Sections are then cut as slowly as possible, with a continuous movement; jerks must be avoided. If the knife and block have been prepared properly, it is not difficult to cut good sections slowly, but when the knife is blunt or the LVNC is insufficiently hard, the sections may crumble unless cut fairly quickly. Some nitrocellulose methods (so-called wet methods) need the block to be covered with 70 per cent alcohol when sections are cut, but if the block has been prepared according to the schedule given above, it will almost always be easier to cut sections from it dry. Occasionally, however, a block may be encountered which yields only very finely wrinkled and corrugated sections; this will sometimes do better if wetted. It is usual to cut sections at a thickness of 15–20 μ; it is difficult to cut them thinner than 10 μ; sections thicker than 20–25 μ are rarely called for.

When the sections have been cut, they are transferred, one at a time, to a shallow container of 70 per cent alcohol, where they are flattened by stroking them gently against the bottom of the vessel with a pair of soft brushes. Once flat the sections tend to stay flat and can be transferred to a jar of 70 per cent alcohol in which they can be stored indefinitely, so long as evaporation is prevented.

The nitrocellulose techniques do not lend themselves to the production of serial sections. A small series may, however, be collected in a row of numbered bottles. If a large series is needed the sections should be collected in a pile with a numbered piece of paper between each. Paper should be chosen which does not go soft in 70 per cent alcohol and does not leave fibres on the sections; cheap toilet paper is suitable.

When numerous sections have to be cut from a block, this may need to be left on the microtome stage for an interval. If this interval is likely to exceed 10–15 minutes, the block should be covered with a piece of cloth soaked in cedarwood oil to prevent drying.

When the block is removed from the block-holder, it may be stored indefinitely in cedarwood oil. Many blocks can be put into a single large vessel if each is labelled with paper or card. The labels will remain legible if written in indelible India ink; they may be fastened to an unimportant part of the LVNC by an office stapling machine.

Staining

Nitrocellulose sections are generally stained by transferring them from one reagent to the next on a bent glass rod. Brushes are unsuitable, since they are apt to carry too much fluid from container to container. Since nitrocellulose sections are thicker than those usually produced by the paraffin technique, it is better not to attach the sections to slides before staining them since this prevents the reagents from reaching one side. If, however, it is thought desirable to attach a section to a slide, this can be done by flattening it on to the slide, blotting, and then softening the LVNC with ether vapour until it sticks.

Most of the staining methods that are used for paraffin sections can be used for nitrocellulose sections. Several stains were originally intended for nitrocellulose sections rather than paraffin. These include the Loyez and Weigert-Pal methods for myelin, and Schmorl's stain for bone canaliculi. Other staining methods can be used just as they would be used for paraffin sections; these include the Marchi method for degenerate myelin, the Perls method for ferric iron, the von Kóssa method for calcium salts, Best's carmine stain for glycogen, and the simple trichrome methods such as Masson's.

Many staining methods rely on differentiation to achieve the correct result. These include toluidine blue, cresyl fast violet, and nuclear haematoxylin methods (such as Ehrlich's and Weigert's), all of which give excellent results so long as the differentiation is carefully controlled. When haematoxylin is combined with a counterstain of the van Gieson type, care should be taken not to linger over the dehydration of the section.

On the other hand, it is very difficult to get good results from staining methods that rely on critical differentiation. With special care it may be possible to achieve satisfactory results with such methods as the complicated trichrome stains, luxol fast blue, methasol fast blue, and reticulin impregnations, but none of these is really suitable for nitrocellulose sections. Phosphotungstic acid haematoxylin will work provided that mercuric chloride is used as mordant (see Note vi, p. 254). No satisfactory results can be obtained with gallocyanin chrome alum or the per-iodic acid Schiff reaction.

Finishing off

When the sections have been stained, they need to be dehydrated, cleared and finally mounted. Like paraffin sections, they are mounted in synthetic resin (e.g. D.P.X.) or in Canada balsam. Nitrocellulose sections differ from paraffin sections, however, in one important respect, which is that the process of flattening the sections on to slides has to take place during dehydration. So long as the sections are in a watery solution, they are unruly and will not lie flat. When they ultimately reach the clearing agent, they again become rigid, and cannot be flattened. The flattening must be done during the intermediate stage, when the sections are in a strong concentration of alcohol, which makes them soft, pliable, and sticky. Sections are therefore handled as follows: bent glass rods are used until they reach strong (96 per cent) alcohol; the sections are then flattened on to the slides; all subsequent treatment takes place on the slides. To flatten the sections, each one is taken from 96 per cent alcohol by introducing a slide into the alcohol, catching the section between the slide and a glass rod, and withdrawing it. With practice, it is possible to orientate the section on the slide in whatever direction is required. After removal, the section is flattened with a soft brush until no wrinkles remain. The section is now adherent to the slide but the bond is not strong, so that careful handling is necessary at each subsequent stage.

Reagents are always run gently on to the centre of the section from a Pasteur pipette. They are removed as follows: a piece of tough smooth paper is placed over the slide. The paper must be larger than the slide; cheap toilet paper is usually used, with its shining side towards the section. The slide and paper are then gripped by the thumb and forefinger of one hand and the fluid is removed by the thumb and forefinger of the opposite hand, which move away from the gripped end like a squeegee. The section is sandwiched between slide and paper and will not be displaced during this procedure. The paper is then peeled off very gently and the next reagent added without delay.

The following sequence is satisfactory for dehydration, mounting and clearing. Stages 1–5 are carried out by transferring the section from one vessel to the next. Stages 7–12 are carried out on the slide as described above. At every stage the reagent should be allowed to act for about $\frac{1}{2}$ minute.

1. 50 per cent alcohol.
2. 70 per cent alcohol.
3. 80 per cent alcohol.

4. 90 per cent alcohol.
5. 96 per cent alcohol.
6. Mount the section on a slide. Do not blot after doing so.
7. Alcohol and chloroform in equal parts.
   This mixture is used, instead of undiluted alcohol, to complete dehydration because it does not dissolve the LVNC.
8. Alcohol-chloroform mixture II.
9. Alcohol-chloroform mixture III.
10. Carbol-xylene (p. 286).
11. Xylene I.
12. Xylene II.
13. Wipe the ends and back of the slide, removing most of the xylene, but do not allow the section to dry.
14. Mount.

T

CHAPTER 19

Frozen Sections

General notes. Cryostat: Freezing; Operating the cryostat; Fixation of sections; Rapid haematoxylin and eosin staining; Cryostat mishaps and faults in technique; Comparison with paraffin sections. Other freezing microtomes; Handling loose frozen sections; Urgent frozen sections. Special staining of frozen sections.

WHEN a piece of tissue is frozen solid, sections may readily be cut from it. This technique is used in circumstances where conventional processing and wax (or nitrocellulose) embedding would be unsatisfactory.

First, some tissue components are removed or altered by conventional processing. Thus, frozen sections are used when lipids are to be preserved for demonstration (e.g. by dyes of the Sudan type). Most of the histochemical methods for enzymes demand frozen sections and so do fluorescent antibody techniques. Many neurohistological methods were developed for use with frozen sections; some of these cannot be used on paraffin or nitrocellulose sections.

Secondly, sections may be produced much more rapidly by freezing than by any other method, so that frozen sections are used for urgent diagnostic work (e.g. during the course of a surgical operation).

Thirdly, wax and nitrocellulose do not provide enough support for certain very dense tissues such as tendons and decalcified teeth. It is easier to cut frozen sections from material of this type, and the sections obtained are flatter.

Tissue for frozen sections does not need to be fixed before sections are cut. For many histochemical enzyme techniques and fluorescent antibody techniques, it must be fresh and unfixed; urgent sections are commonly prepared from unfixed tissue. On the other hand, tissue is usually fixed before frozen sections are cut for the demonstration of lipids, for neurohistological methods, and when the tissue is very dense. Fixation in formalin solutions is satisfactory; alcoholic fixing fluids are inconvenient because of their low freezing point which makes it very difficult to freeze the tissue unless the alcohol is washed out. Mercuric chloride produces tissue that becomes brittle when frozen; the mercury salt attacks knife edges; the removal of mercuric fixation deposit may present problems.

Fixed tissue is more difficult to section than fresh tissue, especially when the sections are cut in a cryostat. This may be due to the swelling effect that formalin has on tissue, with a consequent increase in the amount of water in the block. The problem will be solved if the fixed tissue is treated for some hours (preferably overnight) with dextran or gum-sucrose. We have had satisfactory results with dextran, using a preparation that is supplied for intravenous therapy ('Dextravan 110'). This consists of an aqueous solution of 6 per cent dextran (m.w. 110,000) and 0·9 per cent sodium chloride. Gum-sucrose, which is recommended by Bancroft (1967), is an aqueous solution of 1 per cent gum acacia and 30 per cent sucrose.

Cryostat

The easiest way to produce frozen sections is by means of a cryostat. The alternative is a freezing microtome or an ordinary microtome with freezing attachments; these instruments are discussed below. Several types of cryostat are available, and these vary in detail, but basically each consists of a refrigerated cabinet containing a microtome which can be operated by controls outside the cabinet. The rocker microtome is particularly suitable, since low temperatures have no effect on its pivoting movement, whereas frost is apt to make the sliding movement of other types of microtome stiff. It is rarely necessary to cut frozen sections from pieces of tissue that are too large for the rocker microtome. If, however, large frozen sections are required, a cryostat may be equipped with a rotary microtome or even with a motor-driven sledge microtome. The cabinet in which the microtome is mounted is usually maintained at a temperature of − 20°C, but different types of specimen need lower or higher temperatures, so that some form of temperature control should be included. Often there is a particularly cold chamber within the main cabinet; this may be used for freezing pieces of tissue rapidly.

The cryostat requires little routine maintenance. Frost will slowly accumulate within the cabinet, especially if it is left open. Moderate amounts of frost do not affect the rocker microtome, except for the advancing mechanism; this should be wound upwards and downwards to its full extent each day before the cryostat is used. Full defrosting of the cabinet is needed every two months or so; this may be hastened by using a hair-dryer or other warm air blower. After defrosting and drying, the microtome should be cleaned and oiled. A special low temperature lubricating oil (e.g. Shell 'Clavis 17') must be used.

In order to prevent sections from rolling up as they are cut, the cryostat is fitted with an anti-roll plate. This consists of a piece of glass that is held a short distance away from the knife edge. A piece of an ordinary (76 × 25 mm.) glass slide is suitable; wider slides can be used for unusually wide pieces of tissue. The plate is held away from the knife by thin strips of adhesive cellulose tape (e.g. 'Scotch tape') on the edges of the slide. An anti-roll plate is prepared from a suitable length of glass slide with an end free from chips. Cellulose tape is attached to the edges and folded over the sides, excess being trimmed off with a razor blade (Fig. 10). These strips form cushions which hold

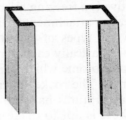

Fig. 10

the plate about 50 microns away from the knife, allowing the sections to pass between them. The plate checks the sections if they curl. Although the section touches the plate, it bounces off and remains in contact with the knife. Occasionally sections may remain attached to the plate rather than the knife; if this occurs, the anti-roll plate may be sprayed with polytetrafluoroethylene (Teflon) in the form of an aerosol to make it smoother. The position of the anti-roll plate in relation to the knife edge is of critical importance. The edge of the plate must be slightly higher than the knife edge and almost directly above it, so that the block of tissue just avoids fouling the plate. The face of the plate must be parallel with the cutting bevel of the knife, not with the knife blade (Fig. 11).

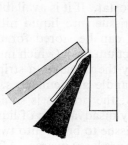

Fig. 11

The knife in common use with a rocker microtome has two slightly concave surfaces. Knives with integral handles are best avoided, since they are not easy to fit onto an automatic sharpening machine. Automatic sharpening is far better than hand honing for cryostat work because it is difficult to use the anti-roll plate properly if the knife edge is not straight; hand honing inevitably removes more metal from the middle than the ends of the knife. It is sometimes stated that knives for cryostat use are not improved by stropping; in our experience, however, stropping improves the edge of the knife so long as a proper stropping device is fixed to the back of the blade.

Freezing

For satisfactory results, tissue must be frozen rapidly. If this is done, innumerable submicroscopic ice-crystals form: if freezing is slow the ice forms a smaller number of large crystals which displace the tissue constituents, leaving clefts which ruin the appearance of the finished section ('ice-crystal artefact'). At the same time as it is cooled, the piece of tissue is attached to the metal block-holder by a drop of water or dextran which freezes solid. Thin pieces of tissue (2–3 mm.) will obviously freeze more quickly than thicker ones.

Some cryostats include a particularly cold chamber which is adequate for rapid freezing: the block-holder is first cooled in this chamber, it is then removed and the tissue is attached by a drop of water, and finally the block-holder with tissue is returned to the cold chamber until it is thoroughly frozen (1–2 minutes).

The alternative is to use a cooling mechanism that is entirely separate from the cryostat. If it is available, the best method of all is to plunge the tissue into liquid nitrogen. This is fairly widely available and can be stored for up to one day in an ordinary domestic vacuum flask (which must not be stoppered). It is convenient to lay the tissue on a strip of metal foil, which makes it easier to handle and enhances cooling. Freezing is almost instantaneous: the process is sometimes referred to as 'quenching'. The only disadvantage of liquid nitrogen is that it may cause pieces of tissue to break into two or more fragments, especially if the pieces are large in area. After it has been cooled, the tissue is attached to a cold block-holder with a drop of water or dextran.

Other cooling mechanisms include: solid carbon dioxide; mixtures of solid carbon dioxide and alcohol or acetone; expanding carbon dioxide gas from a cylinder; and proprietory aerosol sprays (e.g. Arctic Spray). These are usually used to cool the block-holder which, in turn, cools the piece of tissue by conduction. Alcohol and acetone mixtures in particular may have an adverse effect if applied directly to the tissue. A device that makes use of solid carbon dioxide has been described by Barry and Spring (1967). Devices that make use of expanding carbon dioxide gas are available commercially or can be improvised from parts of a freezing microtome.

If it is necessary to cut sections of one or more tiny fragments, these cannot conveniently be attached directly to the surface of the block-holder, as there would be no clearance between block-holder and knife. It is, however, simple to build up successive frozen layers on the block-holder and then attach the fragments, finally flooding the surface with fluid to fill the interstices between them. Water should not be used for this purpose since ice will not cut easily. The dextran solution already mentioned (p. 275) is satisfactory and so are gum solutions and strong sugar solutions.

Operating the cryostat

Cryostats, like all other instruments, cannot be used properly until the operator has gained experience in their use. Although there is no substitute for familiarity, the following points are particularly important or easy to overlook. (1) The instrument should be kept shut whenever possible; if it is left open, the cabinet temperature rises and also frost forms more quickly. (2) When securing the block-holder to the rocker microtome, it is essential to wind the feed arm well down the spindle of the advancing mechanism; this point may be overlooked in cryostats that have the microtome partly concealed at the back of the cabinet. (3) Before operating the cryostat, the linkages, should be checked. In some models a chain connects the external handle to the microtome, and a cord links the microtome handle to the rocker arm. Both of these should pass over pulleys but are apt to slip off, making operation unsatisfactory. (4) Rough cutting of the tissue, to remove superficial excess, must be carried out in fairly small steps (15–25 μ); attempts to slice thick pieces from the surface will often break the joint between tissue and block-holder. (5) The best instrument for removing tissue fragments or unwanted sections from the knife or anti-roll plate is a long-handled brush with a small square end made of stiff bristles (No. 4, Series AA Herkomer). This brush should be wiped frequently with alcohol, acetone, or chloroform to remove grease from the bristles. (6) The knife and anti-roll plate are wiped clean after use, but it is better to avoid handling them when the cryostat is actually being used. If, however, it becomes essential to polish them during use, they may conveniently be re-cooled with a proprietory aerosol spray (e.g. Arctic Spray). (7) The optimum cabinet temperature for one type of specimen is not necessarily suitable for another. The best results with fresh tissues are usually obtained at $-20°C$ to $-25°C$. Fixed tissue, frozen after preliminary soaking in dextran, yields the best results at $-10°C$ to $-14°C$. In special cases (e.g. brain) a temperature as high as $-8°C$ to $-10°C$ may be used.

Collecting sections on slides is very easy. The anti-roll plate is swung out of place and the face of the slide is advanced squarely towards the section as it lies on the knife. As soon as they touch, the section jumps onto the slide. With practice, the slide can be moved relative to the section at the moment of contact and any wrinkles in the section will be stretched out flat. For most purposes, slides are coated with an adhesive such as Mayer's albumin (p. 66) before they are used. Slides must not be too cold or the sections will not be attracted; the lower limit is about 0°C. Coverslips may be used instead of slides; they are held by a rubber suction device. Occasionally it may be necessary to obtain sections loose rather than attached to slides. These are simply allowed to fall down the chute beneath the knife, and are collected in a shallow vessel containing the appropriate reagent. The manipulation of loose sections is described below (p. 285).

Fixation of sections

Once the section is attached to the slide (or coverslip), the next step will depend on whether the tissue has been fixed before being sectioned, also on the purpose for which the sections have been made. Sections from fixed tissue do not need to be fixed again; they should be allowed to become nearly dry ($\frac{1}{2}$–2 minutes) and may then be placed in 70 per cent alcohol. Sections of fresh tissue are usually fixed, although they may be needed unfixed for some purposes (e.g. histochemical or immunological studies). Before they are fixed they should be left in the air until nearly dry ($\frac{1}{2}$–1 minute). We have had satisfactory results from the mercuric-alcohol fixing fluid that is also recommended for smears (p. 324). This fluid consists of a mixture of equal volumes of alcohol and a saturated aqueous solution of mercuric chloride. Those who prefer to avoid mercuric salts may obtain good results using mixtures of alcohol and acetic acid with or without formalin. One typical fluid consists of 5 parts of acetic acid and 95 parts of alcohol; another is 10 parts of formalin, 3 parts of acetic acid, and 87 parts of alcohol. We have preferred the results after mercuric-alcohol; nuclei in particular are fixed well. It is also possible to demonstrate lipids by methods of the Sudan type after mercuric-alcohol fixation, whereas lipids are dissolved in the stronger alcoholic mixtures.

Rapid haematoxylin and eosin staining

There is no reason why cryostat sections should not be stained by a wide variety of methods when time allows. For urgent diagnosis, however, the section is usually stained by a rapid modification of one of the routine haematoxylin and eosin staining schedules. The following makes use of the same reagents as Harris's haematoxylin and eosin method for paraffin sections (p. 99). A bottle containing ammonia is the only additional requirement.

METHOD

1. Fix in any of the above fluids for not less than 1 minute.
2. Rinse in tap water.
3. Harris's haematoxylin 1 minute.
4. Rinse in tap water.
5. Differentiate in acid alcohol 5 seconds.
6. Rinse in tap water.
7. Hold section over a bottle of ammonia until blue.
8. Wash in tap water.
9. Eosin 5 seconds.
10. Rinse in tap water.
11. Dehydrate, clear, and mount.

Cryostat mishaps and faults in technique

Failure to obtain good results from a cryostat may be due to faults in freezing the tissue, faults in the cryostat and its use, or faults in the subsequent handling of the section. To simplify the tracing of faults, it is convenient to group them according to the defects they produce

(i) *Tissue cracks as it is frozen.* Use a thinner piece of tissue. If this still cracks, freeze less abruptly (e.g. by cooling the block-holder and allowing this to cool the tissue).

(ii) *Tissue breaks loose from block-holder.* Use a larger drop between tissue and block-holder. Cut into the face of the tissue in smaller steps.

(iii) *Knife fails to cut tissue.* If the block of tissue will not advance towards the knife, check the mechanical links. If they are sound, make sure that the advancing mechanism is not impeded by frost or at the limit of its travel.

(iv) *Tissue advances but is not cut.* Tighten the knife clamps and block-holder. Examine the joint between the tissue and block-holder. Be sure that the knife is tilted enough. Swing the anti-roll plate away and try again; this shows whether the anti-roll plate is fouling the tissue. Examine the tissue (especially if it is fatty) to ensure that it is frozen solid.

(v) *Sections roll up.* Check that cellulose tape extends to the top of the anti-roll plate. Check that the anti-roll plate is high enough. Ensure that the anti-roll plate is at the correct angle (parallel with the cutting bevel of the knife).

(vi) *Sections thaw when cut.* Cool the knife and anti-roll plate.

(vii) *Sections stick to anti-roll plate.* Cool the anti-roll plate. Remove grease from the anti-roll plate.

(viii) *Sections are puckered.* Sometimes a part of the section appears to be caught. If caught at one end, the section slews; if caught in the middle it assumes a butterfly shape. Sections may pucker for any of the following reasons which should be sought and remedied: debris on the knife edge, a nicked knife edge, a chipped anti-roll plate, a knife of uneven sharpness, a wide block of tissue fouling the cellulose tape.

(ix) *Sections split vertically.* Sometimes the sections split vertically into two or more parts as soon as they are cut; the parts may diverge on the knife blade. When this occurs, clean the front and back of the knife. If this provides no remedy, the knife is probably very blunt. Knives removed from the cryostat cabinet must be dried thoroughly or they will rust.

(x) *Sections are incomplete in width.* The anti-roll plate is not parallel with the knife edge, so that part of it is too high or too low. Sections appear only where the height is correct. Correct setting of the anti-roll plate is particularly difficult when knives have been honed by hand, since these have curved cutting edges.

(xi) *Sections are incomplete in height.* Shorten the cord on the rocker microtome until the rocker arm rises to a sufficient height.

(xii) *Sections wash off slides.* This may occur during fixation or during staining if the slides were put into fixing fluid without adequate drying.

(xiii) *Sections show ice crystal artefact.* This occurs when tissue is not frozen rapidly enough. Thick pieces of tissue are particularly susceptible.

(xiv) *Sections appear fissured.* Sometimes the stained sections are fissured by innumerable fine cracks parallel to the knife edge. This occurs if the tissue was too cold when it was cut. Fixed tissue cut at any temperature is apt to show this fault unless it was soaked in dextran or gum before being frozen.

(xv) *Blurred staining.* Sometimes the tissue may fail to stain sharply, the nucleus in particular being pale and lacking definition. This occurs if the section was allowed to become too dry before fixation.

(xvi) *Pale eosin.* This occurs if the section is not washed thoroughly after treatment with ammonia vapour.

(xvii) *Other staining faults.* Cryostat sections are liable to the same faults as paraffin sections stained with haematoxylin and eosin (see p. 101).

Comparison with paraffin sections

People who are used to paraffin sections may at first be dissatisfied with the microscopic appearances of sections prepared in the cryostat. In general the paraffin sections show sharper demarcation of structures, especially nuclei. With increasing familiarity, however, the cryostat sections will be found just as satisfactory; it is merely a matter of becoming accustomed to a different sort of appearance.

Advantages of cryostat sections fall into two groups. First, rapid results may be obtained with unfixed tissue when a section is required urgently. Secondly, it is possible to demonstrate tissue components that would be destroyed by paraffin processing. Thus cryostat sections are used for the demonstration of lipids, for most kinds of enzyme histochemistry, and for the demonstration of antigens by immunofluorescence techniques. It is sometimes a great advantage to be able to treat several sections from one piece of tissue by different methods; to stain one by haematoxylin and eosin while treating a neighbouring section by an immunological technique, for instance; or to fix several sections in different fixing fluids.

Advantages of paraffin sections again fall into two groups. First, paraffin sections are easier to cut and easier to handle. Thus, the paraffin method will be preferred for large sections, or when perfect sections are required. Large numbers of paraffin sections (e.g. for class teaching sets) are easily produced. Serial sections, which can be prepared comparatively easily by the paraffin method, are more difficult in the cryostat. Secondly, it is easy to store unused paraffin material, either in the form of unstained spare sections or as paraffin blocks. Unused cryostat sections are more difficult to store, and blocks must either be kept sealed and frozen or be processed and embedded in wax. Care must be taken in the preparation of wax blocks from frozen pieces of tissue since rapid thawing will give rise to artefacts. These will be avoided if the tissue is allowed to warm gradually. The piece is transferred from the cryostat cabinet to a refrigerator at 4°C for one hour, after which it may be fixed in a formalin-saline fluid at room temperature without distortion (Aves *et al.*, 1965).

Other freezing microtomes

Before cryostats were available, frozen sections were cut on a freezing microtome (p. 48) or an ordinary microtome fitted with an arrangement for freezing the tissue. The freezing microtome occupies little space and is fairly easy to transport; in most other respects a cryostat is preferable.

A drop of syrupy gum acacia solution is placed between the

block-holder and the tissue, which may be frozen by allowing carbon dioxide gas from a cylinder to expand in the hollow block-holder. The gas should be released in short sharp bursts, since a continuous flow may cause frost to obstruct the tubing. A stream of gas is sometimes directed onto the knife to cool that also.

The alternative cooling device is a thermoelectric module which makes use of the Peltier effect (direct current flowing across a bimetallic junction produces a temperature gradient). In addition to a supply of electricity, a supply of circulating cold water is needed to remove heat from the module. It is essential to start the flow of water before switching on the current, otherwise heat will damage the module, especially its electrical connections.

The carbon dioxide method is quicker and is self-contained, requiring only cylinders of the gas. Thermoelectric modules are much easier to control, so that the tissue may be maintained at a constant temperature. This is important when more than one section is required, because tissue cannot be cut if it is not cold enough, and is likely to fragment if attempts are made to cut it too cold. Using carbon dioxide, it is best to over-cool the tissue and allow it to warm up, hastening the process if necessary by pressing a finger against it.

Sections prepared by either method are usually transferred to a shallow vessel of water. This should be distilled or freshly-boiled water, otherwise dissolved air will form bubbles on the sections. The sections are then either collected on albuminized slides and attached by drying and gentle heat, or are carried through the stains and other reagents loose. It is possible to cool the tissue and the knife by means of modules until a dry section is produced which will jump onto a slide like a cryostat section. The expense of such a system is, however, considerable.

As already stated, the cryostat is preferable to the freezing microtome in almost every respect. The chief drawbacks of the freezing microtome are as follows. It is impossible to cut thin sections. Sections are more difficult to handle unless the knife is also cooled; small fragments present a serious problem; serial sections are almost impossible. Loose-textured tissue, such as lung, needs preliminary treatment with gelatin as described below.

On the other hand, the freezing microtome is relatively small, portable, and cheap. For a few specimens it may be preferable because a wide variation of temperature can be obtained rapidly. Thus, dense firm specimens (such as cartilage and decalcified teeth) are easier to cut when the tissue is only just below freezing point. Using a freezing microtome it is possible to overcool the tissue and then warm the face of the block by finger pressure without melting the joint between tissue and block-holder. The cold atmosphere of the cryostat makes this more difficult.

Gelatin is used to stiffen porous specimens (e.g. lung), or tissue that contains much fat, or tissue that is apt to fragment (e.g. myocardium). Fixed tissue must first be washed well to remove the fixative, impregnated with $12\frac{1}{2}$ per cent gelatin at 37°C for about one day, then with 25 per cent gelatin at 37°C for about one day. It is next embedded in 25 per cent gelatin and cooled. The block is trimmed to a suitable size and fixed for about three days in 15 per cent formalin to harden the gelatin. Sections can then be cut.

Handling loose frozen sections

When sections are stained by transferring them from reagent to reagent on a bent glass rod (section-lifter), they must be free from creases at every stage if uniform staining is to be achieved. The section-lifter is usually prepared from glass rod of about 4 mm. diameter; it is worth trying several shapes, since different workers prefer greater or smaller curves and a larger or smaller knob at the end. Brushes should be avoided as they transfer too much fluid from one vessel to the next. Moreover, sections tend to cling to the bristles.

When a section spends a long time in a reagent, it must be carefully laid flat in the vessel. If only a short treatment is needed, the section is merely lowered into the reagent, taking care that it is carefully balanced on the glass rod without creases. Wide, shallow glass vessels are the most suitable. When a reagent is strongly coloured, there is the danger that the section may be lost in it; a strong source of light below the vessel may then be helpful.

When a section is transferred from an alcoholic reagent to an aqueous one, it should be pushed below the surface and help there for a few moments. If allowed to float, it will be forcibly stretched as an effect of surface tension; this will certainly flatten the section, but may easily cause delicate tissue to break.

When staining is complete, the section is mounted on a clean grease-free slide. This is easily done from a large vessel filled with water almost to the brim. The section is caught between slide and glass rod, and withdrawn from the water. Creases can be removed by lowering first one part of the slide and then another into the water. Depending on the staining method used, the section will be mounted in either an aqueous or a resinous mounting medium. Aqueous media (e.g. Apáthy's, p. 89; glycerin-jelly, p. 89) are relatively straightforward. Water is wiped from the ends and back of the slide, which is then held vertically to allow excess water to drain from the section. When the section is nearly dry, the slide is lowered squarely onto a coverslip charged with the mounting medium. When the medium has set, the preparation should be sealed with a ringing medium (p. 88).

Resinous media (e.g. DPX, p. 86) can only be used if the section is dehydrated and cleared. Once again, excess water is allowed to drain until the section is nearly dry. Alcohol may then be pipetted onto the centre of the section, or the slide may be immersed very gently in alcohol. The section is carefully blotted and treated for a second time with alcohol, and then once with carbol-xylene (25 per cent phenol in xylene) and twice with ordinary xylene, blotting between each stage. Finally the section is mounted in a resinous medium.

Urgent frozen sections

If a cryostat is not available, sections for rapid diagnosis may be prepared as follows. Heat some formalin-saline to about 80°C. Cut or select a piece of tissue about 3–4 mm. thick and not larger than 1 cm. square; place this in the formalin-saline. Do not boil. After about two minutes fixation, attach the tissue to the microtome and cut sections of about 10 μ thickness. Place the sections in distilled water and unroll them if necessary. Mount a suitable section on an albuminized slide, drain off excess water, and dry by gentle flaming. The section may then be stained by the haematoxylin and eosin method that is used for cryostat sections (p. 280), starting at stage 3. If a quicker, simple stain is preferred, use toluidine blue (p. 149).

It is possible to cut frozen sections of fresh unfixed tissue on a freezing microtome. The sections are handled loose and may be stained with toluidine blue or the Geschickter (1930) mixture; they are mounted in 50 per cent glycerol or a 40 per cent glucose solution. The preparations are not permanent. Both the technical procedures and the histological examination present considerable difficulties, and should not be used for urgent diagnosis without extensive practice on unimportant tissue.

Special staining of frozen sections

Although the majority of frozen sections, especially those prepared for rapid diagnosis, are stained by haematoxylin and eosin, there is no reason why other staining methods should not be used for special purposes. In this respect cryostat sections attached to slides are far more versatile than loose sections from a freezing microtome. Any of the methods used with paraffin sections may be applied to cryostat sections. For some purposes cryostat sections are better because a variety of appropriate fixing fluids may be chosen for the different staining methods to be used (including stains for lipids).

Although cryostat sections mounted on slides are generally preferable to loose frozen sections, there are a few methods which demand loose sections. For instance, the Cajal method (p. 256) will not work when sections are attached to slides. For methods of this type, sections may, of course, be cut in a cryostat, so long as they are pushed down the chute into a vessel of fluid.

Loose sections may be used for straightforward staining methods, but they are unsuitable for any method that calls for microscopic control of staining or differentiation. Although the sections are usually thicker and might be expected to need longer at each stage, the reagents have access to both sides of the section and may work rapidly. In practice, therefore, it is virtually impossible to modify a complicated staining method for use with loose sections. Techniques that can, however, be used with loose frozen sections include the following: lipid stains, toluidine blue, methyl violet, and the methods of Perls, Gram, Masson-Fontana, Fouchet, and Schmorl (picro-thionin).

CHAPTER 20

Treatment of Bone and Other Calcified Tissue

General notes. Bone marrow. Large specimens. Teeth. Osteoid tissue. Fixation. Tests for decalcification. Individual methods: Custer's fluid; Trichloracetic acid; Nitric acid; EDTA; Müller's fluid. Undecalcified sections. Ground preparations.

BONE contains a large quantity of calcium salts. These make it hard, so that sections cannot be prepared by ordinary techniques. The same is true of other calcified structures including teeth and a variety of tissues in which calcium salts have been deposited as a result of disease; this happens, for instance, in degenerate arteries and in some tissues infected by tuberculosis.

The usual way of preparing sections from calcified tissue is to *decalcify* it, i.e. to remove the calcium salts and then treat the specimen as though it were a piece of soft tissue. Decalcification is carried out after the tissue has been fixed and before it is dehydrated. Alternative techniques for bone are available but they apply only to special cases. In diseases such as rickets, for instance, the amount of calcium in the bones is reduced; these bones may be sufficiently soft for sections to be cut from paraffin blocks without preliminary decalcification. Sections could be cut more easily from frozen tissue, or from tissue embedded in celloidin, but undecalcified bone of normal density can only be sectioned when embedded in specially hard media such as those used for electron microscopy. Small amounts of calcium salts can be removed chemically from the surface of paraffin blocks although this is a poor substitute for decalcification of the whole piece (p. 313).

Many methods of decalcification have been used, including various acids, chelating agents such as ethylene diamine tetracetic acid (EDTA), electrolysis, and ion-exchange resins. Of these, only EDTA and some of the acids are suitable for routine use, the exact choice depending on the type of specimen to be decalcified. There is no single method that will serve all purposes. Methods that are suitable for the histological study of bone structure will not necessarily be good enough to show the fine cytological detail of the *bone marrow*. Methods that are suitable for thin pieces of bone may be useless for large specimens. All decalcifying fluids cause some loss of histological detail and staining qualities, and this loss is greater when decalcification is rapid. The deterioration is likely to be intolerable if the bone has not been adequately fixed.

Since some deterioration of histological detail is inevitable, the choice of a suitable decalcifying fluid for any particular specimen must be a compromise. If speed is essential the histological quality must suffer: if histological detail is essential the decalcification must be slow and gentle. In any case the tissue should be removed from the decalcifying fluid as soon as decalcification is complete; to leave the tissue in the fluid causes damage to the soft components and especially to the bone marrow. This damage can easily be recognized in sections because the haematoxylin will be pale, muddy, and unpleasantly red, and no attempt to increase the intensity of the haematoxylin by lengthening the staining time will be successful.

Tests which can be used for assessing whether decalcification is complete are described on page 293.

Techniques for bone marrow

When the primary interest is in the cells of the bone marrow rather than the calcified bone, it is possible to obtain pure marrow at necropsy by squeezing a short length of rib in a vice and collecting the extruded marrow on a piece of paper which may then be lowered gently into fixative. Marrow scooped from the shaft of the femur is often sufficiently free from bone to be processed without decalcification. This is better than an extruded specimen if the relationship of cells to each other is important, for instance in cases of tumours of the marrow.

Bone marrow aspirated by sternal puncture is easier to handle if it is fixed and processed in an agar support.

Agar cup method

MATERIALS REQUIRED

Pour a layer of plain agar 1 cm. thick in a Petri dish; allow to cool; cut into cubes of 1 cm. side. Cut a core about 0·7 cm.

U

deep and about 0·5 cm. diameter with a cork-borer. The core may come away in the borer; if not it may be extracted with a needle. The cups may be stored indefinitely in formalin-saline.

METHOD

1. Discharge the sample of aspirated marrow from the syringe into a cup and leave for about 30 minutes to clot.
2. Transfer to Helly's fluid; fix for 24–36 hours; wash in running water 12–18 hours.
3. After washing, trim surplus agar from two opposite sides; dehydrate; clear; impregnate with wax.
4. Embed on one of the trimmed sides, so that sections will be cut along the length of the cylinder of marrow and not across it.

Notes

(i) Cells of different types will be found to have sedimented at different rates, with the largest clumps at the bottom of the cup; hence the advisability of longitudinal sections.

(ii) Sections cut thinner than usual (2–3 μ) provide clearer cellular detail.

If it is necessary to examine bone marrow from other bones such as iliac crest, vertebra, or sternum these will need to be decalcified. In these cases, whenever possible, the hard cortex of the bone should be removed and discarded before decalcification since it adds nothing to the histology of the marrow and would need far longer to decalcify than the remaining piece of spongy bone.

Techniques for large bone specimens

It is sometimes necessary to decalcify a whole bone or a part of the skeleton such as a piece of the vertebral column (p. 297). This is particularly useful when soft structures are concealed within bone, for instance the vertebral arteries which can best be demonstrated by dissecting the cervical vertebrae after decalcification (Yates and Hutchinson, 1961). Another technique suitable for specimens that consist partly of bone and partly of soft tissue is to freeze the well-fixed specimen to $-15°C$ or $-20°C$ and then saw slices from it with a bandsaw. After further fixation the slices can be decalcified with better histological results than those obtained from a bone that was decalcified in its entirety. Sawing a frozen specimen may be the best way of demonstrating a bone tumour in an amputated limb, especially when preparing a museum specimen (Baker, 1940).

Techniques for teeth

It is possible to saw thin slices from teeth with a hacksaw or coping saw, but they are difficult to hold, even in a vice, and difficult to saw cleanly. Moreover, the soft pulp of the tooth is often damaged by the saw. A better method is to decalcify the whole tooth in trichloracetic acid after fixation. Sections may then be obtained from pieces embedded in paraffin or nitrocellulose, although the piece tends to break away from the embedding medium. Good frozen sections may be obtained without so much difficulty and without the need for embedding (Smith, 1962). All decalcifying fluids remove the enamel: in order to retain this, sections must be prepared by grinding.

Techniques for osteoid tissues

The preparation of sections for the demonstration of osteoid tissue presents special problems. Osteoid tissue does not contain any calcium salts whereas bone does. With this important difference, however, the two tissues are extremely similar and cannot be distinguished in histological preparations; each tissue takes up stains for collagen and each is demonstrable by polarized light. It is obvious, therefore, that after the calcium salts have been removed from a specimen, it is not easy to see which parts of it are bone and which parts are osteoid tissue. After routine decalcification, no staining method will distinguish them consistently, although a differential staining effect is sometimes seen in sections stained by haematoxylin and eosin when the intensity of the eosin is greatly reduced. For some reason this is clearer in sections that have spent only a short time in eosin (10 seconds in 0·5 per cent aqueous eosin); it is not so clear if the sections are given full eosin staining followed by attempts to differentiate the stain. At its best this method will show light pink osteoid tissue which is easily distinguished from the slate-coloured bone.

Excellent results are obtained by decalcification in Müller's fluid (p. 299). This takes a long time, even for spongy bone, an may fail entirely to decalcify hard cortical bone such as skull. Unlike most methods for osteoid tissue, decalcification in Müller's fluid can be followed by paraffin embedding.

Bone may be sectioned without decalcification, and when the bone is very soft this presents few problems. Normal bone, however, requires support by something harder than paraffin or nitrocellulose and this in turn needs special equipment to cut it. Frozen sections may be cut from bone impregnated with gelatin (p. 300) and these may be good enough for the recognition of osteoid tissue. Except in practised hands, however, this method is apt to yield no more than a scattered collection of bone splinters. The most satisfactory results are obtained from bone embedded in special media such as are used for electron microscopy (epoxy resins and methacrylate). These cannot be used routinely in most histological laboratories and are beyond the scope of this book.

Histological preparations may be obtained by grinding the surfaces of a slice of bone until it is thin enough for microscopy (p. 301).

Notes on fixation

Bone should be fixed more thoroughly than ordinary tissue for two reasons: (i) fixatives penetrate only slowly into dense bone or cellular bone marrow, and (ii) the piece of bone is transferred straight from fixing fluid to decalcifying fluid without the benefit of additional fixation by alcohol that ordinary tissue gets during dehydration.

For large specimens (e.g. vertebrae), formalin-saline and neutral buffered formalin solution are the only satisfactory fixing fluids. As already indicated, it is better to use small pieces whenever possible. For small pieces the choice of fixing fluids is wider although some are not recommended. For instance the collagen matrix of bone is fairly tough, even after decalcification, so that fluids that harden tissues, such as alcoholic formalin and Carnoy's fluid, should be avoided. Other unsatisfactory fixing fluids are those that penetrate poorly, such as Zenker's fluid or fluids that contain osmium tetroxide.

In some laboratories, mercuric chloride would be unsatisfactory because the X-ray test for complete decalcification cannot be used after it. Apart from this, however, there is no reason for avoiding mercuric chloride and, indeed, good results are obtained with fixing fluids that contain it. Helly's fluid is excellent for bone marrow provided that the piece is thin. Mercuric-chloride-formalin and Susa are satisfactory although no better than formalin-saline and neutral buffered formalin solution which are entirely satisfactory for bone and which are surpassed only by Helly's fluid for the cytological detail of bone marrow.

Satisfactory histological preparations can only be obtained if the piece of tissue selected for fixation and decalcification is thin. The lower limit is usually set by the difficulty of sawing very thin pieces of tissue. Thus, hard bone (e.g. skull) can be sawn thinner than spongy bone; pieces of hard bone may be as thin as 1·5–2 mm. whereas it is rarely possible to saw spongy bone thinner than 3 mm.

Tests for decalcification

These fall into three groups: (1) radiological, (2) chemical and (3) palpation tests in which the altered consistency of the bone is judged by fingering it.

Radiological test

When calcium salts have been removed the specimen ceases to show opaque areas on an X-ray film. The method is the simplest and the surest provided that no mercury salts have been used in the fixing fluid. It is not likely to be available in many routine laboratories.

Chemical test

A method for demonstrating calcium ions in the supernatant decalcifying fluid (Clayden, 1952). Not suitable for all decalcifying fluids.

REAGENTS

A. *0·880 ammonia*

B. *Saturated aqueous solution of ammonium oxalate*

METHOD

1. Put about 5 ml. of supernatant decalcifying fluid in a clean tube with a fragment of litmus paper.

2. Add 0·880 ammonia drop by drop shaking repeatedly until the reaction is alkaline.
3. Add approximately 0·5 ml. of the saturated solution of ammonium oxalate. Leave to stand for 30 minutes.

RESULTS

If the simple addition of strong ammonia produces a cloud of calcium hydroxide, decalcification is not complete.

If ammonium oxalate produces cloudiness or a precipitate, decalcification is not complete.

If the fluid remains clear for 30 minutes, decalcification is complete.

Notes

(i) This test shows whether calcium ions have left the tissue since the last time the fluid was changed. For an accurate end-point the test should be made soon after changing the fluid (e.g. 2 hours for trichloracetic acid).

(ii) The method is unsuitable for decalcifying fluids that contain more than 10 per cent of acid (e.g. Custer's fluid).

(iii) The test will only work if distilled water (not tap water) is used in decalcifying fluids.

Palpation tests

When a piece of bone is decalcified it loses its rigidity, becoming as flexible as a piece of soft tissue of similar density. Thus hard cortical bone, such as skull, comes to resemble cartilage: spongy bone such as the middle of a vertebral body becomes almost as soft as a piece of spleen.

Cortical bone becomes flexible so that, on gentle bending, it has the springy quality of a piece of cartilage or thick celluloid. Moreover, if it has been decalcified in acid it has a translucent appearance like that of cartilage.

Spongy bone may be assessed by gentle squeezing between the thumb and forefinger. The word squeezing suggests more violence than is really required; what is needed is no more than a very gentle depression of the surface. Decalcification is complete when no tiny spicules of bone can be felt. This test should be carried out without gloves as even the thinnest pair destroy the feeling of sharpness of incompletely decalcified spicules. To avoid damage to the skin the specimen should be given a short wash in tap water before it is handled.

Degenerate arteries are decalcified when the wall can be compressed by gentle pressure.

Chalky masses, such as form in old tuberculosis, are difficult to assess by palpation. Chemical or radiological tests would be more suitable for this kind of specimen.

The use of sharp instruments to assess the completeness of decalcification is unsatisfactory. Knives and razor-blades are sometimes advocated, but they cannot provide information about the centre of the specimen without causing damage to it. Needles also cause damage and provide information only about the area tested.

Removal of bone dust

Any specimen that has been sawn will have fine fragments of bone dust packed into the interstices near the sawn surface. These spoil histological sections so that the sawn surface should be trimmed by the removal of a very thin slice (1 mm. or less) with a razor-blade. An alternative is to embed the specimen without trimming but to discard 12–20 sections before collecting any.

Removal of decalcifying fluid

It is commonly supposed that prolonged washing or treatment with an alkali is necessary after every decalcifying fluid. We have not found this to be so after Custer's fluid or trichloracetic acid although washing is necessary after Müller's fluid which contains potassium dichromate. Nitric acid formalin is best removed by repeated changes of 70 per cent alcohol.

Individual methods

Many methods and modifications have been published. Individual problems may require special treatment but we have found that the following selection fulfils the various demands of a routine laboratory.

Custer's fluid

A useful routine method for thin pieces of bone; particularly suitable for bone marrow. (Custer, 1933.)

REAGENT

Custer's fluid

> 20% aqueous trisodium citrate   50 ml.
> Formic acid (technical, 90%)   50 ml.

METHOD

1. Place thin well-fixed pieces of tissue in Custer's fluid. The volume should be about 30 times that of the tissue.
2. Examine daily. If not decalcified, change fluid.
3. Trim to remove bone dust.
4. Transfer to 50% alcohol without preliminary washing.
5. Process and embed in paraffin or nitrocellulose.

Notes

(i) Spongy bone (e.g. from a vertebra) is decalcified in about 18–24 hours. Cortical bone may need 5 days or longer.
(ii) Neither washing in water, nor treatment with alkali is necessary.
(iii) Almost all staining methods give good results.
(iv) The chemical test for decalcification cannot be used.

Trichloracetic acid

As good as Custer's fluid for routine use; better for hard cortical bone and teeth (Smith, 1962).

REAGENT

5 per cent aqueous trichloracetic acid

METHOD

1. Place well-fixed thin pieces of tissue or whole teeth in the fluid. The volume should be about 30 times that of the tissue.
2. Examine once or twice a day. If not decalcified, change fluid daily.
3. Trim to remove bone dust.
4. Transfer to 50% alcohol without preliminary washing.
5. Process and embed in paraffin or nitrocellulose.

Notes

(i) Spongy bone (e.g. from a vertebra) is decalcified in about 12–18 hours. Cortical bone needs 3–4 days. Whole teeth need 3–7 days.

(ii) Neither washing in water nor treatment with alkali is necessary.
(iii) Almost all staining methods give good results.

Nitric acid formalin

A quicker method for thin pieces of tissue; staining results are poorer.

REAGENT

Nitric acid formalin

Formalin	10 ml.
Distilled water	80 ml.
Concentrated nitric acid	10 ml.

METHOD

1. Place thin pieces of tissue in the fluid. The volume should be about 30 times that of the tissue.
2. Examine twice daily. If not decalcified, change fluid daily.
3. Trim to remove bone dust.
4. When decalcified, remove acid with 70% alcohol for several hours.
5. Process and embed in paraffin or nitrocellulose.

Notes

(i) Spongy bone (e.g. from a vertebra) is decalcified in about 6–8 hours. Cortical bone needs about 2 days.

(ii) Old discoloured nitric acid should not be used because it stains the tissue yellowish-brown. The addition of 1 per cent urea to a newly-opened bottle of concentrated nitric acid will prevent this discoloration.

(iii) Stains for tissue structure are often unsatisfactory after decalcification in nitric acid, although reasonable results may be obtained with trichrome stains of the Mallory type.

Nitric acid for large specimens

Suitable for softening whole bones so that they can be dissected. Histological appearances are unsatisfactory.

REAGENT

6 per cent aqueous nitric acid

METHOD

1. Fix thoroughly in formalin-saline. Depending on the size of the specimen this will need ½–3 weeks.
2. Transfer to nitric acid solution. The volume should be about 20 times that of the tissue.
3. Change the decalcifying fluid every second day until decalcification is complete.
4. Wash in running tap water before dissection.

Notes

(i) The method takes several days. The exact time will depend on the size and density of the bone; a specimen of cervical vertebrae is usually decalcified in about 7 days.

(ii) Apart from attempting to cut the specimen, the only satisfactory test for complete decalcification is the X-ray method.

(iii) After this method, staining results are very poor but if histological preparations are required the Notes ii and iii to the previous method should be consulted. Transfer to 50 per cent alcohol, process, and embed in paraffin or nitrocellulose.

EDTA

A slow method which is more suitable for research than for the routine laboratory. (Hillemann and Lee, 1953.)

REAGENT

EDTA

Formalin	10 ml.
Distilled water	90 ml.
Ethylene diamine tetracetic acid (di-sodium salt)	5·5 g.

METHOD

1. Place the well-fixed specimen in the fluid. The volume should be about 30 times that of the tissue.
2. Change the fluid once a week. At the same time examine the specimen for complete decalcification; very small specimens may be examined more frequently.
3. Trim to remove bone dust.
4. Transfer to 70% alcohol, process, and embed in paraffin or nitrocellulose.

Notes

(i) Spongy bone (e.g. from a vertebra) is decalcified in about 5–7 days. Cortical bone will need many weeks or months.

(ii) Ethylene diamine tetracetic acid (EDTA) is also known as Versene or Sequestrene. It removes calcium by chelation; it is not an acid. For this reason no gas bubbles are formed and there is less tendency to disruption of tissue components than with any other decalcifying fluid. The method is particularly suitable when delicate soft tissue is encased within bone (e.g. middle ear).

(iii) All staining methods give good results. In our hands the results with ordinary stains for bone and bone marrow are no better than after Custer's fluid. The results of silver impregnations, however, are said to be better.

Müller's fluid

The only method of decalcification that permits a reliable distinction to be made between osteoid tissue and mineralized bone in histological sections. The method is far too slow to be used for any other purpose.

REAGENT

Müller's fluid

Potassium dichromate	5 g.
Sodium sulphate	1 g.
Distilled water	100 ml.

METHOD

1. Place pieces of well-fixed tissue in about 30 volumes of the fluid. The pieces must be very thin (not more than 2 mm. thick).
2. Examine every second week. If not decalcified, change fluid.
3. Trim to remove bone dust.
4. Remove decalcifying fluid by prolonged washing in running water (36–48 hours).
5. Transfer to 50% alcohol, process. and embed in nitro-cellulose or paraffin.

Notes

(i) Spongy bone (e.g. from a vertebra) is decalcified in about 4 weeks. Cortical bone will need about 3–4 months. These times refer to bone of normal density. The method, however, is particularly useful in skeletal diseases such as rickets and osteomalacia in which the bone is soft. The times would then be correspondingly shorter.

(ii) It is not known what chemical reaction brings about decalcification but the probable explanation is that small amounts of chromic acid are liberated in the tissue. This seems not to occur if the sodium sulphate is omitted. Changing the fluid at more frequent intervals does not seem to accelerate this process and may even inhibit it.

(iii) In sections stained by haematoxylin and eosin, mineralized bone stains slaty blue, osteoid tissue stains pink, and the other tissue components stain as usual. It is not known what components of bone are stained by the haematoxylin; Müller's fluid removes calcium salts, and attempts to demonstrate them (e.g. by von Kóssa's method) are unsuccessful.

(iv) The chemical test for decalcification cannot be used.

(v) Poor staining results usually mean that washing was inadequate so that the decalcifying fluid was not fully removed.

(vi) It is doubtful whether Müller himself appreciated that osteoid tissue can be distinguished from bone after fixation in Müller's fluid. He certainly used chromic acid as a fixative for bone from cases of rickets (Müller, 1858), but the first mention of a mixture of potassium dichromate and sodium sulphate that we can trace is concerned with the fixation of an eye (Müller, 1859). We have been unable to discover exactly when Müller's fluid was first used for the demonstration of osteoid tissue, but this property was certainly known to Pommer (1885).

Undecalcified frozen sections

By cutting frozen sections of gelatin-embedded bone, it is possible to avoid the hardening effect of alcohol. Moreover, frozen gelatin provides more support for the bone during sectioning than paraffin wax would do.

REAGENTS

A. *12½ per cent aqueous solution of gelatin*

B. *25 per cent aqueous solution of gelatin*

C. *15 per cent aqueous solution of formalin*

METHOD

1. Fix well in formalin-saline.
2. Running water overnight.
3. Transfer to 12½% gelatin at 37°C 48 hours.

4. Transfer to 25% gelatin at 37°C 48 hours.
5. Embed in 25% gelatin; allow to cool until solid; trim.
6. Transfer block to 15% formalin to harden for at least 3 days.
7. Cut frozen sections at 15 μ and place in distilled water.
8. Stain by the von Kóssa method to show calcium salts (p. 210) or by haematoxylin and eosin.

Notes

(i) For satisfactory sections the block must be frozen hard; carbon dioxide will reduce the temperature further than a thermoelectric module, and is to be preferred.

(ii) An ordinary freezing microtome may be used but a sledge microtome is better, since it is more rigid. In either case the runners should be lubricated with 'Molyslip Slip G' which reduces play.

(iii) The method is unsuitable for cortical bone.

Ground preparations

Undecalcified preparations of cortical bone or teeth may be obtained by grinding a slice until it is thin enough for microscopy.

METHOD

1. Saw the thinnest possible slice of tooth or cortical bone about 1 sq. cm. in area. The specimen must be thoroughly fixed; this may be done either before or after sawing.
2. (a) Grind the slice by rubbing each face in turn against a fine carborundum stone using water as a lubricant and maintaining heavy pressure with the finger.
   or (b) Grind the slice by rubbing it between two ground glass plates using water as lubricant.
3. When thin enough, wash in warm water.
4. Transfer to 50% alcohol; dehydrate; clear in xylene.
5. Transfer to DPX; leave overnight to impregnate; mount in DPX.

Notes

(i) It is not difficult to obtain preparations as thin as 50 μ. These are suitable for examination with a polarizing microscope.

(ii) If ground preparations are called for frequently, a fossil grinder would be worth while (Friend and Smith, 1962; 1964; 1965).

(iii) The soft tissue in the interstices of the bone is destroyed.

CHAPTER 21

Troublesome Specimens

Large paraffin sections. Small pieces. Serial sections. Extra-rapid paraffin sections. Sections for photography. Double embedding. Eyes. Tough tissue. Finger-nails. Unsuspected calcium in paraffin blocks. Sections which detach during staining.

ALMOST all the material received by a histology laboratory can be handled by the routine techniques described in earlier chapters. A few specimens, however, need particular care if good results are to be obtained. The special precautions necessary for the nervous system and for calcified tissue have been dealt with in separate chapters. The present chapter is concerned with miscellaneous specimens and techniques that call for a modification of routine practice if good results are to be obtained.

Large paraffin sections

When sections are required from a block that is unusually large in area, it is necessary to take particular care that the embedded tissue is flat. A large block-holder is not usually fitted with any device for tilting the block. Moreover, any slight warping or curling of the tissue during fixation, processing, or embedding, may make it impossible to cut a section that includes the whole area of the tissue. For these reasons, it is customary to cut thicker pieces of tissue when the area is large; for instance the tissue will need to be at least 5 mm. thick when it is 4 cm. or more across. Even these thick pieces must be prevented from warping; they need to be kept flat during fixation and processing. Tissue should not stand upright in a jar, or lean against its wall. On the other hand, a flat-bottomed vessel has the drawback that the tissue clings to the glass too closely for proper penetration by the reagents. Stiff card (e.g. thick blotting paper) will provide support during fixation. For fixed tissue it is satisfactory to use a bottle or jar with a slightly dome-shaped bottom; this allows reagents to circulate below the tissue, as well as above it.

Thick pieces of tissue cannot be dehydrated, cleared and impregnated as quickly as routine pieces. If such pieces are numerous, it may be worth using an automatic processing machine which has been programmed specially. Smaller numbers should be processed manually.

Manual processing schedule for large pieces

1. 50% alcohol 8 hours.
2. 70% alcohol overnight.
3. 80% alcohol 8 hours.
4. 90% alcohol overnight.
5. Alcohol I 4 hours.
6. Alcohol II 4 hours.
7. Alcohol III overnight.
8. Cedarwood oil I 4–6 hours.
9. Cedarwood oil II overnight (see Note ii).
10. Benzene 10–15 minutes (see Note iii).
11. Wax I 2 hours.
12. Wax II 3 hours.
13. Wax III 3 hours.
14. Embed in fresh wax.

Notes

(i) This schedule is suitable for very large pieces (up to 0·7 cm. thick). If the pieces are thinner, the times may be reduced.

(ii) Cedarwood oil should render the tissue translucent (i.e. should *clear* it in the true sense of the word). If it is not translucent, the tissue should remain longer in cedarwood oil until it is. Cedarwood oil is a specially suitable clearing agent for large pieces but is expensive. If a cheaper clearing agent is needed, trichloroethylene (or carbon tetrachloride or chloroform) should be used. Stages 8-10 would then be modified as follows:

8. Alcohol ⎱
   Trichloroethylene ⎰ equal parts 4 hours.
9. Trichloroethylene I 4 hours.
10. Trichloroethylene II overnight.

(iii) Benzene removes the excess of cedarwood oil from the surface of the tissue, and thus improves wax impregnation.

Automatic processing schedule for large pieces

Each of the following stages should last for 4 hours if pieces are moderately large, or 6 hours if they are large.

1. 50% alcohol.
2. 70% alcohol.
3. 80% alcohol.
4. 90% alcohol.
5. Alcohol I.
6. Alcohol II.
7. Equal parts of alcohol and trichloroethylene (see Note ii).
8. Trichloroethylene I.
9. Trichloroethylene II.
10. Trichloroethylene III.
11. Wax I.
12. Wax II.
13. Embed in fresh wax.

Notes

(i) When an automatic processing machine is used for longer than 24 hours, the intervals on the second and subsequent days must be the same as those on the first. In practice, it is simplest to use equal intervals throughout the schedule.

(ii) Chloroform or carbon tetrachloride may be used in place of trichloroethylene at stages 7–10.

Large blocks cannot be cut on rotary or rocker microtomes. Sledge microtomes are used; these may need to be fitted with specially large block-holders. To avoid vibration, the tissue should be fixed directly over the supporting pillar of the block-holder. Extra care is needed to ensure that the wax block is securely mounted on its holder. To do this it is necessary first to make the wax block perfectly flat; this can be done by rubbing it against a hot, flat object—such as a large block-holder that has been flamed. The block-holder and the block are then flamed gently and pressed together until the wax has solidified. Before sections are cut, the block must be left to become thoroughly hard; it is better not to accelerate this hardening by freezing the block, since this may cause the wax to crack in the neighbourhood of the block-holder. Moreover, some microtomes will be unsatisfactory if a cold block-holder is attached to them at room temperature, either because of a loose fit or because expansion will give rise to sections of inconstant thickness as the block-holder warms up.

Cutting the sections should present no particular problem, but the ribbon will usually need to be broken into individual sections before being floated on warm water. This is best done with a sharp scalpel. The sections are then mounted on suitable slides and dried in the usual way.

Small pieces

It is always worth tinting these before attempting to process them. Acid fuchsin in the fixing fluids, or picric acid in one of the dehydrating alcohols will do this well. One way to handle tiny fragments is to put them into melted agar, which is then allowed to solidify, trimmed, and treated as though it were a piece of tissue of reasonable size. Suitable moulds for the melted agar can be made by standing several tubes of various sizes in a Petri dish and pouring wax around them. After the tubes have been removed, a mould of suitable size is filled with cool melted agar, the fragments of fixed tissue are added, and the agar allowed to solidify. The whole wax mould is then removed and the agar plug pushed out.

Alternatively, the tissue may be processed in a glass centrifuge tube, being deposited by centrifuging between each change of reagent. After the last change of wax the tube is broken to leave the tissue in solid wax. Instead of centrifuging the reagents, they may be filtered. When this is done, the tissue is finally embedded in a glass tube which can be broken to leave a block.

Serial sections

In the routine laboratory it will rarely be necessary to cut serial sections, although they may be needed for research purposes. The term serial sections means that every section is saved and mounted on a slide. Depending on the size of the block of tissue, one or several sections may be mounted on each slide, but in any case the slides must be labelled in such a way that the order is clear. There are two purposes for which serial sections may be required: either so that the three-dimensional structure of the specimen may be visualized, or so that a tiny feature shall not be overlooked. It is unfortunate that the term serial sections is often misunderstood; we have encountered people who suppose that it means no more than 'many sections', or 'sections from two or more levels in the block', or 'keeping every tenth (or twentieth, etc.) section', or 'a section from each of many blocks'. When (for instance) a gynaecologist requests

X

serial sections of a cervix, he rarely if ever appreciates that each millimetre of tissue will produce 200 sections of 5 μ thickness, so that it would need anything up to 6000 sections to include the entire cervix. Before undertaking to produce serial sections it is wise to verify that every single section from the block or specimen is really required. Often a set of 30 or 50 serial sections will provide abundant information about fine histological structure and, if the specimen is a small one, these sections may be accommodated on as few as three to five slides. When the problem is to demonstrate (or exclude) the presence of a tiny feature, it may be useful to bear in mind that anything larger than 100 μ (0·1 millimetre) can be discovered by saving every twentieth section.

The two main practical problems in the preparation of serial sections are: firstly, the need for every section to be a good one and, secondly, the importance of keeping the series in the correct order at every stage. If these two requirements are appreciated, it will be clear that the routine practice of section cutting (p. 61) needs to be modified in the following ways:

1. Choose a part of the laboratory away from any disturbing influences and free from draughts.
2. Take particular care to have a sharp well-stropped knife.
3. Be sure that the knife and block-holder are securely clamped, and use a microtome that shows no signs of wear.
4. Leave plenty of wax at each end of the tissue when trimming the block: this improves ribboning and also provides a margin by which the sections can be handled.
5. Cut a small piece off one corner of the block so that the ribbons will be easy to orientate (Fig. 12).

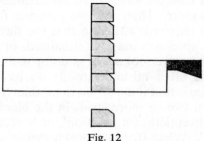

Fig. 12

6. Cut the sections with an even pressure to avoid any tendency for the sections to be alternately thick and thin.

7. If it should be necessary to stop cutting for an interval, or if the knife is moved, retract the block to avoid the danger of cutting a very thick section when work is resumed.

8. As ribbons are obtained, lay them in order on a black surface, holding them in place with pins through the wax if necessary.

9. Divide the ribbon into suitable lengths (one or several sections according to size) by cutting it with a scalpel before placing the pieces on a water-bath or on the slide on a hot-plate.

10. Take care to mount all sections or groups parallel to the edge of the slide and all in the same direction, so that they are either all towards or all away from the diamond marks (Fig. 13).

11. Before using the slides, mark each one with a diamond in such a way that the sequence is obvious.

12. Take precautions against loss of sections during staining by using an adhesive and by drying the slides in an incubator for a generously long time (overnight).

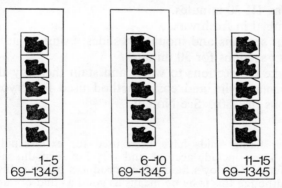

Fig. 13

Extra-rapid paraffin sections

Although the cryostat has largely superseded rapid paraffin methods, it may occasionally be necessary to produce paraffin sections in a hurry. By using the following method, it is possible to produce a stained section within 3–4 hours of receiving the fresh tissue. Stages 1–8 are carried out at 58–60°. Where possible, the reagents should be warmed to this temperature beforehand. Screw-capped vessels should be used to reduce evaporation.

METHOD (stages 1–8 at 58–60°C)

1. Fix a thin piece (2–3 mm.) in Carnoy's fluid (p. 20). Thinner pieces would fix more rapidly, but are apt to warp. When the entire specimen is very thin, it should be laid on a piece of wooden spatula which provides support during fixation.
2. After 10–15 minutes the surface of the piece becomes firm, so that it is no longer liable to warping. Cut a thin slice (1 mm.) from the surface (or remove the specimen from its wooden support) and continue fixation for a further 20–30 minutes.
3. Equal parts of alcohol and chloroform 20 minutes.
4. Chloroform I 20 minutes.
5. Chloroform II 20 minutes.
6. Paraffin wax I (56°C melting-point) 15 minutes.
7. Wax II 30 minutes.
8. Wax III 30 minutes.
9. Embed in fresh wax.
10. Cut sections and mount on slides, using an adhesive.
11. Dry sections for 30 minutes.
12. Take the sections to water and stain them by the rapid haematoxylin and eosin method used for cryostat sections (p. 280). See Note ii.

Notes

(i) Other fixing fluids have been used for extra-rapid paraffin sections. These include acetone and very hot formalin-saline. We have preferred Carnoy's fluid which produces a better histological picture, although this is by no means as good as that obtained using leisurely processing methods. Cytoplasm is apt to be damaged and red blood corpuscles are ruined by Carnoy's fluid; nuclei are excellent.

(ii) If time permits, the routine haematoxylin and eosin methods (Harris, p. 99, or Ehrlich, p. 101) may be used with better results. Alternatively, any other staining method may be used so long as the fixing fluid has not destroyed the relevant tissue component.

Sections for photography

Reasonably satisfactory photographs can be made from any good histological section. For excellent results, however, three points require particular care: the section must be perfect; the stain must be appropriate; dust and dirt must be avoided.

The section must be free from lines, cracks, and wrinkles. For high-power photographs it must be no thicker than $5\,\mu$. There must be no tendency for the section to lift off the slide.

Staining should be strong but precise. The principal objects must be conspicuously demonstrated; methods in which all the colours are pale should be avoided. Grocott's method for fungi, for instance, is preferable to Gridley's. Counterstains should be heavy enough to appear in the picture but must not obscure the principal objects. In some instances it may be necessary to use less counterstain than usual; in others the counterstain should be slightly increased. Eosin, for instance, should be fairly heavy for both monochrome and colour photography. When a choice of methods exists, it is better to use one with sharply contrasting colours.

Dust and dirt must be avoided at every stage. In particular, slides and coverslips must be polished with care, sections must be mounted on slides from perfectly clean water, and adhesives should be used sparingly and should not be applied to the slide with a finger, since this is apt to leave a deposit of squames.

Black and white photographs that are intended for publication should be printed on glossy paper and should show more contrast than photographs taken for ordinary record purposes. This is because some contrast is lost during the preparation of half-tone blocks and their subsequent printing. The magnification of all photographs should be recorded, above all when they are intended for publication.

Double embedding

For certain specimens, good results are obtained by the combined use of nitrocellulose and paraffin wax. After impregnation with nitrocellulose, the tissue is embedded in wax, so that thin sections may be cut as easily as those from an ordinary wax block. Specimens that benefit from this treatment fall into two broad categories. First, tough solid tissue which tends to break loose from a simple wax block during section cutting, and secondly, delicate specimens which are apt to fall apart during processing, section cutting, or staining. The method has been used for bone, finger-nails, brain, eyes, and specimens that contain sutures or plastic prostheses.

Double embedding was devised by Kultschitzky (1887) who used origanum oil. This was replaced with chloroform by Ryder (1887), but otherwise the method is virtually unchanged.

METHOD

1. Fix and dehydrate the specimen, using a schedule appropriate to its size.
2. Equal parts of alcohol and ether overnight.
3. Nitrocellulose (approximately 2 per cent; see Note i) in a mixture of equal parts of alcohol and ether 1–4 days depending on size.
4. Remove the specimen with forceps and drop it into chloroform. Leave overnight.
5. Impregnate and embed in paraffin wax in the usual way.

Notes

(i) Weak nitrocellulose may be prepared by diluting the stronger solution used for the ordinary nitrocellulose method (p. 266).

(ii) Occasionally it may be difficult to flatten sections when they are mounted on slides. In this case, 85 per cent alcohol should be used instead of water.

(iii) In some staining methods, the nitrocellulose will cause a light background staining. A few methods (e.g. per-iodic acid Schiff) are unsatisfactory.

Eyes

The histological examination of the eye presents difficulties. Fixing fluids penetrate relatively slowly through the dense outer layer (sclera), so that the important inner layers (retina and choroid) of an unopened eye are liable to be imperfectly fixed. On the other hand, the retina is very delicate and very easily detached, so that it is hazardous to cut an eye before fixation, and in any event all subsequent handling calls for great care.

Since there is no one perfect method, it may be best to vary the approach according to the type of disease requiring investigation. When the macroscopic appearances are particularly important, the eye should be fixed thoroughly in formalin-saline or neutral buffered formalin solution and then cut. A clean cut should be made near to the midline of the eye but slightly to one side of it, so that the optic nerve and the pupil are together in one of the pieces. A multiple razor-blade may be used. As an alternative, the well-fixed eye may be frozen to $-20°C$ overnight and then cut with a sharp strong knife. When this is done, the pieces are returned to an ice-cold formalin fixing fluid where they may be examined with a dissecting microscope. If cut unfrozen, the retina is apt to become detached: on the other hand freezing may give rise to ice-crystal artefact in histological sections.

When an urgent report is required, it may be thought necessary to cut the eye as soon as it arrives in the laboratory. This is only likely to occur when the eye is believed to contain a tumour. In such cases it is worth while holding the eye against a strong light and inspecting the contents through the pupil; the site of the tumour is usually obvious as an opacity in one part of the globe. A cut can then be made through the tumour and a piece selected for fairly rapid fixation and processing, while the remaining larger piece can be used for the more leisurely preparation of a complete section. When eyes contain tumours, there is less tendency for the retina to detach.

Occasionally, in cases of disease of the retina and choroid, the need is for excellent fixation of the inner layers. With eyes of this type, we have had good results by injecting fixing fluid into the globe. First a fairly wide needle (standard wire gauge 16, or similar) is inserted into the globe and then a fine needle (e.g. standard wire gauge 23). The posterior part must be avoided; points midway between the edge of the cornea and the equator are suitable since the anterior part of the retina is detached less easily. A syringe is then attached to the fine needle and formalin-saline is introduced. Great pressure must be avoided. At first the vitreous drops slowly out of the wide needle, but before long it is dilute enough to flow freely. When about 20 ml. of formalin-saline have been used, the syringe is refilled with Helly's fluid to wash out the formalin-saline. About 20 ml. of Helly's fluid are used; the wide needle is removed; and finally, with continued gentle pressure on the syringe, the fine needle is removed. The eye is then placed in Helly's fluid for

24–36 hours before being cut in the way already described. The dichromate in Helly's fluid must be removed from the tissue by washing, but this should not be done in running water; several changes of formalin-saline over a period of 24–36 hours will give good results. Eyes should never be injected with fixing fluid when they contain blood-clot or a tumour.

At some stage during processing, a piece should be cut from the opposite side so that no bubbles will be trapped when the specimen is embedded. This piece can be almost as large as that removed by the first cut, although the specimen is easier to handle and less liable to warping when only a small piece is removed. It is usually most convenient to allow the specimen to harden before making the second cut; we have usually waited until it was in fairly strong alcohol (80 per cent or more).

When time is not important, excellent results are obtained by embedding in nitrocellulose (Chapter 18, p. 264). Quicker results are obtainable with the double embedding method described above. For either of these techniques, use a dehydrating schedule similar to that previously described (the first seven stages of manual processing schedule I, p. 30). For ordinary paraffin sections, we have used a special schedule for eyes, restricting the time in alcohol to avoid excessive hardening. When this is done, cedarwood oil should be used for clearing. A hardened paraffin wax (e.g. Ralwax I) is an additional aid to satisfactory section cutting.

The schedule that we recommend is as follows:

1. 50% alcohol 1 hour.
2. 70% alcohol 1 hour.
3. 80% alcohol 1 hour.
4. 90% alcohol 1 hour.
5. Alcohol I 1 hour.
6. Alcohol II 1 hour.
7. Alcohol III 1 hour.
8. Cedarwood oil overnight.
9. Benzene 5–10 minutes.
10. Paraffin wax I 15 minutes.
11. Wax II 45 minutes.
12. Wax III 45 minutes.
13. Embed in fresh wax.

Note

This schedule is not suitable for eyes that contain massive tumours or clots.

Softening technique for tough tissue

This is useful for close-packed smooth muscle (e.g. uterus), and especially useful for tissue that contains much keratin or collagen. After thorough fixation, the tissue is transferred to a 4–6 per cent aqueous solution of phenol which will gradually soften it. A piece of uterus will be softened overnight, but a piece of keratinized skin from the sole of the foot or a very keratinized tumour may need 2–3 days. After a good wash in water, the tissue is dehydrated and cleared in the usual way.

Sometimes it is not realized that the tissue is particularly tough until it has been embedded in paraffin wax. In this case it may not be possible to cut sections unless the tissue is subjected to a softening agent. At this stage, the best fluid to use is 4–6 per cent phenol dissolved in a mixture of equal parts of glycerol and 70 per cent alcohol. The paraffin block is supported in a shallow trough of this solution. If the block is treated overnight and then washed well, it is usually possible to cut a few good sections from its surface.

Finger-nails

Occasionally it may be necessary to cut sections of a finger-nail or toe-nail, with or without the adjacent soft tissues. Unless softened with phenol by the method described above, the nail is unlikely to cut easily. Even after softening, it will tend to become detached from the surrounding wax unless the block has been prepared by the double embedding technique, using nitrocellulose as well as paraffin (p. 309). When the sections have been cut they will be difficult to flatten unless they are floated on fairly hot water (almost as hot as the melting-point of the wax used).

Unsuspected calcium in paraffin blocks

However much care is taken in the selection of pieces of tissue for processing, an occasional piece will be found to contain calcium salts when an attempt is made to cut sections. In theory such tissue could be returned through a clearing agent and alcohol to water, decalcified and then taken once more through alcohol and clearing agent to wax. In practice this is time-consuming and leads to excessive hardness of the tissue, even though the calcium salts have been removed.

The alternative is to expose the surface of the tissue to the decalcifying fluid, which will remove enough of the calcium salts for a few sections to be cut. After the surface wax has been removed to expose the tissue, the block (still attached to its holder) is placed face downwards in a small volume of decalcifying fluid; the face should be raised by balancing the block on wooden supports (e.g. pieces of swab-stick). Any acid decalcifying fluid may be chosen. After a short wash in running water, the block is allowed to dry. Usually it is then possible to cut a limited number of sections from the surface of the block before the hard calcium salts are re-encountered. Sometimes, however, surface decalcification causes the tissue to swell and to bulge above the face of the wax. When this happens, the tissue will need to be thoroughly dried and re-embedded before sections can be cut.

Fairly large discrete masses of calcium salts are occasionally encountered (e.g. in old tuberculous lesions). These are usually very resistant to surface decalcification, so that the microtomist is tempted to dislodge them with a needle or a pointed forceps blade. Before doing this, the problem should be discussed with the pathologist, who might otherwise be misled by the holes in the section. When calcified masses have been removed in this way, it is worth while filling the pits with molten wax before cutting sections.

Sections which detach during staining

From time to time, sections give trouble by becoming detached from the slides (washing off) during staining. This is particularly likely to occur when much blood is present (e.g. spleen or blood-clot), and when the sections are subjected to an alkaline solution (e.g. ammoniacal silver). Any section is apt to wash off if it was not dried properly, if no adhesive was used, or if the specimen was inadequately dehydrated, cleared, or impregnated.

There are two ways of dealing with the problem: either the

section can be coated with nitrocellulose, or further sections can be cut and mounted on slides with a stronger adhesive.

For coating sections, a very thin solution of nitrocellulose ($\frac{1}{2}$–1 per cent) must be used; this can be prepared by diluting a thicker solution (p. 266) with a mixture of equal parts of alcohol and ether. The section is dewaxed in xylene and then rinsed in alcohol before being dipped in the very thin nitrocellulose solution. The entire slide should be immersed and then stood vertically to allow the excess nitrocellulose to drain off. The back of the slide may be wiped, but the film should be left covering the whole front surface, otherwise there is a risk of losing the nitrocellulose film complete with section during subsequent staining. After about one minute, the film will have dried by evaporation, and the slide is immersed in 70 per cent alcohol to harden the nitrocellulose. The section is then stained in the ordinary way. After staining, there is no need to remove the nitrocellulose film when applying the coverslip.

When it can be foreseen that a section is likely to wash off the slide, a stronger adhesive may be used. Good results are obtained with gelatin. An aqueous solution of about 0·25 per cent gelatin is prepared and filtered. A small quantity is placed on the slide, and the paraffin section floated on it. After inclining the slide to drain away excess fluid, it is carefully blotted and placed in an incubator at 56°C in an atmosphere of formalin vapour. After drying for at least two hours, the section may be stained in the usual way.

CHAPTER 22

Techniques for Smears

General notes. Making smears. Techniques for fluid. Fixation. Staining: Haematoxylin and eosin; Papanicolaou; Shorr; Leishman; May-Grünwald-Giemsa; Giemsa. Staining membrane filters. Miscellaneous cytological techniques.

SMEARS are made from cells that have been scraped from an accessible part of the body, or from cells that are suspended in fluid. Occasionally it may also be convenient to make smears from a piece of tissue. Smears are preferred to sections when the cells from a particular source may be obtained simply and painlessly, whereas a piece of tissue for sectioning would need operative removal. Moreover, a carefully made smear will include cells from a far wider field than could be covered by a biopsy or even by multiple biopsies. For these reasons, cytology is usually preferred to histology for the examination of cervical and vaginal scrapings, sputum and bronchial aspirates, fluid from body cavities or from cysts, urine, gastric juice, cerebrospinal fluid, prostatic fluid, and scrapings from skin lesions. Smears (usually from the buccal mucosa) are far better than sections for counting Barr bodies to determine chromatin sex. The foregoing smears are usually fixed in fixing fluids similar to those used for histological techniques, and the smears are subsequently stained with haematoxylin and a counterstain.

Another reason for making smears rather than sections is the need for urgent examination of tissue that is soft enough to make thin and even smears, and too soft to be handled easily by rapid histological techniques. Examples of tissue of this consistency are bone marrow and brain. A third reason for preferring smears is the subsequent use of dyes of the Romanowsky type, which give good results only when the smears have first been dried in air and then fixed. Blood films and bone marrow come into this category, as also do conjunctival scrapings for inclusion bodies. In some laboratories this type of stain is also used for other specimens, such as sputum or aspirated fluid.

Making smears

The first essential is to use clean slides. Not only must these be free from greasy substances which make the smears uneven, but they must also be free from dust particles which cling to the cells and protein of the smear. It is wise to keep a stock of slides in spirit; as required these are dried on a fluff-free cloth. The second essential is to know which type of stain will be employed. Romanowsky stains will only work properly on *air-dried* smears, and these are almost always used for blood and aspirated bone marrow. If the marrow has been removed at necropsy, many cells will fragment when the smear is made, although this tendency can be reduced by mixing the specimen of bone marrow with an equal volume of glycerol or albumin before making the smears.

More commonly, however, the smears will be stained by haematoxylin followed by a counterstain. When this is so, it is most important *not* to let the cells dry before they are fixed.

When smears are made before they are sent to the laboratory, the responsibility for selecting suitable material rests on the person who sends them. In this situation, however, the laboratory will often be asked for advice, and may be able to simplify its own task as well as improve the accuracy of the result by giving suitable instructions. It must be emphasized, first of all, that a suitable technique for one type of smear does not necessarily apply to another. Thus, cells scraped or collected in a small volume of fluid (e.g. scrapings from vagina, cervix, skin or conjunctiva, and fluid expressed from the nipple or prostate) will need to be spread fairly thin on the slide. The area covered will depend on the amount of material, so that a cervical smear, will often fill two-thirds of a standard slide whereas material

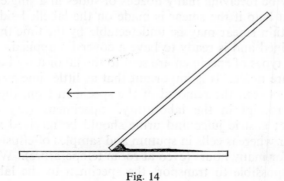

Fig. 14

scraped from the conjunctiva may occupy less than one square centimetre. On the other hand, smears of blood are made by placing a drop on the slide and pulling it out into a smear with the end of a second slide (Fig. 14).

A solid piece of tissue, such as brain, needs yet another technique. This will first need to be flattened by compression between two slides. When the two are slid apart, a smear should be left on each. A similar technique may be used with aspirated bone marrow. It is possible to obtain cells from tissue that is too firm to be squashed. This is done by pressing a freshly cut surface gently but firmly onto the slide. When the tissue is removed, a number of cells are left behind to form what is properly known as an impression preparation rather than a smear, although the subsequent handling will be identical to that of a true smear.

Secondly, it is essential to give clear indications about fixation. The person making the smears must be told whether air-dried or fixed smears are required. For fixed smears, it is not enough to supply fixing agents; it is also necessary to provide simple written instructions for their use. Methods of fixation are described below.

Thirdly, adequate labelling must be ensured. A writing diamond is excellent, but for everyday use it is better to supply slides with ground ends that will accept pencil marks; a hard pencil should be used, since soft pencil marks are apt to smudge. Ordinary (watery) inks and ball-point (greasy) inks must be condemned, since they almost all dissolve during staining. Nor is the plain surname a sufficient identification for a laboratory that may be receiving many dozens of slides in a single day. It is a great help if the smear is made on the labelled side of the slide; a thin smear may be undetectable by the time that it has been stained and is ready to have a coverslip applied.

Other types of specimen are sent to the laboratory before the smears are made. It is important that as little time as possible elapses between the removal of the specimen from the patient and its receipt in the laboratory. Specimens vary in their tolerance; gastric juice and urine should be received within a half-hour whereas cells in sputum and samples of effusions may survive for many hours (even at room temperature). When it is quite impossible to transport the specimen to the laboratory without delay, the cells may be preserved by adding alcohol (an equal volume) or formalin (one part to nine of the specimen). After either of these preservatives have been used, it is, however, impossible to obtain results that are as good as those from a fresh specimen.

When the specimen is received by the laboratory, suitable smears are made. If the specimen consists of a few drops only, these are smeared in their entirety. If, as often happens, the specimen is a large volume of watery fluid, the cells should be concentrated before smears are made (see below). If the specimen is mucoid (e.g. sputum), fragments suitable for smearing are selected with a wire loop or a disposable wooden stick. In order to examine such specimens, they need to be spread out (e.g. in a Petri dish), and viewed against both a dark and a light surface. Attention should be directed to any bloodstained fragment and anything that resembles a scrap of tissue. These must then be smeared, using enough force to disperse any thick lumps. Specimens sent for smearing, and especially samples of sputum, must be regarded as infective and handled with proper precautions. All specimen bottles, Petri dishes, and instruments must be sterilized after use.

Techniques for fluid

The easiest way to concentrate the cells in a specimen of fluid is to centrifuge it. The alternative is to filter the fluid through a membrane that has pores of a suitable size. Before embarking on either of these procedures, however, it is worthwhile considering whether the specimen merits any special treatment. Fluids that benefit from special treatment are: clotted fluids, watery fluids, and fluids that contain much blood.

There are two kinds of clot; fine cobweb-clot, and voluminous gelatinous clot. The latter may be so great that the whole specimen is clotted and no free fluid remains. Clots can, of course, be avoided altogether by the use of an anticoagulant and careful mixing. In our experience, however, any anticoagulant that is convenient to use produces an alteration in the appearance of the stained cells, so that we recommend clean dry bottles. Any clots that form can then be dealt with in the laboratory. The cobweb type of clot is, in fact, most valuable; not infrequently it will be found to contain almost every cell in the ecimen. A clot of this type should be carefully removed, transferred to a rapid-acting fixing fluid, processed, and embedded in paraffin as though it was a fragment of tissue. These clots would not be hardened enough by such fluids as formalin-saline but Susa and Bouin's fluid are excellent. Gelatinous clots are obviously too large for this treatment. This type of clot can, however, be reduced in bulk by shaking or rapping the container until the clot has shrunk to manageable proportions, when it is removed and fixed. After fixation it should be sliced if it exceeds a few millimetres in thickness. We always prepare smears from clotted fluids, as well as making sections of the clot. Comparison of the two is often helpful, especially to anyone more familiar with sections than smears. In addition, the sections will often provide valuable information about the architectural arrangement of neoplastic cells—in acini for instance.

Watery fluids (e.g. urine and cerebro-spinal fluid) are easy to centrifuge, and smears can easily be made from the deposit. The cells are, however, particularly likely to float off the slide during fixation and staining because there is no protein to hold them in place. Such smears will be greatly improved if an adhesive is added to the fluid before it is centrifuged. We use Mayer's egg albumin (p. 66) in the approximate proportion of one drop to every 10 ml. of fluid. An alternative is to make the smears on albuminized slides.

If a specimen of fluid contains much blood, attempts can be made to lyse the red blood corpuscles which are apt to obscure the smears. This can be done by the addition of an equal volume of dilute acetic acid (one part of glacial acetic acid to 99 parts of 0·85 per cent sodium chloride). After centrifugation, the deposit will usually contain many ghosts of red blood corpuscles, but may on occasion contain a large proportion of intact corpuscles. If the deposit is thoroughly resuspended in more of the dilute acetic acid, many of the survivors will be lysed in their turn. After this treatment, smears should be made on albuminized slides, since there is little or no free protein in the suspension.

Most laboratories use a centrifuge to concentrate the cells in specimens of fluid. Because of the risk of breakage, glass tubes should be avoided if possible. If no other type is available, the specimen should be divided between two tubes to minimize the risk of total loss. When plastic tubes are chosen, the problem of subsequent sterilization must be borne in mind. We have used polypropylene tubes which withstand chemical disinfectants or sterilization in an autoclave. Centrifugation should be prolonged and gentle: high speeds will damage many types of unfixed cell. We usually spin fluid for 20 minutes at no more than 800 g (about 2000 rpm in a typical laboratory centrifuge). After discarding the supernatant, it is important to mix the deposit thoroughly before making smears. This is because cells are often deposited in layers and a sample collected at random from an unmixed specimen may contain only one type (e.g. red blood corpuscles). Smears are usually made with a wire loop. Slides need to be free from grease and dust. If the deposit is tiny, only a small area of the slide should be used, since it is very tedious to search a large area for a few isolated cells. Sometimes a deposit may clot, in which case it is best treated as a piece of tissue and processed for the preparation of sections rather than smears. Even when clotting has not occurred, it may be worth while making sections if the deposit is particularly bulky. This is done by resuspending some or all of the deposit in a rapid-acting fixing fluid such as Susa, and centrifuging for a second time. The deposit then forms a small cake which can be treated like a piece of tissue.

The other method of concentrating cells is filtration. Membranes are obtainable which have pores that hold back large cells whilst allowing water, solutes, and small cells such as red blood corpuscles to pass freely. The whole membrane, with the cells on it, is then fixed, stained, and mounted between a slide and coverslip. The method is appropriate for watery fluids (e.g. urine and cerebro-spinal fluid) rather than proteinous fluids which are too viscous to flow easily through the pores. Filtration is achieved either by negative pressure ('Millipore'; 'Membranfiltergesellschaft') or by applying centrifugal force ('Hemming's filter'). The stands for the negative pressure method are relatively large and expensive, so that many laboratories cannot afford duplicates to allow for time spent in cleaning and sterilization. In the Hemming's filter, the membrane is inserted into a metal carrier, each end of which has a rubber washer and screw thread of a suitable size for a bijou bottle. One bottle is filled with fluid, the other is empty, and the

Y

whole device is loaded into a centrifuge with the empty bottle downwards. Fluid is driven from the top bottle to the bottom by centrifugal force, leaving the cells on the membrane. The disadvantage of this method is the limited volume of fluid that can be filtered. The apparatus is, however, small and relatively cheap.

Whichever method is used with membrane filters, it is important not to apply too much force, since this not only spread-eagles the cells on the membrane but also causes parts of the cytoplasm to be forced into the pores. When the pressure is removed, the cytoplasm may not escape from the pores as the cell begins to round up; the effect produced is reminiscent of a skin that shrunk when pinned out to dry. If the negative pressure method is used, the partial vacuum should not exceed 25 mm. of mercury negative pressure. Hemming's filters should be centrifuged relatively slowly (at about 1000 rpm which produces a centrifugal force of not more than 200 g); filtration will be complete in 3–4 minutes if the fluid is watery, even when a few drops of albumin have been added to improve the adhesion of cells to the filter membrane. When filtration is complete, the membrane is transferred to a fixing fluid. We have not investigated the possibility of drying the membrane for subsequent staining by Romanowsky methods.

Fixation

The majority of smears are fixed as soon as they have been made. The main exception to this rule is blood films and similar smears that will be stained by Romanowsky methods. These smears are allowed to dry in the air and will keep for some days at least until they are stained. Smears for bacteriological examination may occasionally be handled in a histological laboratory (e.g. from a necropsy); these are usually fixed by heat and kept dry until they are stained. More rarely, smears of material may need to be examined for spermatozoa. These smears are usually dried in air without the use of heat. Unlike most dry smears they are satisfactory if stained by haematoxylin and eosin after brief fixation in alcohol.

For smears that are to be stained by haematoxylin and most other histological stains, wet fixation is essential if good results are to be obtained. Wet fixation means immersing the smear in fixing fluid before any drying has occurred. For best results, the smear must be dropped into the fluid. If it is lowered gently a great many cells float off the smear; often cells are lost from parts of the slide which then shows alternate thick and thin bands (Naylor, 1958). When smears have to be transported, it may be inconvenient to send them in containers of fluid and, in any event, it is illegal to send alcoholic fluids through the post. It is often recommended that the smears should first be thoroughly fixed and then allowed to dry for transport. However, we have greatly preferred the results when the cells have been preserved by a fixing agent that dries up, coating and protecting the cells during transport.

Alcohol

Undiluted spirit (74° OP) is a satisfactory fixing fluid for most kinds of smear. In our experience, smears should be fixed for several hours. Smears may, however, be stained after no more than 15 minutes, although when this is done the cells are more likely to be detached during staining. On the other hand, the smears do not appear to deteriorate in this fluid if stored for several weeks, provided that evaporation of the alcohol is prevented.

Notes

(i) Before alcohol is re-used for fixing smears, it should be filtered, otherwise there is a risk of cells that have floated off one smear becoming attached to another.

(ii) We have found that smears fixed in alcohol are indistinguishable from those fixed in equal parts of alcohol and ether. Since ether is relatively expensive and much more inflammable, we therefore use alcohol on its own whenever a method specifies alcohol-ether.

(iii) Alcohol is a particularly suitable fixing fluid for smears that are to be stained by the Papanicolaou method. For haematoxylin and eosin, a mercuric fluid (see below) is better.

(iv) Membrane filters may be fixed in alcohol.

(v) Some staining methods (e.g. trichrome stains and phosphotungstic acid haematoxylin) give only mediocre results after fixation in alcohol. Stains for fat are quite unsatisfactory since alcohol dissolves most lipids.

(vi) If alcohol is supplied (e.g. to clinics) the users must be warned that it is inflammable. Its transmission through the post is prohibited.

Alcoholic mercuric chloride

Better than alcohol for smears that are to be stained by haematoxylin and eosin and most histological special stains.

Saturated aqueous solution of mercuric chloride   50 ml.
Alcohol   50 ml.

Smears should preferably be fixed for 6 to 18 hours. Fixation can, however, be as short as 15 minutes although the results are less satisfactory. Smears do not deteriorate if stored in this fluid for some weeks. Evaporation must, of course, be prevented. Deposits of mercury pigment are conspicuous after 1–2 days but these can be removed without difficulty (p. 84).

Notes

(i) Mercuric chloride and alcohol have often been combined in fixing fluids and numerous formulae have been published. Sometimes acetic acid has been added. After comparing the results of fixation by many different mixtures, we recommend this one.

(ii) This fluid is suitable for membrane filters.

(iii) A great variety of staining methods give good results after fixation in this fluid. As well as haematoxylin and eosin, the following methods work well: trichrome stains, phosphotungstic acid haematoxylin, mucus stains including per-iodic acid Schiff, Best's carmine, Feulgen, Gram, Perls, and Masson-Fontana for melanin. In addition it is possible to use fat stains (e.g. Sudan) since this fluid removes little or no lipid.

(iv) The Papanicolaou stain can be used after this fluid but the results are poor compared to those after fixation in alcohol.

(v) The fluid should be changed often since the alcohol evaporates and the mercuric chloride is lost by attachment to protein.

(vi) Like any other solution that contains mercuric chloride, this fluid attacks most metals. It is also very poisonous.

Polyethylene glycol fixing agent

The solvent is allowed to evaporate, leaving the polyethylene glycol ('Carbowax'), which preserves the cells by forming a dry protective coat. The smears can then be transported easily by post or otherwise. Polyethylene glycol has been recommended for this purpose for many years (Sills, 1953; Sills and Garret, 1957); the formula given below is that of Higgins (1963) and is very satisfactory.

Polyethylene glycol 1500 ('Carbowax' 1500)	6 g.
Distilled water	10 ml.
Glacial acetic acid	0·6 ml.
Alcohol	200 ml.

Dissolve the polyethylene glycol in the water with the aid of gentle heat, then add the acetic acid. Finally add the alcohol, mix well, and dispense into small plastic dropping bottles. It would be illegal to send this mixture through the post. It is, however, perfectly satisfactory to mail the mixture of polyethylene glycol, water and acetic acid with instructions to the recipient to add an appropriate amount of methylated spirit.

METHOD

As soon as the smear has been made and before it begins to dry, lay the slide flat (smear uppermost) and add enough fixing mixture to cover the entire smear. Leave until the solvent has evaporated (usually 10–15 minutes). The smear may then be transported by post or otherwise. In the laboratory the coating of polyethylene glycol dissolves in the first watery or alcoholic reagent used.

Notes

(i) It is important to allow ample time for the solvent to evaporate. Heat should not be used to hasten this process, since it spoils the appearance of the stained cells.

(ii) At least one of the evaporating mixtures available commercially (Ortho 'Cytofixative') appears to be similar if not identical to this mixture. Other manufacturers supply fluids and aerosols, but we have not found any that we prefer to this formula.

(iii) After fixation by this method, the appearances of stained smears are very similar to those fixed in alcohol. The Papanicolaou method gives excellent results; haematoxylin and eosin staining is tolerable though less satisfactory than following alcoholic mercuric chloride; lipids are not preserved.

(iv) The method is particularly suitable for use at a distance from a laboratory, and is ideal for cervical and vaginal cytology. It is also very satisfactory for the demonstration of Barr bodies which are rendered conspicuous by the acetic acid in the mixture.

(v) Smears of watery fluid in which cells are few may be fixed by this method without the cells floating into the fixative, as they are apt to do when the slide is plunged into a large volume of fixing fluid.

(vi) Once dry, smears may be kept for a long period (at least several months) without deterioration.

(vii) The method is not suitable for membrane filters.

Staining

As already mentioned, smears that have been fixed while wet are stained by haematoxylin and a counterstain, whereas smears that have been allowed to dry before being fixed are stained by a Romanowsky method. When haematoxylin is used, the counterstain is nearly always either eosin or the Papanicolaou method. The favourite Romanowsky methods are May-Grünwald-Giemsa and Leishman. Diluted Giemsa stain is occasionally used for inclusion bodies.

In addition, almost any histological special staining method may be used for wet fixed smears; we have been successful with trichrome methods, phosphotungstic acid haematoxylin, Heidenhain's iron haematoxylin, mucin stains including the per-iodic acid Schiff reaction, Best's carmine, Perls's method, the Masson-Fontana method, and stains for nucleic acids. Fat stains (e.g. Sudan) may be used provided that the fixing fluid has not dissolved the lipids.

Haematoxylin and eosin

Widely used by cytologists whose basic training has been histological rather than haematological. Suitable for all wet-fixed smears, although less satisfactory for cervical and vaginal smears than the Papanicolaou method (see below).

REAGENTS

A. *Carazzi's haematoxylin* (p. 106)

B. *1 per cent hydrochloric acid in 70 per cent alcohol*

C. *0·5 per cent aqueous solution of eosin* (yellowish; water and alcohol soluble)

METHOD

1. Take smears to water (see Note ii).
2. Carazzi's haematoxylin 10 minutes.
3. Running tap water for at least 5 minutes (see Note iii).
4. Differentiate in acid alcohol 5–10 seconds.
5. Blue in running tap water for at least 10 minutes (see Note iii).
6. Eosin 5–10 minutes.

7. Running tap water 5 minutes.
8. 50% alcohol 3–5 minutes.
9. Dehydrate slowly, clear and mount (for full instructions
   see page 87).

RESULTS

Nuclei; bacteria: *blue*.
Red blood corpuscles; eosinophil leucocytes: *red*.
Cytoplasm of other cells: *shades of pink*.

Notes

(i) After comparing many haematoxylin mixtures, we have preferred Carazzi's because the chromatin detail is fine and the haematoxylin does not colour cytoplasm or mucus. Anyone wishing to
experiment with alternatives is recommended to try Harris's and
Mayer's mixtures which give results that are nearly as good.

(ii) Smears fixed in alcohol (or alcohol-ether mixture) should be
rehydrated gently, spending about a minute in 70 per cent alcohol
and 50 per cent alcohol before being placed in water. Attempts to
hasten this process cause cells to be lost from the smear.

Smears fixed in alcoholic mercuric chloride will only require treatment with 50 per cent alcohol before being washed in water. If
smears have spent more than about 24 hours in alcoholic mercuric
chloride, they should be treated with iodine and sodium thiosulphate
(p. 85) to remove fixation deposit.

Smears fixed in polyethylene glycol fixing agent should be placed
in water for 5 to 10 minutes to remove the protective coat before they
are stained.

(iii) In regions where the tap water is neutral or acid (soft water),
Scott's tap water substitute should be used at stages 3 and 5 (p. 100).

(iv) In some places the tap water removes eosin from the smears
unusually rapidly. When this occurs, calcium chloride should be
added to the eosin (p. 101).

(v) If staining machines are used, it may be preferable to avoid the
use of running water (p. 99).

The Papanicolaou method

The favourite method for cervical and vaginal smears. The
colours are attractive and may be useful, although they are not
reliably consistent. Cytoplasm appears translucent, which is a
decided advantage over haematoxylin and eosin for smears that
include large numbers of overlapping cells. In the original
method (Papanicolaou, 1942), the staining solutions were

prepared from alcoholic stock solutions. We have had more consistent results by following Koss and Durfee (1961) who use aqueous stock solutions which are less affected by evaporation.

REAGENTS

A. *Haematoxylin stock solution*

Haematoxylin	1 g.
Alcohol	10 ml.
Potassium alum (aluminium potassium sulphate)	20 g.
Distilled water	200 ml.
Mercuric oxide	0·5 g.

Dissolve the haematoxylin in the alcohol. Dissolve the alum in the water, using heat. Mix the two solutions; heat to boiling-point; add the mercuric oxide. Cool rapidly by immersing the flask in cold water.

B. *Haematoxylin working solution*

Dilute stock solution with an equal volume of distilled water. The diluted solution is ready for use immediately, and will keep for 2–3 days. The stock solution will keep for 3–4 months.

C. *0·25 per cent solution of hydrochloric acid in distilled water*

D. *OG 6*

10% aqueous solution of orange G	50 ml.
Ethanol	950 ml.
Phosphotungstic acid	0·15 g.

After it has been filtered, the solution is ready for use and keeps well provided that evaporation is prevented.

E. *EA 36* (see Note v)

10% aqueous solution of eosin	45 ml.
10% aqueous solution of Bismarck brown	10 ml.
10% aqueous solution of light green	9 ml.
95% ethanol	to 2000 ml.
Phosphotungstic acid	4 g.
Saturated aqueous solution of lithium carbonate	20 drops
Glacial acetic acid	25 ml.

Mix thoroughly. After it has been filtered the solution is ready for use and will keep for some weeks.

METHOD I (manual staining)

1. Take smears to water (see Note vi).
2. Haematoxylin 6 minutes.
3. Distilled water 1–2 minutes.
4. Hydrochloric acid solution 4–10 seconds.
5. Running tap water 5–10 minutes (see Note ii).
6. Rinse in 50% alcohol.
7. Rinse in 70% alcohol.
8. Rinse in 80% alcohol.
9. Rinse in 90% alcohol.
10. OG 6 solution 2–3 minutes.
11. Rinse in alcohol.
12. EA 36 solution 3–4 minutes.
13. Rinse in alcohol I.
14. Rinse in alcohol II.
15. Clear and mount (for full instructions see page 87).

METHOD II (automatic staining machine)

Before loading slides into the machine, remove polyethylene glycol fixing agent if that has been used (see Note vii).

1. 70% alcohol 1 minute ⎫
2. 50% alcohol 1 minute ⎬ See Note vii.
3. Tap water 1 minute ⎭
4. Haematoxylin 6 minutes.
5. Distilled water 1 minute.
6. Hydrochloric acid solution 10 seconds.
7. Tap water 1 minute ⎫
8. Tap water 4 minutes ⎬ See Notes ii and iii.
9. Tap water 4 minutes ⎭
10. 50% alcohol 1 minute.
11. 70% alcohol 1 minute.
12. 80% alcohol 1 minute.
13. 90% alcohol 1 minute.
14. OG 6 solution 6 minutes.
15. Alcohol 1 minute.

16. Alcohol 1 minute.
17. EA 36 solution 12 minutes.
18. Alcohol 1 minute.
19. Alcohol 1 minute.
20. Xylene 1 minute.
21. Xylene 2 minutes.
22. Xylene until mounted.

RESULTS

Nuclei: *blue*.

Superficial ('cornified') cell cytoplasm: *usually orange-red*.

Intermediate and basal ('non-cornified') cell cytoplasm: *usually green or bluish-green*.

Endocervical cell cytoplasm: *blue or greenish-blue*.

Trichomonas vaginalis: bluish-grey or greenish-grey, sometimes with pink granules.

Bacteria: *usually pale bluish-grey*.

Red blood corpuscles; fungi: *variable; pink or green*.

Notes

(i) The haematoxylin mixture differs from Harris's haematoxylin in only two respects. It does not contain acetic acid, and it is used at half the concentration of Harris's formula. In many laboratories a stock solution of Harris's haematoxylin is prepared without acetic acid. This may then be diluted for cytological use or may be used for histological staining when acetic acid is added.

(ii) In regions where the tap water is neutral or acid (soft water), Scott's tap water substitute should be used at stage 5 of the manual method and at stages 7, 8 and 9 of the automatic method. For Scott's tap water substitute see page 100.

(iii) The automatic method given above is for a staining machine not equipped with arrangements for washing the slides in running tap water. If, however, the machine is so equipped, stages 7, 8 and 9 should be replaced by a single wash in running tap water for 5–10 minutes.

(iv) Pure absolute alcohol (ethanol) is recommended for the preparation of the OG 6 and EA 36 staining solutions. Industrial methylated spirit is less satisfactory although it may be used at all other stages of the staining method.

(v) EA 36 is sometimes referred to as EA 50. The formula given here differs from the original which did not contain acetic acid. We have had consistently better results after adding acetic acid, which is also added by at least one manufacturer of ready-mixed stain.

(vi) Smears fixed in alcohol (or alcohol-ether mixture) should be rehydrated gently, spending about a minute in 70 per cent alcohol and 50 per cent alcohol before being placed in water. Attempts to hasten this process cause cells to be lost from the smear. Smears fixed in polyethylene glycol fixing agent should be placed in water for 5 to 10 minutes to remove the protective coat before they are stained.

(vii) The automatic method given above is suitable for smears received in alcohol (or alcohol-ether mixture). Smears fixed by polyethylene glycol fixing agent can be added at stage 1 after soaking in 80 per cent alcohol for 5–10 minutes to remove the protective coat. When it can be foreseen that every smear will be received in polyethylene glycol fixing agent, stages 1, 2 and 3 can be replaced by a single soak in tap water for 5–10 minutes.

(viii) Staining times in OG 6 and EA 36 are longer than those stated in the original published method. We have found that these longer times give better and more consistent results.

Common faults

(i) Poor results are usually attributable to exhausted reagents. It is essential to change all the solutions at frequent intervals and it may be necessary to replace loss by evaporation even more often. The hydrochloric acid solution should be changed daily. When a machine is used with static tap water, this should be replaced after every batch of slides. The rinsing water at stage 5 of the automatic method should be changed daily. Other reagents will usually need replacing about twice a week.

(ii) If one end of the slide is unstained or the colours are incorrect, the level of fluid in one of the vessels is too low.

(iii) Incorrect haematoxylin staining will occur if the haematoxylin solution is stale, if the hydrochloric acid solution is exhausted, or if the tap water is insufficiently alkaline because it needs to be changed or because the water itself is too soft.

(iv) The colours will often be too red when the EA 36 solution is made without acetic acid.

(v) The green colour will be inconsistent unless the EA 36 stock solutions and working solution are well mixed before use. This is because the green dye tends to gravitate to the bottom of the container.

(vi) Granules or crystals of precipitated stain occur when the haematoxylin is not filtered before use and when the OG 6 is allowed to evaporate excessively.

(vii) Occasionally it is difficult to remove all the water from a very thick smear by the ordinary use of dehydrating and clearing agents. These smears need a longer time in dehydrating alcohol and will benefit from clearing in carbol-xylene (25 per cent phenol in xylene) for 5 to 10 minutes, followed by the routine treatment with xylene.

Shorr's stain

Used for vaginal smears when the primary interest is the assessment of hormone activity (Shorr, 1941).

REAGENT

Shorr's stain

Ethanol	200 ml.
Distilled water	200 ml.
Biebrich scarlet (water soluble)	2 g.
Orange G	1 g.
Fast green FCF	0·3 g.
Phosphotungstic acid	2 g.
Phosphomolybdic acid	2 g.
Glacial acetic acid	4 ml.

Mix by shaking; filter. The stain is ready for use immediately and keeps well.

METHOD

1. 50% alcohol 1–5 minutes.
2. Shorr's stain 1–2 minutes.
3. Rinse in 70% alcohol.
4. Rinse in 90% alcohol.
5. Rinse in alcohol I.
6. Rinse in alcohol II.
7. Clear and mount.

RESULTS

Superficial ('cornified') cell cytoplasm: *orange-red*.
Intermediate and basal ('non-cornified') cell cytoplasm: *green*.
Nuclei: *dark brownish-red*.

Notes

(i) This method is the third that was published by Shorr and is therefore known sometimes as S3.

(ii) Pure absolute alcohol (ethanol) is recommended for the preparation of this stain; industrial methylated spirit is less satisfactory.

(iii) Shorr's stain is not an alternative to the Papanicolaou method since the emphasis is on cytoplasm rather than nuclei. It has often been suggested that this stain should be used after haematoxylin but in our experience most if not all of the haematoxylin is removed by

Shorr's stain. All the haematoxylin mixtures that we have tested give poor results, including the zinc haematoxylin mixture (Papamiltiades, 1953) that was recommended specifically for use with Shorr's stain by Pundel (1957).

Leishman's stain

Used for air-dried smears of blood or bone marrow (Leishman, 1901). Excellent rapid results are obtainable but the method does not lend itself to automatic staining machines.

REAGENTS

Leishman's stain

> Leishman's stain powder   1·5 g.
> Methanol (pure, acetone-free)   1000 ml.

Dissolve by intermittent shaking over several hours. Ready for use the following day, the stain will keep for many months in well-stoppered bottles.

METHOD

1. Cover the smear with undiluted stain and leave for $\frac{1}{2}$ to 1 minute.
2. Add freshly-distilled water or phosphate buffer (pH 6·8) and mix by blowing on the slide. The amount added should be about twice as much as the original volume of stain used. Allow the diluted stain to act for 5 to 10 minutes.
3. Wash thoroughly with freshly-distilled water (or buffer), preferably by allowing the water to cascade down the inclined slide.
4. Blot dry. Examine under direct oil-immersion or rinse with xylene and mount, preferably in a neutral mounting medium.

Notes

(i) Buffered distilled water (pH 6·8) may conveniently be made by using commercially produced buffer tablets.

(ii) When the method is used for smears in which cells are very few (e.g. deposit from centrifuged cerebro-spinal fluid), the time in diluted stain may need to be greatly reduced. As little as one minute will often suffice.

May-Grünwald-Giemsa stain

A very popular stain for air-dried smears of blood and bone marrow. The method makes use of the stain described by May and Grünwald (1902) followed by that described by Giemsa (1904) in his third publication on the subject. The composite method differs from both of the original descriptions in many details. In its present form it is suitable for use in automatic staining machines.

REAGENTS

A. *May-Grünwald stock solution*

            May-Grünwald stain powder   3 g.
            Methanol (pure, acetone-free)   1000 ml.

Dissolve by warming to 50°C; allow to cool; shake intermittently over several hours. The stain is ready for use the following day after filtration. It keeps well.

B. *May-Grünwald working solution*

May-Grünwald stock solution   2 parts
Buffered distilled water (pH 6·8)   1 part

Must be freshly prepared every day.

C. *Giemsa stock solution*

            Giemsa stain powder   7·5 g.
            Glycerol   500 ml.
            Methanol (pure, acetone-free)   500 ml.

Dissolve the stain in the glycerol at 56°C for 1 to 2 hours, shaking intermittently. Add the methanol, mix, and leave for seven days. The stain is then ready for use after filtration and keeps well.

D. *Giemsa working solution*

Giemsa stock solution   1 part
Buffered distilled water (pH 6·8)   9 parts

Must be freshly prepared every day.

METHOD

1. Methanol 5-10 minutes.
2. May-Grünwald working solution 5–10 minutes.

3. Giemsa working solution 10–20 minutes.
4. Rinse in several changes of distilled water buffered to pH 6·8 (see Note ii).
5. Blot dry. Examine directly by oil-immersion or rinse in xylene and mount, preferably in a neutral mounting medium.

Notes

(i) Buffered distilled water (pH 6·8) may conveniently be made by using commercially produced buffer tablets.

(ii) After it has been stained, the smear is differentiated by the buffered water. The degree of differentiation may be controlled by microscopic examination, by simple inspection, or, with experience, by time alone.

Giemsa stain for inclusion bodies

Suitable for trachoma and related inclusion bodies in air-dried conjunctival scrapings.

METHOD

1. Methanol 2 minutes.
2. Giemsa working solution (as used in the previous method) 1 hour.
3. Rinse in methanol 4 seconds.
4. Differentiate in freshly-distilled water or buffer (pH 6·8) 2–5 minutes.
5. Dehydrate, clear and mount (for full instructions see p. 87).

Staining membrane filters

Most cytological and histological staining methods may be used for membrane filters. The filters are not attached to slides before they are stained, but are transferred from one vessel to the next with forceps. When large numbers of filters need to be stained, this may be done by placing each one in a capsule of the type used for tissue on an automatic processing machine. Batches of this kind can then be stained automatically with results that are more consistent than those obtained manually.

After they have been stained, membrane filters should be

dehydrated, cleared, and mounted in a resinous medium. These final stages require extra care because the membrane is relatively thick and cannot be dehydrated and cleared quickly.

Miscellaneous cytological techniques

Innumerable methods and variations have been published. We have had limited experience with some of these. The following notes are intended merely as a guide for further reading for anyone who wishes to make practical use of these special techniques.

Fluorescence microscopy has been used since von Bertalanffy *et al.* (1956) first described their technique for staining smears with acridine orange. The same authors published a fuller account with colour pictures two years later (von Bertalanffy *et al.*, 1958). The method remains unchanged to the present day. It may be useful for the identification of malignant cells in aspirated fluid, and it has a place in research (Wied and Manglano, 1962), but it is not as good as the Papanicolaou method for the routine examination of gynaecological smears (Löwhagen *et al.*, 1966) or sputum (Papageorgiou and Wolters, 1966).

The examination of circulating blood for malignant cells has been undertaken by many workers in many different ways. The fact that so many methods have been proposed is itself an indication that none of them is entirely satisfactory. Moreover there is no universal agreement about the significance of abnormal cells in blood even when they have been demonstrated. The 'cautionary note' published by the National Cancer Institute (Nadel *et al.*, 1963) is as true today as when it was written. Techniques that have been used include: lysis of red corpuscles, differential filtration through membranes of different pore size, centrifugation in albumin or silicone density gradients, and the removal with magnets of phagocytes that have been allowed to ingest particles of iron. For a review of these and other methods and a full list of references, the reader is advised to consult Goldblatt and Nadel (1965).

Mucoid specimens such as sputum or gastric juice may be concentrated if the mucin is lysed enzymatically. Enzymes that have been used include papain (Rosenthal and Traut, 1951), trypsin (Farber *et al.*, 1953; Chang *et al.*, 1961), and hyaluronidase (Knudtson, 1963).

Assessment of chromatin sex by the demonstration of Barr bodies is not difficult when smears stained with haematoxylin are used. The counterstain may be eosin, although we have preferred the Papanicolaou stain. However, several special stains have been advocated for this purpose; these include cresyl violet (Moore and Barr, 1955) thionin (Klinger and Kurt, 1957), and Biebrich scarlet combined with fast green (Guard, 1959).

CHAPTER 23

Preparation of Museum Specimens

Preservation. Display. Preparation technique. Common faults.
Other methods for routine use. Use of gelatin. Haemosiderin.
Lipids. Amyloid. Suppression of bile staining. Cleared specimens.
Injected specimens. Dry bones.

MUSEUM specimens are of no value unless they are adequately
preserved and suitably displayed. Many techniques have been
recommended for the preparation of museum specimens. Some
of these are virtually interchangeable; others are intended only
for overcoming unusual problems or preparing specimens in
special ways. Most laboratories will find it convenient to use a
single method for general purposes and to use special techniques only occasionally. We give details below of a basic
method that has proved convenient and reliable. Mention of
special techniques will be found later in the chapter.

Preservation

A preservative must suppress micro-organisms and must prevent destruction of tissue by autolysis. Since the tissue is very
often soft, it is an advantage if the preservative will also harden
it. Almost all the routine histological fixatives have these
properties, but unfortunately they also destroy the colour of the
specimen sooner or later. It is usual, therefore, to employ three
stages in the preparation of a specimen, namely fixation, colour
restoration, and preservation. In practice the only suitable
fixative is formalin, since all the others bleach the tissue so much
that the colour can never be restored.

Display

Because preparation includes the use of a fixative which
hardens the tissue, the specimen must be placed in the right
position *before* it is fixed. Attempts to alter the shape of a fixed
specimen are rarely satisfactory. Before fixation, therefore, it
may be necessary to fill the lumen of an organ with fixing fluid,
or with moistened cotton-wool. For other specimens it may be
appropriate to pin the organs on a sheet of cork or expanded

polystyrene which will float on the surface of the fixing fluid and allow the suspended organs to fix without distortion. As an alternative a cake of wax may be used—this could even be prepared to a special shape for a particular problem; care must, however, be taken that contact with the wax is not so extensive as to prevent access of fixing fluid to the tissue. For all pinning it is, of course, necessary to use rustless pins.

However much care is taken in arranging the specimen, it will nearly always be necessary to trim it when it is hardened. This should be done as early as possible, especially when the specimen is bulky, since the centre is unlikely to be as well fixed as the outside, and may even be somewhat autolysed. To cut a thick slice from such a specimen will show a misleading difference between the edge and the centre. It is usually satisfactory to cut a thin slice from the surface after a day or so in fixing fluid. The use of a rotary meat-slicer has been advocated for this purpose (Hall, 1944) but a sharp, long-bladed knife is perfectly adequate. In any event, all trimming must be completed before the colour is restored because, once again, only the surface of the specimen is properly recolorized.

It is almost universal practice to use polymethyl methacrylate (Perspex) jars for mounting specimens since these are lighter in weight than glass, less fragile, optically clearer, and easier to seal. Moreover, they can be prepared or bought in the exact size needed for each specimen. Perspex jars withstand all ordinary preserving fluids, although exceptional specimens which are mounted in alcohol or oil of wintergreen must be housed in glass since these substances attack acrylics. Perspex can also be obtained coloured or opaque; occasionally it is useful to mount a specimen against such a background to draw attention to a particular feature, or to conceal the other side of the tissue when it is damaged or imperfectly fixed, or contains irrelevant and misleading features.

Preparation technique

This is basically similar to the Kaiserling method, although it should be pointed out that Kaiserling himself published three different methods at different times. For details of these and many other methods the reader is advised to consult the book by Edwards and Edwards (1959).

REAGENTS

A. *Fixing fluid*

Neutral buffered formalin solution (p. 17) or Kaiserling (1897) Solution I:

Potassium acetate	30 g.
Potassium nitrate	15 g.
Formalin	200 ml.
Distilled water	1000 ml.

B. *Colour restoring fluid*

Kaiserling (1897) Solution II:
80% alcohol

C. *Mounting fluid*

Kaiserling (1900) Solution III:

Potassium acetate	200 g.
Glycerol	300 ml.
Distilled water	900 ml.

METHOD

1. The specimen should be obtained with a minimum of damage. Remove surplus tissue and wash away contaminating blood with saline. At all costs avoid contact with water since haemolysis will cause discoloration of the final mounting fluid. Position the specimen carefully.
2. Fix thoroughly. This will need no more than a few days if the specimen is thin (e.g. an opened piece of intestine) but is likely to take several weeks for a large solid specimen (e.g. a liver or brain). The fixing fluid should be changed frequently. As soon as the surface of the specimen is hard enough, it should be trimmed to its final form. When cutting a face on a specimen it is important to make a single sweeping cut; jerky movements produce ridges or furrows.
3. Wash in running tap water for ½ to 2 hours depending on the size of the specimen.
4. Restore the colour. This can only be done correctly by observing the specimen frequently whilst it is in the colour restoring fluid. Agitate the fluid and examine the specimen

frequently. A thin specimen may need only 20 minutes; a large specimen may take several hours. Do not leave the specimen too long or the colour will disappear again and cannot then be restored.

5. Rinse for a few minutes in running tap water.
6. Transfer to mounting fluid.
7. Fasten the specimen in a jar of suitable size, fill the jar with mounting fluid, remove bubbles, and seal.

Jars can be bought ready-made or put together from pieces of Perspex sheet joined by ethylene dichloride or chloroform. Full descriptions of methods for making jars and mounting specimens are given by Gordon (1951) and Hackett and Norman (1952). Briefly the procedure for mounting is as follows. When the jar is complete except for one side or end, a label may be fixed inside it with ethylene dichloride or chloroform. The specimen is suspended from Perspex lugs attached to the inside of the jar or, more often, it is stitched to a Perspex centre plate which is itself retained in position by Perspex lugs attached to two edges of the jar. The jar is then filled with mounting fluid almost to capacity. Unnecessary air bubbles will be avoided if the mounting fluid is heated and cooled just before it is added. The last side or end of the jar is then attached but before this is done a small hole (about 3 mm. diameter) is drilled in one end of the jar above the fluid level. After the last joint is hard, the jar is filled with mounting fluid through this hole using a narrow tube. For most specimens, especially porous ones, this is not done until all air bubbles have been removed. The object is to leave no air inside the jar. Finally, the small hole is closed with a Perspex plug sealed with ethylene dichloride or chloroform, or with a thin Perspex plate.

Specimens prepared by this technique will keep their colour well for many years if not exposed to direct sunlight. If necessary they can be taken down, washed, recolorized, and remounted. Histological preparations from old specimens preserved by this method are remarkably good; almost any histological stain may be used except the per-iodic acid Schiff method which seems to be affected by the glycerol in the mounting fluid even if the tissue is washed thoroughly.

Common faults

(i) *The mounting fluid is discoloured.* Brown discoloration is inevitable when the specimen contains much melanin or chromaffin pigment. Bile will discolour the mounting fluid green, although this can be minimized by the use of special techniques (see below). The commonest cause of discoloration is blood pigment from lysed red blood corpuscles. Haemolysis occurs when specimens are allowed to dry or are washed in water before they are fixed, or when they are fixed inadequately. Occasionally discoloration may be unavoidable because the specimen itself contains haemolysed blood (e.g. a lung infarct). Some specimens shed intact red blood corpuscles into the mounting fluid. These settle to the bottom, but are apt to be stirred up when the jar is handled. Gelatin may be used to prevent the detachment of red blood corpuscles (see below).

(ii) *The mounting fluid is turbid.* Droplets of fat may leave the specimen and accumulate as a scum at the top of the jar. When the specimen is handled, this fat will be scattered and may adhere to other faces of the jar. The fault occurs particularly when the mounting fluid has been warmed but not properly cooled before it is added. Special care is needed when the specimen contains much fat (e.g. breast; fatty bone marrow).

Glycogen produces an opalescent milkiness throughout the mounting fluid. Specimens of liver and some ovarian tumours may show this appearance. Fungi occasionally grow in the mounting fluid. They produce a mat of fine filaments at the bottom of the jar. This disperses when the jar is handled and obscures the specimen. Such specimens should be remounted and a few small crystals of thymol added to the mounting fluid.

(iii) *The colour is uneven.* Part of the surface will be brown and glazed if the specimen was allowed to dry before fixation, or if the specimen was not entirely immersed in fixing fluid. Slightly sunken grey patches are caused when the specimen came so close to the wall of the container during fixation that fluid was excluded. The commonest cause of unevenness of colour is the removal of too much surplus tissue after fixation or after colour restoration.

(iv) *The specimen is distorted.* This is almost always due to insufficient care during fixation. If the specimen is fixed in the wrong position, it will rarely be possible to correct this later; cavities should be filled with fluid or moist cotton wool, but excessive packing may flatten the surface, ruining the normal pattern of the tissue. During fixation, specimens should not be packed with, or covered by, textiles with a coarse woven pattern since this may cause a persistent impression on the surface of the tissue.

(v) *The colours are too pale.* All specimens tend to lose some of their colour with the passage of years. This occurs more rapidly in strong light, especially in direct sunlight. The process is probably more rapid when a large air bubble is present in the jar. Some specimens are too pale when first mounted. These may have been fixed badly, having spent too long in fixing fluid or been subjected to an unnecessarily strong formalin solution. Alternatively the time in colour restoring fluid may have been too long or too short. Some museums contain old specimens that are bleached quite white. These are usually mounted in alcohol; all efforts to restore colour will be unavailing.

Other methods for routine use

As already indicated, the method given above is one of innumerable variants that make use of the basic Kaiserling principle of colour restoration by alcohol. In addition to all these variants, two techniques are available that use entirely different methods of colour restoration. The older of these makes use of carbon monoxide (coal gas) which is bubbled through the fluid in which the specimen is immersed until a suitable colour is obtained. This is now rarely if ever used because of its inherent dangers. The other method makes use of sodium hydrosulphite to restore the colour. The first account of colour restoration by sodium hydrosulphite was published by Pulvertaft (1936), who used it for a special purpose. It was applied to specimens of all types by Wentworth, and the method is known by his name. We have little experience of Wentworth's method, which appears to give excellent results in the hands of its originator (Wentworth, 1938; 1939; 1957), but has been criticized by some writers on the grounds that the colours, although vivid, are unrealistic.

Use of gelatin

Gelatin may be used to fill the cavity of a thin-walled viscus or cyst so that it will not collapse. This is particularly necessary when the viscus or cyst needs to be opened to display the lining. For special purposes the gelatin may be coloured before being used; varicose veins, for instance, show a satisfactory appearance when filled with a mixture of gelatin and India ink.

Gelatin is useful as a paint or dip to prevent red blood corpuscles or other small fragments becoming detached from the specimen. Provided that a thin layer is used, it will not be visible. For special purposes it may be desirable to embed parts of a specimen in gelatin. Thus gall stones may be secured in a layer of gelatin within an opened gall bladder.

In all cases the specimen should be rinsed in water after fixation. The gelatin is then applied and allowed to cool before the specimen is returned to the fixing fluid, which will render the gelatin insoluble. For most purposes a simple solution of gelatin in water is sufficient. For filling spaces or embedding stones this should be fairly thick (about 10 per cent) but for painting surfaces it should be thin (about 2 per cent). When translucency is important, it is better to use arsenious acid gelatin, which is prepared as follows. Add 20 g. of arsenious oxide (arsenic trioxide) to one litre of distilled water in a flask with a reflux condenser. Boil in a fume cupboard for 1–2 hours. Add water to restore the volume to one litre and then add 120 g. of gelatin. Re-heat to just below boiling point (a steamer is suitable), and filter through a coarse paper. Add 100 ml. of glycerol and then, drop by drop, add a weak (0·5 per cent) aqueous solution of Victoria blue until the whole of the mixture is tinged with blue. Dispense into bottles and store in the dark; the mixture keeps well. As required, the gelatin mixture is melted by heat. Immediately before use add 1 ml. of formalin to every 200 ml. of the mixture to render the gelatin insoluble.

Haemosiderin

Specimens that contain haemosiderin may be coloured blue by potassium ferrocyanide using a simple modification of the Perls histological method. The fixed specimen is washed in running tap water and then in distilled water. It is transferred to a mixture of equal parts of a 4 per cent aqueous solution of potassium ferrocyanide and a 13 per cent aqueous solution of hydrochloric acid (the exact strengths and proportions are not important). After about 15 to 20 minutes it is rinsed in distilled water, washed for several hours in running tap water, and mounted. Most authorities recommend 5 or 10 per cent formalin-saline as a mounting fluid but we have obtained satisfactory results with the mounting fluid that we use for ordinary specimens. In several months the colour will begin to fade; when necessary it can be restored by opening the specimen to the air or adding a few drops of hydrogen peroxide.

Lipids

After fixation, the specimen is washed well in running tap

water and rinsed in 70 per cent alcohol. It is then stained in Herxheimer's reagent for 20 to 30 minutes (Herxheimer, 1903). Excess dye is removed by a brief wash in 70 per cent alcohol, and the specimen is washed in running tap water for several hours before mounting. Once again, we have had satisfactory results with the mounting fluid that we use for ordinary specimens although most authorities recommend 10 per cent formalin-saline.

Herxheimer's reagent is prepared as follows:

Acetone	100 ml.
Alcohol	70 ml.
Distilled water	30 ml.
Sudan III	to saturation
Sudan IV	to saturation

Heat the solvents in a water-bath to about 56°C. Add the dyes (about 0·5 g. of each) and allow to cool. Filter before use.

Amyloid

This may be demonstrated either by iodine or by Congo red. For the iodine method (Boyd, 1922), the fixed specimen is washed well in water and then transferred to a mixture of 99 parts of Lugol's iodine (p. 84) and 1 part of concentrated sulphuric acid. Maximum contrast develops within an hour or two. The specimen is again washed in running tap water very well (overnight), and then transferred directly to liquid paraffin, in which it must remain for several weeks until it appears bright. It is finally mounted in fresh liquid paraffin.

For the Congo red method, the fixed specimen is washed in water and treated with a 1 per cent aqueous solution of Congo red for about one hour. It is then transferred to a saturated aqueous solution of lithium carbonate for 2 minutes, after which it is differentiated in 80 per cent alcohol to remove the dye from everything except the amyloid. At this stage careful inspection is needed; differentiation may take anything from 5 minutes to 1 hour. After a rinse in water, the specimen is finally mounted in the routine mounting fluid (p. 340).

Suppression of bile staining

If a specimen contains much bile pigment, there is no method whereby this can be completely prevented from discolouring the mounting fluid. There are, however, two ways of minimizing such discoloration. When the specimen has already been fixed in formalin-saline or a fluid of the Kaiserling type such as that given on page 340, it is recolorized in the usual way, rinsed in water, and then transferred to a 10 per cent aqueous solution of calcium chloride in which it should be left overnight. After a brief rinse in water, it is then mounted in the routine mounting fluid (p. 340). This method can equally well be applied to specimens that have already been mounted; these are removed from their museum jars, the colour is restored if necessary, and they are then soaked in calcium chloride solution before being re-mounted in fresh mounting fluid.

When the specimen is received before it has been fixed, bile staining will be minimized if it is prepared according to the method of Jores (1913). In this method, colour is largely pre-served by the fixing fluid so that, when fixation is complete, the specimen is merely washed well in running tap water and moun-ted in the routine mounting fluid. It is common to see one of the items in the formula for Jores's fixing fluid referred to as 'artificial Karlsbad salts'. In chemical terms the formula is:

Sodium sulphate	22 g.
Potassium sulphate	1 g.
Sodium chloride	9 g.
Sodium bicarbonate	18 g.
Formalin	50 ml.
Saturated aqueous solution of chloral hydrate	50 ml.
Distilled water	1000 ml.

Cleared specimens

If the water in a piece of tissue is replaced by something of higher refractive index, the tissue becomes comparatively translucent so that more of its internal structure can be seen. It is then referred to as a cleared specimen. Clarity is further increased if the red blood corpuscles in the specimen are de-stroyed or bleached. Clearing is often used to demonstrate the skeleton (e.g. in a human or animal embryo), especially if the bones are made even more conspicuous by the use of a stain. The technique is also suitable for demonstrating structures such as blood-vessels or air-passages that can be injected with opaque (and preferably with coloured) substances before the specimen is cleared. Many substances of high refractive index have been recommended for the clearing of specimens but in practice glycerol has the merit of being readily available and inoffensive as well as suitable for specimens that are to be mounted in Perspex jars.

The method given below for the preparation of a cleared specimen to demonstrate the skeleton of an embryo is that of Dawson (1926). It will be obvious, however, that it can easily be modified for other purposes; for instance the omission of potassium hydroxide will leave the larger blood-vessels conspicuous by virtue of their content of red blood corpuscles, or the alizarin will be omitted if the preparation is intended to reveal structures other than bones (e.g. an injected specimen). The original method specified fixation in 95 per cent alcohol, but entirely satisfactory results are obtainable after a formalin-saline mixture. Fixation must be thorough; the time needed will depend on the size of the specimen. The specimen is then treated with a 1 per cent aqueous solution of potassium hydroxide until the bones are clearly visible through the soft tissues. It is then transferred to the staining solution which consists of 1 part of alizarin red S in 10,000 parts of 1 per cent aqueous potassium hydroxide solution. This will stain the bony parts of the skeleton a strong purple-red colour overnight; if the colour is too weak, the stain can be renewed and left for a further day. The specimen is then transferred to a mixture of 1 part of potassium hydroxide, 20 parts of glycerol, and 79 parts of water. This mixture will remove the stain from all the soft tissues within a day or two. Thereafter it is treated with increasingly strong solutions of glycerol, and should spend not less than one week in each of the following: 30, 50, 75 per cent, and undiluted glycerol. It must remain in undiluted glycerol until quite clear, when it is mounted in fresh glycerol.

Injected specimens

When museum specimens were preserved in alcohol, they quickly became bleached, so that it was necessary to add artificial colour. This was usually done by introducing red pigment into the blood-vessels. Modern museum specimens are usually prepared in a way that preserves their natural colours. It is, however, still necessary in special instances to use an injection technique to demonstrate a particular feature. The basic requirements are: the substance injected must be fluid enough to enter the specimen easily; once in place it must set quickly; it must not be dissolved or decolorized by any of the fluids that will later be used to prepare and mount the specimen; it must not be brittle or easy to dislodge. In practice, injections are made with an insoluble pigment mixed with either gelatin or synthetic latex. For some purposes it may be convenient to choose a pigment that is radio-opaque, or to incorporate a third, radio-opaque, substance in the mixture.

Pigments that have been used include vermilion (red mercuric sulphide), chrome yellow (lead chromate), and India ink, among many others, but it is more convenient to purchase stable pigments of suitable colours (Chromopaque) from specialist suppliers. When gelatin is used, this may be in the form already described or in an alkaline solution. Alkaline gelatin (metagelatin) has the merit that it does not require heating, since it is fluid at room temperature; it can, nevertheless, easily be hardened by formalin solutions. Synthetic latex (Neoprene) was first used for the injection of specimens by Lieb (1940). It readily solidifies in weak acid to form a tenacious but flexible mass. Since this mass is resistant to corrosive chemicals, Neoprene is particularly suitable for the production of corrosion casts of vessels or viscera, which are readily prepared by treating the injected specimen with concentrated hydrochloric acid at 56°C overnight and washing away the remaining fragments of tissue with a jet of water.

Whenever possible, the specimen should be injected before it has been fixed. When the injection is made into blood-vessels, it is common practice to start by flushing out blood and small clots. When the final colour is unimportant, or a corrosion cast is to be prepared, plain water is suitable for this; otherwise saline should be used. The injection may be made using artificial pressure or by a gravity feed arrangement. When small vessels need to be filled, it is necessary to apply artificial pressure, either to the vessel that contains the injection mass, or by means of a syringe. For large volumes, a Higginson syringe is preferable to one of hypodermic type. The most satisfactory cannula for a small vessel is a piece of plastic tubing which can be threaded inside the vessel and tied tightly; after injection the plastic tube can be closed with a screw clamp. When the injection mass is of the gelatin type, a small volume of formalin (1 part to 200) should be added just before use to convert the gelatin to an insoluble gel; this is particularly necessary when large vessels or cavities are injected, even when the entire specimen will next be placed in a formalin fixing fluid. For fuller practical accounts of injection techniques and their special applications, the book by Tompsett (1956) should be consulted.

Dry bones

Occasionally it is desirable to prepare a dry specimen of bone or a part of the skeleton. This is done by first removing the soft tissue, secondly removing fatty constituents, and thirdly bleaching. It is best to start with an unfixed specimen, although fixed specimens may be used provided that more time is devoted to them. Surplus soft tissue is removed by cutting and gentle scraping. The specimen is then macerated in water at 80°C for 2–3 hours, after which most if not all of the soft tissue can be picked off or removed with a nail brush. If some of the soft tissue resists removal, the bone is returned to hot water for a further 2–3 hours and the process repeated as often as necessary. This treatment will not destroy ligaments or loosen teeth. If the specimen is merely dense cortical bone, the process can be hastened by using 10 per cent sodium hydroxide solution at 80°C instead of water, but this must not be used if ligaments are to be preserved or teeth are to remain in place.

When all the soft tissues have been removed, the bone is allowed to dry at room temperature (not in an oven which may cause delicate bones to crack). When dry, the specimen is placed in a fat solvent such as chloroform or carbon tetrachloride for several hours. Often this will need to be changed at least once. The bone is again allowed to dry at room temperature and is then bleached in hydrogen peroxide overnight. After drying once more, the bone may be preserved by painting or spraying its surfaces with varnish.

CHAPTER 24

Special Techniques

Enzyme histochemistry: DOPA-oxidase; Gomori for alkaline phosphatase; Gomori for acid phosphatase; Diazo for alkaline phosphatase; Diazo for acid phosphatase. Autoradiography. Processing for electron microscopy: Osmium; Glutaraldehyde. Staining tissue cultures. Paper mounted sections. Sections for direct projection.

Enzyme histochemistry

Histochemical studies of enzyme activity are used to only a limited extent in routine laboratories. Enzyme methods may become more widely used for diagnostic purposes in the future, but at present the necessity for fresh tissue or special methods of fixation, and the time and skill required are beyond the resources of the average laboratory. We have, however, included in this book a method for DOPA-oxidase and two methods each or alkaline phosphatase and acid phosphatase since these may occasionally be required in routine histological laboratories. For further theoretical information about enzyme histochemistry, as well as practical details of many suitable methods, the reader is recommended to Chayen et al. (1969).

An enzyme is a biological catalyst; that is to say it increases the rate of a chemical reaction but is not itself formed or destroyed by the reaction. The raw material is known as the substrate: substances formed as a result of enzyme reaction are known as products. Enzymes vary in their specificity: some will attack only a particular chemical substance; others attack a wide variety of related substances. Usually an enzyme is given a name that indicates the type of substrate that it attacks, with the suffix -ase added. Thus, succinic dehydrogenase attacks succinic acid, from which it removes hydrogen atoms. A phosphatase will attack a variety of phosphates.

Enzymes consist almost entirely of protein, and therefore stain in the same way as other cell proteins. Thus it is impossible to identify enzymes by simple staining methods. In many instances, however, it is possible to demonstrate sites of enzyme activity. In a few cases the product of the reaction is evident;

thus DOPA-oxidase produces an insoluble melanin-like pigment. More often, one of the products can be demonstrated by chemical means; thus phosphates have been demonstrated by capturing the newly-formed phosphate with heavy metals such as calcium or lead, and in turn demonstrating the heavy metal. In such a case it is, of course, essential that the phosphate reacts instantly with the heavy metal, before it has had time to diffuse, otherwise the method will not indicate the sites of enzyme activity with precision. For the same reason it is essential that the metallic phosphate precipitate is completely insoluble. When an enzyme is not entirely specific, but can be made to attack a variety of substrates, it may be possible to provide it with an artificial substrate which yields easily demonstrable products. This is the basis of the diazo methods for phosphatase in which the substrate is α-naphthyl phosphate. When the phosphate is removed, the remaining part of the molecule reacts instantly with the salt of an azo dye to yield an insoluble coloured substance.

DOPA-oxidase

Scope

A method for demonstrating enzymes that oxidize dihydroxyphenylalanine (DOPA). The tissue is incubated with DOPA and a dark deposit of melanin-like oxidation products marks the site of enzyme activity. The method is used in the study of melanin-forming cells in the skin and other sites; it is also valuable for non-pigmented melanomas. Tissue must be fresh or briefly fixed in formalin. We have used the method of Becker, Praver and Thatcher (1935) modified by preliminary fixation.

Reagents

A. *Substrate*

0·1% dihydroxyphenylalanine in 0·1 M phosphate buffer at pH 7·3-7·5 (see Note i).

B. *Bouin's fluid* (p. 20)

Method

1. Fix thin (2 mm.) pieces of tissue in neutral buffered formalin solution for about one hour.

2. Running tap water about 5 minutes.
3. Substrate at 37°C for one hour.
4. Fresh substrate at 37°C for 12–15 hours.
5. Running tap water 5 minutes.
6. Bouin's fluid at least 12 hours.
7. Dehydrate, clear, impregnate and embed in paraffin wax.
8. Cut sections 5–8 μ thick, mount on slides and dry.
9. Sections to water.
10. Counterstain as required (see Note iv).
11. Dehydrate, clear, and mount.

RESULTS

Sites of DOPA-oxidase activity: *dark brown to black.*
Other structures: according to counterstain used.

CONTROLS

(*a*) To inhibit enzyme activity add potassium cyanide to the substrate in 1 mM concentration.
(*b*) For a positive control use fresh skin.

Notes

(i) The pH must be correct. At higher pH (e.g. 7·7) there is much non-specific blackening: at lower pH (e.g. 6·8) enzyme activity is greatly reduced.
(ii) Fresh substrate is used because the first batch is apt to become acid.
(iii) Cryostat sections may be used. These may be cut from tissue fixed briefly in a formalin fixing fluid. Alternatively unfixed tissue may be used, in which case the sections are briefly fixed. Cryostat sections should be treated with substrate at 37°C for 2–4 hours and examined microscopically from time to time.
(iv) Suitable counterstains include neutral red, haematoxylin and eosin, and trichrome stains. The counterstain should be light.

Gomori for alkaline phosphatase

SCOPE

A method for alkaline phosphatase (i.e. phosphatase that is active in an alkaline medium). Suitable for cryostat sections or for tissue fixed in alcohol or acetone. The newly-formed phosphate is instantly precipitated as calcium phosphate. This is converted to cobalt phosphate which is in turn converted to

the black pigment cobalt sulphide. The method is slightly
modified from the original (Gomori, 1939).

REAGENTS

A. *Substrate mixture*

3% aqueous sodium β-glycerophosphate	10 ml.
2% aqueous sodium diethyl barbiturate (barbitone sodium)	10 ml.
2% aqueous calcium chloride (anhydrous)	20 ml.
5% aqueous magnesium sulphate	1 ml.
Distilled water	5 ml.

   The pH should be 9·4.

B. *2 per cent aqueous cobalt nitrate*

C. *0·5 per cent ammonium sulphide in distilled water*

METHOD

1. Fix thin (1–2 mm.) pieces of tissue in alcohol or acetone
   at 0–4°C for 18–24 hours. The fluid should be changed
   at least once during this time.
2. Clear in benzene.
3. Impregnate and embed in paraffin wax (see Note i).
4. Cut sections and mount them on slides. Dry at 37°C for
   no more than 2–3 hours (see Note ii).
5. Sections to water.
6. Substrate mixture at 37°C for 1–6 hours (see Note iii).
7. Running tap water 1 minute.
8. Cobalt nitrate 5 minutes.
9. Rinse in distilled water.
10. Weak ammonium sulphide 1–2 minutes.
11. Running tap water 2–3 minutes.
12. Counterstain if required (see Note v).
13. Dehydrate, clear, and mount.

RESULTS

   Sites of alkaline phosphatase activity: *black*.
   Other structures: according to counterstain used.

CONTROLS

(*a*) omit glycerophosphate from the substrate.
(*b*) for a positive control use fresh kidney.

   2 A

Notes

(i) Temperature in wax must not rise above 56°C and the time should not exceed 1½ hours.

(ii) Paraffin blocks may be stored at 4°C without loss of enzyme activity. Paraffin sections, however, lose this activity within a day or two.

(iii) The optimum time of incubation will vary from one specimen to another. When possible a number of sections should be incubated so that one of them can be removed every half-hour or so.

(iv) Cryostat sections may be used. If unfixed, these will require 10–60 minutes in substrate. Alternatively the sections may be fixed briefly in cold alcohol or cold dilute aqueous formalin, in which case incubation should continue for ½–4 hours.

(v) Suitable counterstains include neutral red and aqueous eosin.

Gomori for acid phosphatase

SCOPE

A method for acid phosphatase (i.e. phosphatase that is active in an acid medium). Suitable for cryostat sections or for tissue fixed in acetone. The newly-formed phosphate is instantly precipitated as lead phosphate which is then converted to the black pigment lead sulphide. The method is modified from that of Gomori (1941).

REAGENTS

A. *Substrate mixture*

0·05 M acetate buffer at pH 5·0	250 ml.
Lead nitrate	0·3 g.
3% aqueous sodium β-glycerophosphate	25 ml.

Leave the mixture at 37°C for 24 hours. Add 2–3 ml. distilled water; filter. Use within a few days.

B. *0·5 per cent aqueous ammonium sulphide*

METHOD

1. Fix thin (1–2 mm.) pieces of tissue in acetone at 0–4°C for 18–24 hours. The fluid should be replaced once during this time. 2–4. Exactly as for Gomori's alkaline phosphatase method above.

5. Sections rapidly to water.
6. Rinse in distilled water.
7. Substrate mixture 1–18 hours (see Note iii).
8. Rinse in distilled water.
9. Weak ammonium sulphide 1–2 minutes.
10. Running tap water 2–3 minutes.
11. Counterstain if required.
12. Dehydrate, clear, and mount.

RESULTS

Sites of acid phosphatase activity: *black*.
Other structures: according to counterstain used.

CONTROLS

(*a*) To inhibit enzyme activity add sodium fluoride to the substrate in 10 mM concentration.
(*b*) For a positive control use fresh prostate.

Notes

(i) Temperature in wax must not rise above 56°C and the time should not exceed $1\frac{1}{2}$ hours.

(ii) Paraffin blocks may be stored at 4°C without loss of enzyme activity. Paraffin sections, however, should be used within a few hours.

(iii) The optimum time of incubation varies. Several sections should be incubated so that one may be removed from time to time.

(iv) Cryostat sections may be used. If cut from unfixed tissue, the sections should be fixed in cold (−15°C) acetone for 15–30 minutes followed by acetone at room temperature for 30 minutes. Alternatively cryostat sections may be cut from tissue that was fixed in Baker's formalin-calcium (p. 159) at 0–4°C for 18–24 hours, followed by treatment with gum-sucrose (p. 275) at 0–4°C for 24 hours or longer.

(v) Suitable counterstains include neutral red and aqueous eosin.

Diazo method for alkaline phosphatase

SCOPE

A less laborious method for alkaline phosphatase. Suitable for frozen sections. The method is modified from Menten, *et al.* (1944).

REAGENTS

A. *Substrate mixture*

2% aqueous sodium diethyl barbiturate (barbitone sodium)	25 ml.
Sodium α-naphthyl phosphate	10 mg.
10% aqueous magnesium chloride	0·2 ml.
Fast red TR salt	25 mg.

Dissolve the naphthyl phosphate in the barbitone; add the magnesium chloride; mix well. Finally add the fast red, mix well, filter, and use at once (see Note i).

B. *Carazzi's haematoxylin* (p. 106).

METHOD

1. Fix thin pieces of tissue in cold (0–4°C) formalin-calcium (p. 159) for 12–24 hours.
2. Cut frozen sections.
3. Substrate mixture at room temperature 10–15 minutes.
4. Wash well in distilled water.
5. Carazzi's haematoxylin 1 minute.
6. Tap water 5 minutes.
7. Mount in glycerin-jelly (p. 89).

RESULTS

Sites of alkaline phosphatase activity: *red.*
Nuclei: *grey-blue.*

CONTROLS

(*a*) Omit α-naphthyl phosphate from the substrate.
(*b*) For a positive control use fresh kidney.

Notes

(i) The method must be performed without delay once the substrate has been prepared. Fast red TR loses its activity after 20 minutes or so in solution.

(ii) Many other diazonium salts may be used. If a blue colour is preferred, fast blue RR gives good results.

(iii) A modification for smears of blood was published by Kaplow (1955).

Diazo method for acid phosphatase

SCOPE

A method for acid phosphatase. Less laborious than Gomori's method but also less precise. Suitable for frozen sections.

REAGENTS

A. *Substrate mixture*

0·1 M veronal acetate buffer at pH 5	20 ml.
Sodium α-naphthyl phosphate	10–20 mg.
Polyvinyl pyrrolidine	1·5 g.
Fast garnet GBC salt	20 mg.

Dissolve the naphthyl phosphate and polyvinyl pyrrolidine in the buffer. Finally add the fast garnet, mix well, filter, and use at once (see Note i).

B. *Carazzi's haematoxylin* (p. 106)

METHOD

1. Fix thin pieces of tissue in cold (0–4°C) 10% aqueous neutralized formalin for 10–16 hours.
2. Cut frozen sections.
3. Substrate mixture at 37°C ½ minute to 1 hour.
4. Tap water 1–2 minutes.
5. Carazzi's haematoxylin 1 minute.
6. Tap water 5 minutes.
7. Mount in glycerin-jelly (p. 89).

RESULTS

Sites of acid phosphatase activity: *reddish-brown*.
Nuclei: *grey-blue*.

CONTROLS

(*a*) To inhibit enzyme activity heat a section at 80°C for 10–15 minutes.
(*b*) For a positive control use fresh prostate.

Notes

(i) The method must be performed without delay once the fast garnet has been dissolved.

(ii) Other diazonium salts may be used: fast red ITR gives good results.

Autoradiography

If a section contains radioactive substances, these can be demonstrated by their effect on photographic emulsion. Radioactive particles affect the emulsion in the same way as the light rays of conventional photography. The photographic emulsion is applied either in the form of a thin gelatin sheet ('stripping film') or as a coat of melted sensitized gelatin. It is processed in the same way as a photographic negative. Before and after exposure to the section it must be handled in the dark or with a suitable safelight; after exposure the affected silver particles must be treated with a suitable reducing agent (photographic 'developer') and the unaffected silver salts removed by a photographic 'fixer'.

The pattern of affected silver grains is examined microscopically and indicates the radioactive sites. By staining the section while leaving the emulsion on it, the type of cell responsible for the radioactivity can be identified. If the emulsion is of uniform thickness, it is possible to measure the quantity of radioactivity released during the period of exposure.

Not every radioactive source is suitable: to produce results it must emit particles that have sufficient penetrating power to escape from the section and enter the emulsion. Particles with too much energy, on the other hand, tend to pass right through the emulsion without leaving many altered silver grains in their path. Furthermore, a source must be used that has a suitable rate of disintegration (half-life). If this is too great, the exposure will need to be unduly prolonged, whereas a substance with a half-life of only minutes or hours will have decayed before the section can be prepared. Tritium (radioactive hydrogen) is one of the substances commonly used for autoradiography: it has the additional advantage that it is readily incorporated into a wide variety of organic substances suitable for biological investigation.

Obviously the results will be blurred or inaccurate unless the following precautions are taken: the section must be thin, there must be no gap between section and emulsion, the emulsion must be thin, and the emulsion must not move after it has been exposed.

REAGENTS

A. *Adhesive*

    Gelatin   1 g.

    Chrome alum (chromium potassium sulphate) 0·1 g.

    Water   200 ml.

B. *Stripping film*

    Kodak AR 10 *or* AR 50.

  or *Liquid emulsion.*

    Kodak NTB 2 nuclear track emulsion (see Note i).

C. *Anhydrous calcium sulphate* (see Note ii).

D. *Developer* (D 19B)

Metol	2·2 g.
Sodium sulphite (anhydrous)	72 g.
Hydroquinone	8·8 g.
Sodium carbonate (anhydrous)	48 g.
Potassium bromide	4 g.
Distilled water	1000 g.

Dissolve the salts separately; mix in the order given; filter before use.

E. *Stop bath*

Chrome alum (chromium potassium sulphate)	20 g.
Sodium metabisulphite	20 g.
Distilled water	1000 ml.

This solution keeps well.

F. *Fixing bath*

30% aqueous sodium thiosulphate	50 ml.
Stop bath (above)	25 ml.

Mix shortly before use. The stock solution of sodium thiosulphate keeps well.

METHOD (Stages 5, 6, 8, 9 and 10 in the dark room)

1. Fix tissue in a simple fluid, avoiding mercury and chromium. Process and embed in paraffin wax (see Note iii).

2. Cut thin sections (2–$5\,\mu$) and mount them on prepared slides. The slides must be carefully cleaned, dipped in adhesive, and allowed to dry before use. Dry the mounted sections thoroughly.
3. Sections to water.
4. Wash well in distilled water.
5. In a darkroom, at least one metre away from a Wratten No. 2 safelight,
   either: Incise and detach a piece of stripping film and float this on distilled water at 22–$25°C$ for 2–3 minutes until it is completely flat. Float the film with its emulsion downwards and ensure that it is wider than the slide. Insert the slide beneath the film and withdraw them obliquely together so that the film overhangs both edges of the slide and is in close contact with the section,
   or: Melt a small quantity of liquid emulsion at 40–$45°C$ (see Note iv) and dip the slide in it. Wipe the back of the slide and stand it vertically to drain.
6. Allow the gelatin layer to dry thoroughly in the dark (2–3 hours). Pack the slides in a light-proof box in which there is a small quantity of anhydrous calcium sulphate.
7. Store the box in a refrigerator at $4°C$ for the necessary length of time (see Note v).
8. In the darkroom (Wratten No. 2 safelight), remove the slides and develop the emulsion at 17–$18°C$ 2–$2\frac{1}{2}$ minutes.
9. Stop bath 5 minutes.
10. Fixing bath 10 minutes.
11. Wash well in distilled water, changing the water several times.
12. Counterstain as required (see Note vi).
13. Dehydrate, clear, and mount.

RESULTS

Sites of radioactivity: *small black granules above the section.*

Notes

(i) Stripping film is uniform in thickness and suitable for precise measurements: liquid emulsion forms a layer of variable and unknown thickness. On the other hand, the liquid emulsion makes closer contact with the section.

Of the two stripping films, AR 10 is the thinner emulsion and will be preferred for very accurate results; AR 50 is more sensitive so that results are obtained more quickly.

(ii) Anhydrous calcium sulphate for drying purposes is obtainable from Hopkin and Williams, Ltd., who sell it as Drierite.

(iii) The amount of radioactive substance in most specimens is small, but nevertheless they should be handled with proper precautions and reagents disposed of with care. For general guidance see *Code of Practice for the Protection of Persons Exposed to Ionising Radiations in Research and Teaching* (1964).

(iv) Liquid emulsion is expensive and needs to be stored in the dark at 4°C. It is convenient to dispense it into small containers in advance and to use the smallest vessel that will hold a slide.

(v) The time is dependent on the radioactive substance used. It is wise to make several preparations so that they can be removed at intervals. Days or weeks will usually be needed, so that it is wise to arrange the slides with the emulsion downwards to prevent contamination by dust. Sections must not be packed too close or the radioactivity may contaminate neighbours.

(vi) Counterstains should not be heavy. Possibilities include Carazzi's haematoxylin and eosin, neutral red, pyronin and methyl green, and the Feulgen reaction. Alternatively the section may be stained before it is coated with emulsion.

(vii) When electric incubators or water-baths are used in a dark-oom, the indicator bulbs should be removed and the thermostats rovered to conceal electric sparks.

Processing tissue for electron microscopy

Very few routine laboratories have access to an electron microscope, so that a full account of its use would be out of place in this book. There is, however, an increasing tendency to rely on the electron microscope for the diagnosis of certain diseases, especially those of the kidney. Tissue must be absolutely fresh, and the final result depends to a great extent on its initial treatment, so that all routine laboratories should be prepared to undertake the fixation and processing of specimens of tissue destined for electron microscopy, even though they are unable to section or examine it. For this reason, we have included suitable methods below.

The principles involved in preparing tissue for the electron microscope are analogous to those of conventional processing but the details are entirely different. The chief problems that have to be solved are the preservation of intracellular structures, the preparation of very thin sections, and the choice of an embedding medium that will withstand the high vacuum and high temperature in the electron microscope itself.

First, the tissue must be fixed with extreme care in view of the magnifications at which it will be examined ($\times 2000$ to $\times 100,000$). Thus small pieces of tissue are selected to ensure uniform penetration, and buffered isotonic fluids are used to avoid destruction of the cells. Secondly, the tissue is dehydrated and (usually) cleared. Thirdly, it is embedded in a much firmer medium than paraffin wax or nitrocellulose in order that very thin sections may be prepared. These must be no thicker than 500–1000 Å (0.05–$0.1\ \mu$) and are produced on a specially rigid and precise microtome (ultramicrotome) using a knife made from broken plate-glass or from a diamond. It is convenient to use an embedding medium from which thicker sections suitable for optical microscopy can also be cut. For examination in the electron microscope, the sections are finally mounted on metal grids.

Sections are not stained with dyes, since the electron microscope does not depend on variations of colour. Structures are distinguishable in an electron microscope when they scatter the electron beam to a greater or lesser extent than their surroundings. A component that allows electrons to pass freely will be distinguishable from one that prevents their passage by scattering them in all directions. Electrons are scattered by substances of high atomic weight, so that these may be used to enhance contrast provided that they have varying affinities for various tissue components. The most useful substance for this purpose is osmium (in the form of osmium tetroxide) which readily becomes attached to the lipid parts of cellular and intracellular membranes. Other metals that have been used include uranium, lead, tungsten, manganese and chromium. Usually the piece of tissue is treated with metal before being processed, but in some methods the sections are treated as well or instead. When used on unprocessed tissue, the metal is either incorporated in the primary fixing fluid or in a secondary fixing fluid.

To be satisfactory for occasional use in non-specialist laboratories, a technique must be relatively straightforward and must not demand special equipment or complicated time schedules. The method given below consists basically of fixation in buffered osmium (Palade, 1952) followed by embedding in Epon by a method modified from Finck (1960). When osmium is used as a fixative, the tissue must be processed forthwith; there is no convenient stage at which it can be left overnight or over a weekend. It is therefore common practice to use glutaraldehyde (Sabatini, Bensch, and Barrnett, 1963) as a primary fixative, and to store the tissue until it can conveniently be processed. For this reason we have included glutaraldehyde as an optional primary fixative, to be followed by secondary fixation in osmium. This sequence should be used if time is likely to elapse between taking the specimen and its receipt in the laboratory, or if it is not convenient to process the tissue at once. The results are not quite as good as those obtained with primary fixation in osmium.

Primary osmium fixation

REAGENTS (see Note i)

A. *Phosphate buffer* (pH 7·2–7·4)

2·26% aqueous sodium dihydrogen phosphate (NaH$_2$PO$_4$.H$_2$O)	83 ml.
2·52% aqueous sodium hydroxide	17 ml.

B. *Buffered osmium fixing fluid*

Phosphate buffer	45 ml.
5·4% aqueous glucose	5 ml.
Osmium tetroxide	0·5 g.

Adjust to pH 7·2–7·4. Osmium tetroxide dissolves very slowly but heat must not be used. Store at 4°C where the solution will keep for a few days.

C. *Propylene oxide*

D. *Impregnating mixture*

Epon 812	10 ml.
DDSA (dodecenyl succinic anhydride)	18 ml.
HHPA (hexahydrophthalic anhydride)	1 ml.

Melt the HHPA at 55°C and then transfer all the reagents to an incubator at 37–40°C. Measure the quantities in warm all-glass syringes and mix them by vigorous stirring with a glass rod in a polythene beaker. This mixture keeps for several days (see Note iii).

E. *Embedding mixture*

Impregnating mixture to which is added 1% of the accelerator BDMA (benzyl dimethylamine). This mixture must be freshly prepared.

METHOD (stages 10–14 at 37–40°C; stage 15 at 55–60°C)

1. Fix very small pieces (not greater than one millimetre cubes) of very fresh tissue in buffered osmium at 4°C for 1–2 hours. (See Note ii).
2. Wash well with distilled water.
3. 30% alcohol 10 minutes.
4. 50% alcohol 10 minutes.
5. 70% alcohol 10 minutes.
6. 90% alcohol 10 minutes.
7. Alcohol 10 minutes.
8. Repeat with fresh alcohol.
9. Propylene oxide 30 minutes.
10. Equal parts of propylene oxide and impregnating mixture at 37–40°C for 15 minutes in an unsealed vessel.
11. Impregnating mixture 1 hour.
12. Impregnating mixture 1–2 days. Replace the impregnating mixture once during this time (see Note ii).
13. Embedding mixture 1 hour.
14. Embedding mixture overnight.
15. Arrange the tissue in fresh embedding mixture in a suitable container and transfer to an incubator at 55–60°C for 2–3 days (see Note iv).

Notes

(i) The constituents of Epon resin must be handled with care, since some of them are carcinogenic. The vapour of osmium tetroxide is toxic as well as the solution.

(ii) Fixation time depends on the compactness of the tissue. Two hours should never be exceeded; most tissue (e.g. kidney) is well-fixed in $1\frac{1}{2}$ hours. Similarly, the time in impregnating mixture (stage 12) depends on the type of tissue.

(iii) Syringes and other vessels that have contained Epon resin or its constituents must be cleaned in acetone and dried immediately after use. When possible, disposable plastic vessels should be used. Surplus resin must not be poured into drains.

(iv) Stages 1–9 can be carried out in any small glass vessel. Whatever is used for later stages of the method will need to be discarded.

Shallow metal-foil trays are convenient. The final stage (hardening) may also be carried out in a metal-foil tray: alternatively small moulds may be used. Trays are easier to manage, especially when the orientation of the specimen is important, and bubbles can readily be dislodged. On the other hand the final block will need trimming with a saw. Disposable plastic moulds or carefully dried gelatin drug capsules (size 0 or 00) produce smaller blocks but do not permit orientation of the specimen.

Primary glutaraldehyde fixation

REAGENTS

A. *Buffered glutaraldehyde fixing fluid.*

Stabilized 25% glutaraldehyde solution (see Note i)	16 ml.
Phosphate buffer at pH 7·2–7·4 (as used in the osmium method above)	84 ml.

B. *Buffered sucrose*

Sucrose	6·5 g.
Phosphate buffer (pH 7·2–7·4)	100 ml.

Store at 4°C.

METHOD

1. Fix small pieces of very fresh tissue in buffered glutaraldehyde at room temperature for 2–24 hours.
2. Wash in buffered sucrose to remove glutaraldehyde. This requires at least three hours and the sucrose should be changed twice during that time.
3. Either store the tissue in buffered sucrose at 4°C, or transfer it directly to buffered osmium fixing fluid and proceed according to the method above.

Notes

(i) Stabilized glutaraldehyde may be purchased from TAAB Laboratories.

(ii) Although pieces must be small, they may be slightly larger than those used for primary osmium fixation. When such pieces are used, they must be trimmed before secondary fixation in osmium.

(iii) Workers with small animals can obtain particularly good fixation by perfusing the anaesthetized animal with buffered glutaraldehyde before removing the pieces.

(iv) Although glutaraldehyde fixation is usually followed by secondary osmium fixation, it is possible to process tissue after fixation in glutaraldehyde alone. This method is appropriate for certain histochemical techniques: it does not provide satisfactory sections for the study of cell structure.

Staining tissue cultures

Tissue cultures may be stained by many routine histological methods although sometimes their staining reactions differ from those of other sections or smears. With haematoxylin and eosin, for instance, many methods are apt to give blue cytoplasm; for satisfactory results Carazzi's haematoxylin (p. 106) is recommended.

Cells in tissue culture are sometimes grown in suspension: more often in monolayers. When they are suspended, the cells are handled in the same way as other specimens of fluid (p. 319). Monolayers are either grown on coverslips or on the inside of roller-tubes. Coverslips are comparatively simple to fix and stain by conventional methods. Roller-tubes, on the other hand, require special handling. The most satisfactory technique (Cheatham, 1954) is to impregnate the monolayer with nitrocellulose, allow this to dry, and then peel it off the inside of the tube and remove it together with the layer of cells. Several staining methods are suitable, and some of these are most conveniently performed before the cells are removed from the tube. The method below uses haematoxylin in the tube followed by an eosin counterstain after the monolayer has been removed. Alternative staining methods include phloxine (in the tube) followed by tartrazine (outside), and Feulgen (in the tube) followed by a counterstain (outside).

REAGENTS

A. *Alcoholic mercuric chloride* (*p.* 324) *or neutral buffered formalin* (p. 17)

B. *Carazzi's haematoxylin* (p. 106)

C. *1 per cent hydrochloric acid in 70 per cent alcohol*

D. *Alcohol-ether mixture* (equal parts)

E. *5 per cent nitrocellulose* in a mixture of equal parts of alcohol and ether. This may be prepared by diluting a stronger solution (p. 266).

F. *0·5 per cent aqueous eosin*

G. *Alcohol-chloroform mixture* (equal parts)

H. *Carbol-xylene* (p. 286)

METHOD

1. Pour off the culture fluid and submerge the roller-tube in fixing fluid overnight (see Note).
2. Wash well in several changes of tap water.
3. Fill the tube with Carazzi's haematoxylin for 10–15 minutes.
4. Wash well in several changes of tap water during 5 minutes.
5. Acid-alcohol 5–10 seconds.
6. Wash well in several changes of tap water during 5–10 minutes.
7. Alcohol 1–2 minutes.
8. Repeat with fresh alcohol.
9. Alcohol-ether 1–2 minutes.
10. Fill the tube with nitrocellulose, cork, and leave for 1–2 hours.
11. Decant the nitrocellulose and stand the tube vertically upside-down to drain for about 30 minutes.
12. Leave the tube horizontal until the nitrocellulose film is hard (usually overnight).
13. Submerge the tube in cold tap water for 30 minutes. During this time the film begins to detach.
14. Extract the film with forceps, place it in water, and cut out an area containing cells.
15. Eosin 5–10 minutes.
16. Wash in tap water 1–2 minutes.
17. Dehydrate, clear, and mount. Treat the piece of nitrocellulose film as though it were a nitrocellulose section (p. 273), using alcohol-chloroform and carbol-xylene.

Note

When the tissue culture has been made to demonstrate the growth of a virus, the culture fluid must be poured off with care and disinfected. The tube is submerged in alcoholic mercuric chloride or formalin solution to destroy infectivity as well as to fix the cells.

Paper mounted sections

Thick sections of a whole organ can be mounted on strong paper as an alternative to the preparation of museum specimens. Paper mounted sections are convenient for filing and are particularly suitable for demonstrating the pattern or texture of the organ. Although originally developed for whole lungs, the method has been applied to other specimens. Tissue with an intrinsic colour makes good preparations, but it is also possible to use a limited number of stains, including Perls's method and myelin stains of the Loyez type. Thick sections are cut from a slice of tissue impregnated with gelatin. The sections are then mounted on paper. This method is considerably modified from the original (Gough and Wentworth, 1949a and b).

REAGENTS

A. *Impregnating gelatin*

Gelatin	250 g.
Cellosolve (ethylene glycol monoethyl ether)	40 ml.
Capryl alcohol	5 ml.
Distilled water	850 ml.

Add the gelatin to the hot water; cool and add the other reagents.

B. *Mounting gelatin*

Gelatin	75 g.
Glycerol	70 ml.
Cellosolve (ethylene glycol monoethyl ether)	40 ml.
Distilled water	850 ml.

Prepare in the same way as the impregnating gelatin.

METHOD

1. Fix the specimen thoroughly in neutral buffered formalin solution (see Note i).
2. Cut a slice 1·5 to 2 cm. thick and return it to the fixing fluid for several days.
3. Running tap water for 3 days.
4. Impregnating gelatin at 60°C under reduced pressure (see Note ii).

5. Transfer to fresh impregnating gelatin at 37°C for 2 days.
6. Embed by allowing the gelatin to cool in a suitable mould prepared from stiff paper or metal-foil.
7. Remove the gelatin block and press it onto a heated block-holder. Hold the block in place with a weight until it is firmly attached; then cool it at $-15°C$ for several hours (preferably overnight).
8. Attach the block-holder to the microtome and remove excess superficial gelatin. Cut sections as the surface thaws; if necessary assisting it to thaw by rubbing with a warm cloth. Sections of lung should be about $400\,\mu$ thick; more solid organs about $300\,\mu$.
9. Transfer the sections to neutral buffered formalin solution for 1–2 days.
10. Wash in cold water for 1–2 hours.
11. Flood a sheet of Perspex with warm mounting gelatin. Place the section on this after removing the excess of gelatin from its edges. Cover the section with a sheet of Whatman's No. 1 filter paper and squeegee lightly to remove excess gelatin and all air bubbles.
12. Drain away the excess mounting gelatin and then leave the preparation flat until firm. Dry by using moderate heat (a film drying cabinet is suitable). When thoroughly dry, peel the paper from the Perspex.

Notes

(i) Hollow organs should be filled with fixing fluid. Lungs may be distended by filling them through the main bronchus from a reservoir 1 to 1·5 metres above the specimen.

(ii) Reduced pressure is conveniently obtained by using a vacuum embedding container. If this is not available, the specimen in warm gelatin may be placed in a vacuum desiccator, where the gelatin will usually remain fluid long enough for all bubbles to escape.

(iii) If the section requires staining, this should be carried out between stages 10 and 11.

Sections for direct projection

As an alternative to low-power photography, it is often convenient to mount a section directly on a lantern slide. When it has been stained, the section is mounted in plenty of resinous medium, covered with a second lantern slide, allowed to dry, and finished with binding tape. The method is useful for sections

2 B

of tissue showing a coarse pattern or containing a fairly large lesion.

Since the pieces of tissue are usually larger than those used for ordinary paraffin sections, they need processing more slowly (p. 303). Sections must be free from imperfections and preferably thicker than usual ($10\,\mu$).

Stains should be strong and should be differentiated by examining their macroscopic appearance. Fine detail is of no value, so that some counterstains are better omitted (e.g. haematoxylin in the per-iodic acid Schiff method or in elastic stains). When the specimen is suitable, good results can be obtained with one or more of the following: haematoxylin and eosin (preferably Ehrlich's haematoxylin), per-iodic acid Schiff, alcian blue, trichrome stains, elastic stains, myelin stains, and the methods of van Gieson, Perls, von Kóssa, and Marchi.

Two or more sections can be combined on a single slide and these need not be stained by the same method. Since the finished lantern slide consists of two plates of glass, it is possible to use each half for mounting a separate section and to stain the two halves by different methods, finally mounting them face-to-face to produce a composite lantern slide (Eade, *et al.*, 1969).

CHAPTER 25

Using The Optical Microscope

Cleaning the microscope. Lighting systems. Measuring with the microscope.

As its title suggests, this chapter is concerned with the practical use of the optical microscope. We have laid particular stress on cleaning the microscope and setting up the illumination, because it has been our experience that these points usually receive too little attention. As a result, many microscopes in routine use do not give a satisfactory performance. We have also included a few notes on the use of the microscope for making measurements, because many routine users seem to have little understanding of this aspect of microscopy. No attempt has been made to deal with the theory of the microscope: for this the reader is recommended to the simple accounts by Hartley (1962), Casartelli (1965) and Barer (1968).

Microscopes get less attention than they deserve because any deterioration is usually so gradual as to pass unnoticed in day-to-day use. There are, in fact, only two places where sudden catastrophic failure may occur. One of these is the lamp bulb which will burn out with no warning. The other is the nosepiece clip which breaks after long use, usually giving warning by gradually losing its springiness so that the nosepiece rotates too freely. Whenever a microscope is in constant use, the user is strongly recommended to keep a spare lamp bulb and also a nosepiece clip with suitable screws ready to hand.

When the performance deteriorates gradually, three possibilities should be considered. These are: dirty lenses, misalignment so that the optical axis is not straight, and incorrect focusing of the light source. If these faults are sought and corrected periodically, the effort will be amply repaid by the optical and aesthetic rewards obtained. The same attention should be given to a new or unfamiliar microscope before any attempt is made to assess its merits.

Cleaning the microscope

Most of the components of the optical system remain clean

for months without attention, but a few parts are particularly liable to become dirty and need to be cleaned more often. These are the top surfaces of eyepieces, the bottom of objectives, the top surface of the condenser and the mirror. Eyepieces become dusty if the microscope is left uncovered; they are also liable to be coated by a thin film of grease from eyelashes. The bottom of objectives may be coated by grease from a finger applied carelessly when the nosepiece is being rotated. Other deposits at this site may include immersion oil and occasionally a thin film or streak of mounting medium (balsam or D.P.X.) from a newly mounted slide; these transparent films may not be obvious until the lens is viewed with a magnifying glass in a good light. The top of the condenser may collect dust and also minute chips of glass; these are broken from the edges and corners of slides by stage clips that are allowed to spring sharply into place. Because of the likelihood that these glass chips will scratch the lens surface, the condenser must be cleaned by blowing or gentle brushing before being rubbed with even the softest tissue. The mirror collects dust. It may be cleaned with no special precautions except when a surface-aluminized or surface-silvered mirror is provided, as it may be when the illumination is built in. In this case, special care is needed to avoid scratching the delicate metallic coating; gentle mopping with tissues soaked in alcohol and then with dry tissue is the most that is permissible.

When cleaning any of the optical components of the microscope, it is essential to avoid all forms of fibrous or starchy textiles; a soft camel-hair brush will remove dust particles, and a piece of lens tissue or well-washed soft and thin cotton may be used to remove grease. The surface may be moistened by condensation from the breath, or by clean water. Obstinate grease marks can usually be removed successfully with diluted alcohol; stronger grease solvents (e.g. xylene) should be handled with caution since they may soften the cement in which the lenses are mounted.

Sometimes the microscope image is marred because dust particles appear to be superimposed on it. As an aid to the location of this dust, the best plan is to proceed as follows. First move the slide to make sure that the dust is not there. Secondly rotate the eyepiece; if the dust particles rotate they are on one of the eyepiece lenses. Thirdly, if the dust is still undetected, alter the focus of the condenser; if the image of the dust vanishes it is on the condenser, mirror, or lamp; if it persists it is in the objective. Fourthly, if the mirror is adjustable, move it slightly; if the dust moves it is on the lamp or the mirror itself. More rarely the microscope image appears to have a fibre or thread superimposed upon it. This can usually be located in the way already described, but occasionally the fibre will be found to be caught in the edge of an iris diaphragm so that it projects into the path of light. Gently opening and closing the iris diaphragms will readily locate such a fibre.

When cleaning the optical system of a microscope, the components should be dismantled as little as possible. It is better to return an unsatisfactory component to the supplier, or to call for the services of an expert, than to venture into unfamiliar territory. Such items as high-power objectives and, above all, binocular prism systems should not be dismantled by the inexperienced. Dust or opacity in a compound lens or prism is very rarely due to a fault between the various glass elements. When, however, attention to the accessible surfaces does not remove the dust or opacity, the defect is probably attributable to crystallization of the cement between two elements, or the growth of fungi within the lens. Faults like these can only be remedied by an expert.

The mechanical parts of the microscope also need to be cleaned from time to time, but once again it is better not to dismantle unfamiliar components. In general, it is comparatively easy to dismantle and reassemble nineteenth-century and early twentieth-century microscopes, since these were assembled by hand from blocks of solid brass. Many modern microscopes, however, include mechanical components that were assembled with the use of special tools. Most modern iris diaphragms, for instance, should be dismantled only by the expert. If the microscope is protected against dust when not in use, it will need cleaning and lubricating only occasionally. A piece of rag soaked in xylene is useful for removing dirty oil, but all the xylene must be wiped away before new oil is applied. The parts requiring lubrication are: bearings that house rotating axles (e.g. the coarse adjustment spindle), pivots (e.g. stage clips and many fine adjustments), and slides (e.g. those permitting the condenser mounting to slide up and down on the microscope stand). The actual teeth of cogwheels, or rack and pinion mechanisms, do not need lubricant since this collects dust and grit which is likely to grind away the surfaces of the teeth until they fail to mesh firmly with each other. In choosing a lubricant, the best plan is to follow the instructions of the microscope manufacturer. In general we have preferred to use light machine oil at frequent intervals. The alternative is thin grease; this is particularly popular for old microscopes, where it may confer a temporary improvement in performance by reducing the play in the worn mechanical stage or other moving part. Grease does not need to be renewed as often as oil; this sometimes produces a false sense of security so that the microscope receives no attention for a long time. It is then found that every trace of grease has been squeezed out of the working parts and has dried up in gummy brown nodules along their edges.

Lighting systems

For satisfactory results the source of light must be correctly aligned (centred) and correctly focused. The exact method of doing this depends on the type of light source, but in every case it is the light, the mirror and the condenser that must be brought into line, since the eyepiece and objective lenses are already in an alignment that cannot be altered. For most purposes, it is worth paying particular attention to the illumination of the field of the high-power ($\times 40$ lens), because it is at this power that the difference between perfect and imperfect illumination is most conspicuous. If, by chance, the low-power lenses are not centred on exactly the same field as the high-power, the illumination at low powers may be slightly imperfect, but the loss of quality is unlikely to be noticeable. Three lighting systems are in common use: a simple lamp bulb, a focusing spotlight separate from the microscope, and a spotlight built into the microscope.

When a simple lamp bulb is used, possibly with a piece of opal glass in front of it, the source is easily aligned and focused by manipulating the substage condenser, iris diaphragm, and mirror to obtain so-called critical illumination (better termed source-focused illumination) in which the source is focused on the object. Proceed as follows:

1. Select a section that includes an artery (or other conspicuous object); position this centrally in the field of the high-power lens. Return to the low-power lens without moving the section. Once the object is in focus, do not touch the focusing screws again and do not move the section.

2. Partly close the iris diaphragm and lower the condenser until the edge of the iris is sharp; this can be verified by opening and closing it slightly.

3. Adjust the condenser centering screws until the iris is centred on the artery. With an old microscope it may be worth verifying that the iris opens symmetrically; if not, do not centre it in the fully closed (pin-hole) position but partly open.

4. Open the iris and raise the condenser, at the same time moving the mirror until the lamp bulb (or opal glass in front of it) is in focus and is centred on the artery. If necessary make a mark on the bulb or glass to do this. The illumination is now both aligned and focused.

5. Return to the high-power lens and verify that the artery is in the centre of the field. Remove the eyepiece and inspect the upper lens of the objective. Partly close the iris until the outer one-quarter of this lens is dark; when the eyepiece is replaced, this partial closure of the iris will be found to have improved the clarity of the image without destroying more than a fraction of its brightness.

6. If the image of the lamp (or opal glass) is obtrusive when the microscope is used, the condenser should be lowered just enough to remove the image of the light source.

The method of source-focused illumination, using a simple lamp bulb, may be satisfactory for routine microscopy, but it suffers from two major drawbacks. First, it is difficult to fill the field of low-power objectives with light, so that the method is unsatisfactory for scanning large sections. Secondly, it is difficult to obtain uniform illumination of the whole field at any power, so that photography is difficult. For these purposes in particular, but also for convenience in general use, the method of Köhler illumination is preferred. Köhler illumination requires a focusing spotlamp, consisting of a lamp with its own condenser and iris diaphragm. These are known as the lamp condenser and lamp iris to avoid confusion with the substage condenser and substage iris attached to the microscope. For correct Köhler illumination, there are two conditions to fulfil: first the lamp must be focused on the substage iris; secondly the microscope must be focused on the lamp iris. When the spot-lamp is separate from the microscope, proceed as follows:

1. Remove any filters and opal glass screens from the lamp housing and shine the beam on the microscope mirror.

2. Close the substage iris and direct the light beam onto it by moving the mirror.

3. Focus the lamp condenser until the image of the lamp filament on the substage iris is sharp.

4. Select a section with an artery (or other conspicuous object). Centre this in the high-power field as before and then return to low-power.

5. Lower the substage condenser until the substage iris is in focus; centre this in the same way as before.

6. Open the substage iris and close the lamp iris. Raise the substage condenser until the image of the lamp iris is sharp. Open the lamp iris just enough to fill the field with light.

7. Return to the high-power lens; remove the eyepiece and inspect the upper lens of the objective. Close the substage iris until the outer one-quarter of this lens is dark.

8. Replace any filters or opal glass screens that may be required, but avoid placing a gelatin filter or polarizing film in the substage filter-carrier, since heat will be focused at this point as well as light.

When the light source is built into the microscope, it is almost always provided with a lamp condenser and lamp iris for Köhler illumination. Most manufacturers fix the position of the lamp condenser and mirror, so that the lighting should remain correctly aligned until the lamp bulb is changed. When this is done, it will be necessary to centre the bulb until the image of its filament falls in the centre of the substage iris. With built-in illumination it is, of course, still necessary to focus the condenser until a sharp image of the lamp iris is obtained in the plane of the section. It may also be necessary to centre the condenser.

Measuring with the microscope

It is relatively easy to make accurate measurements with a microscope. Histological sections, however, differ from living tissue in many respects, so that when a section is measured the results must be interpreted with caution. Tissue shrinks during processing and may be compressed when sections are cut; for these reasons it may be necessary to compare the size of the section with that of the original piece of tissue. It must also be remembered that the whole of a structure may not be included within the thickness of a section so that, for instance, measurement of average nuclear diameter is very difficult. It is also unwise to rely on the accuracy of the advancing mechanism of the microtome; many sections cut at a supposed 5μ are in reality about 7μ thick.

Provided that the differences between histological sections and fresh tissue are borne in mind, it is possible to make linear measurements, or area measurements, or to calculate the relative amounts of two or more constituents of a tissue.

Linear measurements are made with eyepieces that have been suitably modified. The simplest modification is the incorporation of a graticule (ruled scale or grid). A more elaborate modification is the provision of two hair lines that can be separated by a calibrated wheel. For special purposes an image-shearing eyepiece is obtainable which produces twin images in contrasting colours; these images can be separated by rotating a calibrated wheel. Whatever eyepiece measuring device is used, it must first be calibrated to discover its relationship to actual linear distances on the section. This is done with a stage micrometer (ruled slide) and must be recorded for each objective. When used in another microscope, the eyepiece measuring device must be re-calibrated since objectives from different manufacturers vary considerably in their magnifying power even when both are marked $\times 10$ or $\times 40$. Once the eyepiece measuring device has been calibrated, it is a simple matter to make linear measurements. We have used graticules for comparing the diameters of muscle fibres in sections of biopsy material, for determining what proportion of the nuclei in a smear exceed a certain diameter, and for discovering the maximum diameter of abnormal nuclei in sections.

To measure the area of an object in a section, it is almost always necessary to reproduce its outline. This is most conveniently done by projecting an image onto paper or card and outlining it in pencil. The area within the pencil line can then be measured with a planimeter. Another possibility is to project the outline on squared paper, when a close approximation to the area can be made by counting squares. A third possibility is to cut out an area outlined on thick card and weigh it. Instead of projection, the outline can be made with a camera lucida. A better way is to photograph the section and measure the photographic image with a planimeter or by weighing. In every case it is necessary to draw or photograph the image of a stage micrometer at the same magnification. When the area is too large for even the low-power lens of the microscope, a photographic enlarger makes a satisfactory projector.

When the problem is to determine the relative amounts of the various components of a tissue, it is possible to measure them by one of the methods just described. Since only proportions are required, however, it is considerably easier to use a special graticule known as an integrating eyepiece. This consists of a number of points; a record is made of how many points fall on each of the tissue components. Provided that enough fields are counted, the results are very accurate. A second type of integrating eyepiece is available to determine how much of a surface is of a particular type; for instance, what proportion of the surface of bone trabeculae is covered with osteoid tissue. For a discussion of the use of integrating eyepieces and many other aspects of measurement in histology, the reader should consult Dunnill (1968).

References

ADAMS, C. W. M. (1956). Stricter interpretation of the ferric ferricyanide reaction with particular reference to the demonstration of protein-bound sulphydryl and di-sulphide groups. *J. Histochem. Cytochem.* **4**, 23.

ADAMS, C. W. M. & SWETTENHAM, K. V. (1958). The histochemical identification of two types of basophil cell in the normal human adenohypophysis. *J. Path. Bact.* **75**, 95.

ANDERSON, J. (1929). *How to Stain the Nervous System.* Edinburgh: Livingstone.

APÁTHY, S. (1892). Erfahrungen in der Behandlung des Nervensystems für histologische Zwecke. *Z. wiss. Mikrosk.* **9**, 15.

APÁTHY, I. (1897a). A késtartó szeréperöl a mikrotomiában kapcsolatban egy új fajtanak léirásával. *Ért. érdél. Múz.-Egyes. Orvos.-Term.-Tumom. Szakoszt.* **19**, 32.

This article was published simultaneously in Hungarian and German. Although bound together, the two languages maintain separate page numbers, each beginning at 1. As an additional complication, the journal was issued in two distinct halves; Orvosi szak (=Ärztliche Abtheilung) and Természettudományi szak (=Naturwissenschaftliche Abtheilung). The article in question is in the latter. The above reference is to the Hungarian text, which contained the illustrations in the copy consulted. The same article, in the same number of the same journal, but printed in German, is shown in the succeeding reference. The forename Istvántól in Hungarian is recorded in German as Stefan.

APÁTHY, S. (1897a). Ueber die Bedeutung des Messerhaltes in der Mikrotomie. *Sitzungsberichte der Medicinisch-naturwissenschaftlischen Sektion des Siebenbürgischen Museumvereins (II Naturwissenschaftliche Abtheilung),* **19**, 11.

APÁTHY, S. (1897b). Ein neuer Messerhalter und die Aenderung der Neigung des Messers durch Keile. *Z. wiss. Mikrosk.* **14**, 157.

AUMONIER, F. J. & SETTERINGTON, R. (1967). Some notes on the mounting of histological sections. *Proc. R. microsc. Soc.* **2**, 428.

AVES, E. K., JONES, G. R. N. & CUNNINGHAM, G. J. (1965). Storage of frozen sections in paraffin blocks. *J. clin. Path.* **18**, 383.

BAKER, J. R. (1944). The structure and chemical composition of the Golgi element. *Q. Jl microsc. Sci.* **85**, 1.

BAKER, J. R. (1946). The histochemical recognition of lipine. *Q. Jl microsc. Sci.* **87**, 441.

BAKER, J. R. (1958). *Principles of Biological Microtechnique*. London: Methuen.

BAKER, J. R. (1966). *Cytological Technique*, 5th ed. London: Methuen.

BAKER, S. L. (1940). A freezing method for preparing museum specimens composed of bone and soft tissue. *Bull. int. Ass. med. Mus.* **20**, 42.

BANCROFT, J. D. (1967). *An Introduction to Histochemical Technique*. London: Butterworths.

BARER, R. (1968). *Lecture Notes on the Use of the Microscope*, 3rd ed. Oxford: Blackwell.

BARKA, T. & ANDERSON, P. J. (1963). *Histochemistry*. New York: Hoeber.

BARRETT, A. M. (1944a). A method for staining sections of bone marrow. *J. Path. Bact.* **56**, 133.

BARRETT, A. M. (1944b). On the removal of formaldehyde-produced precipitate from sections. *J. Path. Bact.* **56**, 135.

BARRY, D. H. & SPRING, B. J. (1967). An apparatus for rapid attachment of frozen tissue to cryostat tissue carriers. *Stain Technol.* **42**, 147.

BECKER, S. W., PRAVER, L. L. & THATCHER, H. (1935). An improved (paraffin section) method for the dopa reaction. *Archs Derm. Syph.* **31**, 190.

BENNHOLD, H. (1922). Eine spezifische Amyloidfärbung mit Kongorot. *Münch. med. Wschr.* **69**, 1537.

VON BERTALANFFY, L., MASIN, F. & MASIN, MARIANNA (1956). Use of acridine-orange fluorescence technique in exfoliative cytology. *Science, N.Y.* **124**, 1024.

VON BERTALANFFY, L., MASIN, MARIANNA & MASIN, F. (1958). A new and rapid method for diagnosis of vaginal and cervical cancer by fluorescence microscopy. *Cancer, N.Y.* **11**, 873.

BEST, F. (1906). Über Karminfärbung des Glykogens und der Kerne. *Z. wiss. Mikrosk.* **23**, 319.

BIELSCHOWSKY, M. (1904). Die Silberimprägnation der Neurofibrillen. *J. Psychol. Neurol., Lpz.* **3**, 169.

BIELSCHOWSKY, M. (1909). Eine Modifikation meines Silberimprägnationsverfahrens zur Darstellung der Neurofibrillen. *J. Psychol. Neurol., Lpz.* **12**, 135.

BOUIN, P. (1897). Études sur l'évolution normale et l'involution du tube séminifère. *Archs Anat. microsc.* **1**, 225.

BOYD, W. (1922). The preservation of amyloid specimens. *Bull. int. Ass. med. Mus.* **8**, 77.

BRAIN, E. B. (1966). *The Preparation of Decalcified Sections*. Springfield: Thomas.

BUSCH, C. K. (1898). Ueber eine Färbungsmethode secundärer Degenerationen der Nervensystems mit Osmiumsäure. *Neurol. Zentbl.* **17**, 476.

CAJAL, S. RAMON Y (1913). Sobre un nuevo proceder de impregnación de la neuroglia y sus resultados en los centros nerviosos del hombre y animales. *Trab. Lab. Invest. biol. Univ. Madr.* **11**, 219.

CAJAL, S. RAMON Y (1916). El proceder del oro-sublimado para la coloración de la neuroglia. *Trab. Lab. Invest. biol. Univ. Madr.* **14**, 155.

CARAZZI, D. (1911). Eine neue Hämatoxylinlösung. *Z. wiss. Mikrosk.* **28**, 273.

CARLETON, H. M. (1926). *Histological Technique.* London: Oxford University Press.

CARLETON, H. M. & DRURY, R. A. B. (1957). *Histological Technique,* 3rd ed. London: Oxford University Press.

CARLETON, H. M. & LEACH, E. H. (1938). *Histological Technique,* 2nd ed. London: Oxford University Press.
    For 4th ed. see Drury and Wallington.

CARNOY, J. P. (1887). Conférence donnée à la société Belge de microscopie. *Cellule,* **3**, 229.

CARR, L. B., RAMBO, O. N. & FEICHTMEIR, T. V. (1961). A method of demonstrating calcium in tissue sections using chloranilic acid. *J. Histochem. Cytochem.* **9**, 415.

CARSON, FREIDA, KINGSLEY, W. B., HABERMAN, S. & RACE, G. J. (1964). Unclassified mycobacteria contaminating acid-fast stains of tissue sections. *Am. J. clin. Path.* **41**, 561.

CASARTELLI, J. D. (1965). *Microscopy for Students.* London: McGraw-Hill.

CASSELMAN, W. G. B. (1959). *Histochemical Technique.* London: Methuen.

CATER, D. B. (1953). *Basic Pathology and Morbid Histology.* Bristol: Wright.

CHANG, J. P., ANKEN, M. & RUSSELL, W. O. (1961). Sputum cell concentration by membrane filtration for cancer diagnosis. *Acta cytol.* **5**, 168.

CHAYEN, J., BITENSKY, LUCILLE, BUTCHER, R. G., & POULTER, L. W. (1969). *A Guide to Practical Histochemistry.* Edinburgh: Oliver and Boyd.

CHAYEN, J. & DENBY, E. F. (1968). *Biophysical Technique.* London: Methuen.

CHEATHAM, W. J. (1954). *in* J. F. Enders and T. C. Peebles. Propagation in tissue cultures of cytopathogenic agents from patients with measles. *Proc. Soc. exp. Biol. Med.* **86**, 277.

CHESTERMAN, W. & LEACH, E. H. (1949). Low viscosity nitro-cellulose for embedding tissues. *Q. Jl microsc. Sci.* **90**, 431.

CLAYDEN, E. C. (1952). A discussion on the preparation of bone sections by the paraffin wax method with special reference to the control of decalcification. *J. med. Lab. Technol.* **10**, 103.

CLAYDEN, E. C. (1962). *Practical Section Cutting and Staining*, 4th ed. London: Churchill.

Code of Practice for the Protection of Persons Exposed to Ionising Radiations in Research and Teaching (1964). London: H.M. Stationery Office.

COLE, E. C. (1943). Studies on haematoxylin stains. *Stain Technol.* **18**, 125.

Colour Index (1956). 2nd ed. Bradford: Society of Dyers and Colourists *and* Lowell: American Association of Textile Chemists.

CONN, H. J. (1961). *Biological Stains*, 7th ed. Baltimore: Williams and Wilkins.

CORNIL, V. (1875). Sur la dissociation du violet de méthylaniline et sa séparation en deux couleurs sous l'influence de certains tissus normaux et pathologiques, en particulier par les tissus en dégénérescence amyloïde. *C.r. hebd. Séanc. Acad. Sci., Paris* **80**, 1288.

CRUICKSHANK, B., DODDS, T. C. & GARDNER, D. L. (1968). *Human Histology*, 2nd ed. Edinburgh: Livingstone.

CULLING, C. F. A. (1963). *Handbook of Histopathological Techniques*, 2nd ed. London: Butterworths.

CURTIS, F. (1905). Nos méthodes de coloration élective du tissu conjonctif. *Archs Méd. exp. Anat. path.* **17**, 603.

CUSTER, R. P. (1933). Studies on the structure and function of bone marrow. III. Bone marrow biopsy. *Am. J. med. Sci.* **185**, 617.

DADDI, L. (1896). Nouvelle méthode pour colorer la graisse dans les tissus. *Archs ital. Biol.* **26**, 143.

DAWSON, A. B. (1926). A note on the staining of the skeleton of cleared specimens with alizarin red S. *Stain Technol.* **1**, 123.

DIVRY, P. & FLORKIN, M. (1927). Sur les propriétés optiques de l'amyloïde. *C.r. Séanc. Soc. Biol.* **97**, 1808.

DIXON, K. C. (1959). Oxidized tannin-azo method for protein in tissues. *Am. J. Path.* **35**, 199.

Documenta Geigy (1962). 6th ed. Ed. Diem, K. New York: Geigy Pharmaceutical.

DONIACH, I. (1960). Diseases of endocrine organs. In *Recent Advances in Pathology*, 7th ed. Ed. Harrison, C. V. London: Churchill.

DRURY, R. A. B. & WALLINGTON, E. A. (1967). *Carleton's Histological Technique*, 4th ed. London: Oxford University Press.

DUNNILL, M. S. (1968). Quantitative methods in histology. In *Recent Advances in Clinical Pathology*, series five. Ed. Dyke, S. C. London: Churchill.

EADE, KAY C., DISBREY, BRENDA D., & RACK, J. H. (1969). Histological sections for direct projection. *J. Sci. Technol.* **15**, 12.

EDWARDS, J. J. & EDWARDS, M. J. (1959). *Medical Museum Technology.* London: Oxford University Press.

EHRLICH, P. (1886). Fragekasten. *Z. wiss. Mikrosk.* **3**, 150.

EINARSON, L. (1932). A method for progressive selective staining of Nissl and nuclear substance in nerve cells. *Am. J. Path.* **8**, 295.

EISENSTEIN, R., WERNER, M., PAPAJIANNIS, S., KONETZKI, W. & LAING, IRIS. (1961). Chloranilic acid as a histochemical reagent for calcium. *J. Histochem. Cytochem.* **9**, 154.

EVANS, R. W. (1966). *Histological Appearances of Tumours*, 2nd ed. Edinburgh: Livingstone.

FAINE, S. (1965). Silver staining of spirochaetes in single tissue sections. *J. clin. Path.* **18**, 381.

FARBER, S. M., PHARR, S. L., WOOD, D. A. & GORMAN, R. D. (1953). Mucolytic and digestive action of trypsin in preparation of sputum for cytologic study. *Science, N.Y.* **117**, 687.

FEULGEN, R. & ROSSENBECK, H. (1924). Mikroskopisch-chemischer Nachweis einer Nucleinsäure vom Typus der Thymonucleinsäure und die darauf beruhende elektive Färbung von Zellkernen in mikroskopischen Präparaten. *Hoppe-Seyler's Z. Physiol. Chem.* **135**, 203.

FEULGEN, R. & VOIT, K. (1924). Über einen weitverbreiteten festen Aldehyd. *Pflügers Arch. ges. Physiol.* **206**, 389.

FINCK, H. (1960). Epoxy resins in electron microscopy. *J. biophys. biochem. Cytol.* **7**, 27.

FISCHLER, F. (1904). Ueber die Unterscheidung von Neutralfetten Fettsäuren und Seifen im Gewebe. *Zentbl. allg. Path. path. Anat.* **15**, 913.

FISCHLER, F. J. & GROSS, W. (1905). Über den histologischen Nachweis von Seife und Fettsäure im Tierkörper und die Beziehungen intravenös eingefuhrter Seifenmengen zur verfettung. *Beitr. path. Anat.* **Suppl.** 7, 326. Festschrift für Professor Julius Arnold.

FLEMMING, W. (1884). Mittheilungen zur Färbetechnik. *Z. wiss. Mikrosk.* **1**, 349.

FONTANA, A. (1912). Verfahren zur intensiven und raschen Färbung des Treponema pallidum und anderer Spirochäten. *Derm. Wschr.* **55**, 1003.

FOOT, N. C. (1924). A technic for demonstrating reticulum fibers in Zenker-fixed paraffin sections. *J. Lab. clin. Med.* **9**, 777.

FRIEND, J. V. & SMITH, G. S. (1962). Routine preparation of calcified tooth sections. *J. med. Lab. Technol.* **19**, 255.

FRIEND, J. V. & SMITH, G. S. (1964). A rapid method of preparing thin (7 micron) calcified tooth sections. *J. med. Lab. Technol.* **21**. 51.

FRIEND, J. V. & SMITH, G. S. (1965). Recent modifications to our technique of preparing thin, flat, polished tooth sections. *J. med. Lab. Technol.* **22**, 4.

GASTON, P. J. (1964). *The Care, Handling and Disposal of Dangerous Chemicals.* Aberdeen: Northern Publishers.

GATENBY, J. B. (1921). *The Microtomist's Vade-mecum*, 8th ed. London: Churchill.

GATENBY, J. B. & BEAMS, H. W. (1950). *The Microtomist's Vademecum*, 11th ed. London: Churchill.

GATENBY, J. B. & COWDRY, E. V. (1928). *The Microtomist's Vademecum*, 9th ed. London: Churchill.

GATENBY, J. B. & PAINTER, T. S. (1937). *The Microtomist's Vademecum*, 10th ed. London: Churchill.

For earlier editions see Lee.

GENDRE, H. (1937). A propos des procédés de fixation et de détection histologique du glycogen. *Bull. Histol. appl. Physiol. Path.* **14**, 262.

GESCHICKTER, C. F. (1930). Fresh tissue diagnosis in the operating room. *Stain Technol.* **5**, 81.

GIEMSA, G. (1904). Eine Vereinfachung und Vervollkommnung meiner Methylenazur-Methylenblau-Eosin-Färbemethode zur Erzielung der Romanowsky-Nochtschen Chromatinfärbung. *Zentbl. Bakt. ParasitKde (Abt. I)* **37**, 308.

GIESMA, G. (1909). Ueber die Färbung von Feuchtpräparaten mit meiner Azur-Eosinmethode. *Dt. med. Wschr.* **35**, 1751.

VAN GIESON, I. (1889). Laboratory notes of technical methods for the nervous system. *N.Y. med. J.* **50**, 57.

GOLDBLATT, S. A. & NADEL, E. M. (1965). Cancer cells in the circulating blood. A critical review II. *Acta cytol.* **9**, 6.

GOLDNER, J. (1938). A modification of the Masson trichrome technique for routine laboratory purposes. *Am. J. Path.* **14**, 237.

GOLODETZ, L. & UNNA, P. G. (1909). Zur Chemie der Haut III. Das Reduktionsvermögen der histologischen Elemente der Haut. *Mh. prakt. Derm.* **48**, 149.

GOMORI, G. (1937). Silver impregnation of reticulum in paraffin sections. *Am. J. Path.* **13**, 993.

GOMORI, G. (1939). Microtechnical demonstration of phosphatase in tissue sections. *Proc. Soc. exp. Biol. Med.* **42**, 23.

GOMORI, G. (1941). Distribution of acid phosphatase in the tissues under normal and under pathologic conditions. *Archs Path.* **32**, 189.

GOMORI, G. (1946). A new histochemical test for glycogen and mucin. *Am. J. clin. Path.* **16**, 177.

GOMORI, G. (1950). Aldehyde-fuchsin: a new stain for elastic tissue. *Am. J. clin. Path.* **20**, 665.

GOMORI, G. (1951). Histochemical staining methods. *Methods in Medical Research* **4**, 1. Ed. Visscher, M. B. Chicago: Year Book Publishers.

GORDON, H. (1951). Method of fabricating museum containers from plastic. *Bull. int. Ass. med. Mus.* **32**, 103.

GORDON, H. & SWEETS, H. H. (1936). A simple method for the silver impregnation of reticulum. *Am. J. Path.* **12**, 545.

GOTHARD, E. (1898). Quelques modifications au procédé de Nissl, pour la coloration élective des cellules nerveuses. *C.r. Séanc. Soc. Biol.* **5**, 530.

GOUGH, J. & WENTWORTH, J. E. (1949a). The use of thin sections of entire organs in morbid anatomical studies. *Jl R. microsc. Soc.* **69**, 231.

GOUGH, J. & WENTWORTH, J. E. (1949b). A comparison of the radiological and pathological changes in coalworkers' pneumoconiosis. *J. Fac. Radiol.* **1**, 28.

GRAHAM, RUTH M. (1963). *The Cytologic Diagnosis of Cancer*, 2nd ed. Philadelphia: Saunders.

GRAM, C. (1884). Ueber die isolirte Färbung der Schizomyceten in Schnitt- und Trockenpräparaten. *Fortschr. Med.* **2**, 185.

GRAY, P. (1954). *The Microtomist's Formulary and Guide.* New York: Blakiston.

GREENBURY, C. L. (1966). Cautionary tale. *J. clin. Path.* **19**, 526.

GRIDLEY, MARY F. (1953). A stain for fungi in tissue sections. *Am. J. clin. Path.* **23**, 303.

GROCOTT, R. G. (1955). A stain for fungi in tissue sections and smears. *Am. J. clin. Path.* **25**, 975.

GUARD, H. R. (1959). A new technic for differential staining of the sex chromatin, and the determination of its incidence in exfoliated vaginal epithelial cells. *Am. J. clin. Path.* **32**, 145.

HACKETT, C. J. & NORMAN, W. A. (1952). Duguid-Young technique for making plastic specimen containers. *Med. biol. Illust.* **2**, 191.

HAGGIS, G. H. (1966). *The Electron Microscope in Molecular Biology.* London: Longmans.

HALE, C. W. (1946). Histochemical demonstration of acid mucopolysaccharides in animal tissues. *Nature, Lond.* **157**, 802.

2 C

HALL, MARY, J. (1960). A staining reaction for bilirubin in sections of tissue. *Am. J. clin. Path.* **34**, 313.

HALL, W. E. B. (1944). A method for preparation of gross demonstration and museum specimens using cross-sectioned tissue. *Bull. int. Ass. med. Mus.* **24**, 12.

HALMI, N. S. (1952). Differentiation of two types of basophils in the adenohypophysis of the rat and the mouse. *Stain Technol.* **27**, 61.

HAM, A. W. (1965). *Histology*, 5th ed. Philadelphia: Lippincott.

HARRIS, H. F. (1900). On the rapid conversion of haematoxylin into haematein in staining reactions. *J. appl. Microsc. Lab. Meth.* **3**, 777.

HART, K. (1908). Die Färbung der elastischen Fasern mit dem von Weigert angegebenen Farbstoff. *Zentbl. allg. Path. path. Anat.* **19**, 1.

HARTLEY, W. G. (1962). *Microscopy*. London: English Universities Press.

HEADDEN, G. F. & MCWILLIAMS, E. (1968). A comparison of embedding waxes. *J. med. Lab. Technol.* **25**, 250.

HEIDENHAIN, M. (1896). Noch einmal über die Darstellung der Centralkörper durch Eisenhämatoxylin nebst einigen allgemeinen Bemerkungen über die Hämatoxylinfarben. *Z. wiss. Mikrosk.* **13**, 186.

HEIDENHAIN, M. (1916). Über neuere Sublimatgemische. *Z. wiss. Mikrosk.* **33**, 232.

HELLY, K. (1903). Eine Modification der Zenker'schen Fixirungsflüssigkeit. *Z. wiss. Mikrosk.* **20**, 413.

HENLE, J. (1865). Ueber das Gewebe der Nebenniere und der Hypophyse. *Z. Ration. Med.* **24**, 143.

HERXHEIMER, G. (1903). Zur Fettfärbung. Bemerkung zu der gleichnamigen Erwiderung des Herrn B. Fischer in No. 15 dieses Zentbl. *Zentbl. all. Path. path. Anat.* **14**, 841.

HIGGINS, J. A. (1963). A non-drying fixative for use in a cervical smear diagnostic postal service. *J. med. Lab. Technol.* **20**, 261.

HIGHMAN, B. (1946). Improved method for demonstrating amyloid in paraffin sections. *Archs Path.* **41**, 559.

HILLEMANN, H. H. and LEE, C. H. (1953). Organic chelating agents for decalcification of bones and teeth. *Stain Technol.* **28**, 285.

HOLZER, W. (1921). Über eine neue Methode der Gliafaserfärbung. *Zentbl. ges. Neurol. Psychiat.* **25**, 360.

HOTCHKISS, R. D. (1948). A microchemical reaction resulting in the staining of polysaccharide structures in fixed tissue preparations. *Archs Biochem.* **16**, 131.

HUECK, W. (1912). Pigmentstudien. *Beitr. Path. Anat.* **54**, 68.

HUGHES, HELENA E. & DODDS, T. C. (1968). *Handbook of Diagnostic Cytology*. Edinburgh: Livingstone.

JAMES, K. R. (1967). A simple silver method for the demonstration of reticulin fibres. *J. med. Lab. Tech.* **24**, 49.

JONES, D. B. (1957). Nephrotic glomerulonephritis. *Am. J. Path.* **33**, 313.

JORES, L. (1913). Ueber eine verbesserte Methode der Konservierung anatomischer Objekte. *Münch. med. Wschr.* **60**, 976.

KAISER, E. (1880). Verfahren zur Herstellung einer tadellosen Glycerin-Gelatine. *Bot. Zbl.* **1**, 25.

KAISERLING, C. (1897). Weitere Mittheilungen über die Herstellung möglichst naturgetreuer Sammlungspräparate. *Virchows Arch. path. Anat. Physiol.* **147**, 389.

KAISERLING, C. (1900). Ueber Konservirung und Aufstellung pathologisch-anatomischer Präparate für Schau- und Lehrsammlungen. *Verh. dt. path. Ges.* **2**, 203.

KAPLOW, L. S. (1955). A histochemical procedure for localizing and evaluating leukocyte alkaline phosphatase activity in smears of blood and marrow. *Blood* **10**, 1023.

KAY, D. (1965). *Techniques for Electron Microscopy*, 2nd ed. Oxford: Blackwell.

KAY, W. W. & WHITEHEAD, R. (1941). The role of impurities and mixtures of isomers in the staining of fat by commercial Sudans. *J. Path. Bact.* **53**, 279.

KIRKPATRICK, J. & LENDRUM, A. C. (1939). A mounting medium for microscopical preparations giving good preservation of colour. *J. Path. Bact.* **49**, 592.

KIRKPATRICK, J. & LENDRUM, A. C. (1941). Further observations on the use of synthetic resin as a substitute for canada balsam. *J. Path. Bact.* **53**, 441.

KLINGER, H. P. & KURT, S. L. (1957). A universal stain for the sex chromatin body. *Stain Technol.* **32**, 235.

KLÜVER, H. & BARRERA, ELIZABETH (1953). A method for the combined staining of cells and fibres in the nervous system. *J. Neuropath. exp. Neurol.* **12**, 400.

KNUDTSON, K. P. (1963). Mucolytic action of hyaluronidase on sputum for the cytological diagnosis of lung cancer. *Acta cytol.* **7**, 59.

KOHN, A. (1898). Ueber die Nebenniere. *Prag. med. Wschr.* **23**. 193.

KOSS, L. G. (1968). *Diagnostic Cytology and its Histopathologic Bases*, 2nd ed. Philadelphia: Lippincott.

KOSS, L. G. & DURFEE, GRACE R. (1961). *Diagnostic Cytology and its Histopathologic Bases*. Philadelphia: Lippincott.

VON KÓSSA, J. (1901). Ueber die im Organismus künstlich erzeug-
baren Verkalkungen. *Beitr. path. Anat.* **29**, Suppl. IV, 163.
KULTSCHITZKY, N. (1887). Zur histologischen Technik. *Z. wiss.
Mikrosk.* **4**, 46.
KULTSCHITZKY, N. (1889). Über eine neue Methode der Hämatoxy-
lin-Färbung. *Anat. Anz.* **4**, 223.
KUPER, S. W. A. & MAY, J. R. (1960). Detection of acid-fast organ-
isms in tissue sections by fluorescence microscopy. *J. Path. Bact.*
79, 59.
KURNICK, N. B. (1952). Histological staining with methyl-green-
pyronin. *Stain Technol.* **27**, 233.
KURNICK, N. B. (1955). Pyronin Y in the methyl-green-pyronin
histological stain. *Stain Technol.* **30**, 213.
LANGERON, M. (1949). *Précis de Microscopie*, 7th ed. Paris: Masson.
LEE, A. B. (1885). *The Microtomist's Vade-mecum*. London:
Churchill.
LEE, A. B. (1890). *The Microtomist's Vade-mecum*, 2nd ed. London:
Churchill.
LEE, A. B. (1893). *The Microtomist's Vade-mecum*, 3rd ed. London:
Churchill.
LEE, A. B. (1896). *The Microtomist's Vade-mecum*, 4th ed. London:
Churchill.
LEE, A. B. (1900). *The Microtomist's Vade-mecum*, 5th ed. London:
Churchill.
LEE, A. B. (1905). *The Microtomist's Vade-mecum*, 6th ed. London:
Churchill.
LEE, A. B. (1913). *The Microtomist's Vade-mecum*, 7th ed. London:
Churchill.
       For later editions see Gatenby.
LEISHMAN, W. B. (1901). Note on a simple and rapid method of
producing Romanowsky staining in malarial and other blood films.
Br. med. J. **2**, 757.
LENDRUM, A. C. (1944). The staining of eosinophil polymorphs and
enterochromaffin cells in histological sections. *J. Path. Bact.* **56**,
441.
LENDRUM, A. C. (1947a). Routine diagnostic technique of the
general morbid anatomist. In *Recent Advances in Clinical Pathology*.
Ed. Dyke, S. C. London: Churchill.
LENDRUM, A. C. (1947b). The phloxin-tartrazine method as a
general histological stain and for the demonstration of inclusion
bodies. *J. Path. Bact.* **59**, 399.
LENDRUM, A. C., FRASER, D. S., SLIDDERS, W. & HENDERSON, R.
(1962). Studies on the character and staining of fibrin. *J. clin.
Path.* **15**, 401.

LENDRUM, A. C. & McFARLANE, D. (1940). A controllable modification of Mallory's trichromic staining method. *J. Path. Bact.* **50**, 381.

LENDRUM, A. C., SLIDDERS, W. and FRASER, D. S. (1969). The similarity of the ageing changes, in the kidney, of amyloid deposit to those of the fibrinous deposits of diabetes mellitus. *Ned. Tijdschr. Geneesk.* **113**, 373.

LEVADITI, C. (1905). Sur la coloration du spirochaete pallida Schaudinn dans les coupes. *C.r. Séanc. Soc. Biol.* **59**, II, 326.

LIEB, ETHEL (1940). Demonstration of vascular tree with Neoprene. *Bull. int. Ass. med. Mus.* **20**, 48.

LIEB, ETHEL (1948). Modified phosphotungstic acid-haematoxylin stain. *Archs Path.* **45**, 559.

LILLIE, R. D. (1928). The Gram stain. *Archs Path.* **5**, 828.

LILLIE, R. D. (1948). *Histopathologic Technic.* Philadelphia: Blakiston.

LILLIE, R. D. (1950). Further exploration of the HIO_4-Schiff reaction with remarks on its significance. *Anat. Rec.* **108**, 239.

LILLIE, R. D. (1951a). Histochemical comparison of the Casella, Bauer, and periodic acid oxidation-Schiff leucofuchsin technics. *Stain Technol.* **26**, 123.

LILLIE, R. D. (1951b). Simplification of the manufacture of Schiff reagent for use in histochemical procedures. *Stain Technol.* **26**, 163.

LILLIE, R. D. (1954). *Histopathologic Technic and Practical Histochemistry,* 2nd ed. New York: Blakiston.

LILLIE, R. D. (1957). Trichoxanthin, the yellow pigment of guinea pig hair follicles and hairs. *J. Histochem. Cytochem.* **5**, 346.

LILLIE, R. D. (1965). *Histopathologic Technic and Practical Histochemistry,* 3rd ed. New York: McGraw-Hill.

LILLIE, R. D. & ASHBURN, L. L. (1943). Supersaturated solutions of fat stains in dilute isopropanol for demonstration of acute fatty degenerations not shown by Herxheimer technic. *Archs Path.* **36**, 432.

LISON, L. (1936). *Histochimie Animale.* Paris: Gauthier-Villars.

LISON, L. (1954). Alcian blue 8G with chlorantine fast red 5B. A technic for selective staining of mucopolysaccharides. *Stain Technol.* **29**, 131.

LISON, L. (1960). *Histochimie et Cytochimie Animales,* 3rd ed. Paris: Gauthier-Villars.

LISON, L. & DAGNELIE, J. (1935). Méthodes nouvelles de coloration de la myéline. *Bull. Histol. appl. Physiol. Path.* **12**, 85.

LONGNECKER, D. S. (1966). A program for automated haematoxylin and eosin staining. *Am. J. clin. Path.* **45**, 229.

LÖWHAGEN, T., NASIELL, M. & GRANBERG, INGRID (1966). Acridine orange fluorescence cytology in detection of cervical carcinoma. *Acta cytol.* **10**, 194.

LOYEZ, M. (1910). Coloration des fibres nerveuses par la méthode à l'hématoxyline au fer après inclusion à la celloïdine. *C.r. Séanc. Soc. Biol.* **69**, 511.

MALAPRADE, L. (1934). Étude de l'action des polyalcools sur l'acide periodique et les periodates alcalins. *Bull. Soc. Chim. Fr.*, **5** series, **1**, 833.

MALLORY, F. B. (1897–8). On certain improvements in histological technique. *J. exp. Med.* **2**, 529.

MALLORY, F. B. (1900–1). A contribution to staining methods. *J. exp. Med.* **5**, 15.

MALLORY, F. B. (1938). *Pathological Technique.* Philadelphia: Saunders.

MALLORY, F. B. & PARKER, F. (1939). Fixing and staining methods for lead and copper in tissues. *Am. J. Path.* **15**, 517.

MARCHI, V. & ALGERI, G. (1885). Sulle degenerazioni discendenti consecutive a lesioni della corteccia cerebrale. *Riv. sper. Freniat. Med. leg. Alien. ment.* **11**, 492.

MARCHI, V. & ALGERI, G. (1886). Sulle degenerazioni discendenti consecutive a lesioni sperimentali in diverse zone della corteccia cerebrale. *Riv. sper. Freniat. Med. leg. Alien. ment.* **12**, 208.

MARSLAND, T. A., GLEES, P. & ERIKSON, L. B. (1954). Modification of the Glees silver impregnation for paraffin sections. *J. Neuropath. exp. Neurol.* **13**, 587.

MASSON, P. (1914). La glande endocrine de l'intestin chez l'homme. *C.r. hebd. Séanc. Acad. Sci., Paris* **158**, 59.

MASSON, P. (1929). Some histological methods. Trichrome stainings and their preliminary technique. *Bull. int. Ass. med. Mus.* **12**, 75.

MAY, R. & GRÜNWALD, L. (1902). Über Blutfärbungen. *Zentbl. inn. Med.* **23**, 265.

MAYER, P. (1883). Einfache Methode zum Aufkleben microskopischer Schnitte. *Mitt. zool. Stn. Neapel.* **4**, 521.

MAYER, P. (1896). Über Schleimfärbung. *Mitt. zool. Stn. Neapel.* **12**, 303.

MAYER, P. (1903). Notiz über Hämateïn und Hämalaun. *Z. wiss. Mikrosk*, **20**, 409.

McFARLANE, D. (1944). Picro-Mallory. An easily controlled regressive trichromic staining method. *Stain Technol.* **19**, 29.

McMANUS, J. F. A. (1946). Histological demonstration of mucin after periodic acid. *Nature, Lond.* **158**, 202.

McMANUS, J. F. A. & MOWRY, R. W. (1960). *Staining Methods. Histologic and Histochemical.* New York: Harper and Row.

MENTEN, MAUD L., JUNGE, JOSEPHINE & GREEN, MARY H. (1944). A coupling histochemical Azo dye test for alkaline phosphatase in the kidney. *J. biol. Chem.* **153**, 471.

MERCER, E. H. & BIRBECK, M. S. C. (1966). *Electron Microscopy*, 2nd ed. Oxford: Blackwell.

MICHAELIS, L. (1901). Ueber Fett-Farbstoffe. *Virchows Arch. path. Anat. Physiol.* **164**, 263.

MOORE, G. W. (1951). Low viscosity nitrocellulose for embedding chrome mordanted tissues of the central and peripheral nervous system. *J. med. Lab. Technol.* **9**, 105.

MOORE, K. L. & BARR, M. L. (1955). Smears from the oral mucosa in the detection of chromosomal sex. *Lancet* **2**, 57.

MÜLLER, H. (1858). Ueber die Entwickelung der Knochensubstanz nebst Bemerkungen über den Bau rachitischer Knochen. *Z. wiss. Zool.* **9**, 147.

MÜLLER, H. (1859). Anatomische Untersuchung eines Microphthalmus. *Verh. phys.-med. Ges. Würzb.* **10**, 138.

NADEL, E. M. and members of the National Cancer Institute, N.I.H. (1963). A cautionary note to those concerned with circulating cancer cells in the blood. *Acta cytol.* **7**, 70.

NAYLOR, B. (1958). The elimination of a 'ribbing' effect observed in cytologic smears. *Am. J. clin. Path.* **30**, 143.

NEELSEN, F. (1883). Ein Casuistischer Beitrag zur Lehre von der Tuberkulose. *Zentbl. med. Wiss.* **21**, 497.

NISSL, F. (1885). Ueber die Untersuchungsmethoden der Grosshirnrinde. *Neurol. Zentbl.* **4**, 500.

NISSL, F. (1894). Ueber eine neue Untersuchungsmethode des Centralorgans speciell zur Feststellung der Localisation der Nervenzellen. *Neurol. Zentbl.* **13**, 507.

OLLETT, W. S. (1947). A method for staining both Gram-positive and Gram-negative bacteria in sections. *J. Path. Bact.* **59**, 357.

OLLETT, W. S. (1951). Further observations on the Gram-Twort stain. *J. Path. Bact.* **63**, 166.

ORCHIN, J. C. (1967). Modern techniques in histology. In *Progress in Medical Laboratory Technique*, vol. 4. Ed. Baker, F. J. London: Butterworths.

PAGE, KATHLEEN M. (1965). A stain for myelin using solochrome cyanin. *J. med. Lab. Technol.* **22**, 224.

PAL, J. (1886). Ein Beitrag zur Nervenfärbetechnik. *Med. Jb.* **1**, 619.

PALADE, G. E. (1952). A study of fixation for electron microscopy. *J. exp. Med.* **95**, 285.

PAPAGEORGIOU, A. & WOLTERS, H. (1966). Acridine orange fluorescence microscopy on specimens from the respiratory tract. *Acta cytol.* **10**, 232.

PAPAMILTIADES, M. (1953). Sur la composition de deux hématoxylines pour les colorations cytologiques. *Acta anat.* **19**, 24.

PAPANICOLAOU, G. N. (1942). A new procedure for staining vaginal smears. *Science, N.Y.* **95**, 438.

PAPPENHEIM, A. (1899). Vergleichende Untersuchungen über die elementare Zusammensetzung des rothen Knochenmarkes einiger Säugethiere. *Virchows Arch. path. Anat. Physiol.* **157**, 19.

PAUL, J. (1965). *Cell and Tissue Culture*, 3rd ed. Edinburgh: Livingstone.

PEARSE, A. G. E. (1950). Differential stain for the human and animal anterior hypophysis. *Stain Technol.* **25**, 95.

PEARSE, A. G. E. (1955). Copper phthalocyanins as phospholipid stains. *J. Path. Bact.* **70**, 554.

PEARSE, A. G. E. (1960). *Histochemistry: Theoretical and Applied*, 2nd ed. London: Churchill.

PEARSE, A. G. E. (1968). *Histochemistry. Theoretical and Applied*, Vol. I, 3rd ed. London: Churchill.

PEASE, D. C. (1964). *Histological Techniques for Electron Microscopy*, 2nd ed. New York and London: Academic Press.

PEREZ-TAMAYO, R. (1961). *Mechanisms of Disease*. Philadelphia: Saunders.

PERLS, M. (1867). Nachweis von Eisenoxyd in gewissen Pigmenten. *Virchows Arch. path. Anat. Physiol.* **39**, 42.

POMMER, G. (1885). Ueber Methoden welche zum Studium der Ablagerungsverhältnisse der Knochensalze und zum Nachweise kalkloser Knochenpartien brauchbar sind. *Z. wiss Mikrosk.* **2**, 151.

POPPER, H. (1941). Histologic distribution of vitamin A in human organs under normal and pathological conditions. *Archs Path.* **31**, 766.

PRUDDEN, J. M. (1885). Fragekasten. *Z. wiss. Mikrosk.* **2**, 288.

PUCHTLER, HOLDE, SWEAT, FAYE & LEVINE, M. (1962). On the binding of congo red by amyloid. *J. Histochem. Cytochem.* **10**, 355.

PULVERTAFT, R. J. V. (1936). Colour fading in chloroma and other museum specimens. *Bull. int. Ass. med. Mus.* **16**, 27.

PUNDEL, J. P. (1957). *Acquisitions Récentes en Cytologie Vaginale Hormonale*. Paris: Masson.

QUINCKE, H. (1880). Zur Pathologie des Blutes. *Dt. Arch. klin. Med.* **25**, 567.

RINEHART, J. F. & ABUL-HAJ, S. K. (1951). An improved method for histologic demonstration of acid mucopolysaccharides in tissue. *Archs Path.* **52**, 189.

Rio-Hortega, P. del (1917). Noticia de un nuevo y fácil método para la coloración de la neuroglia y del tejido conjunctivo. *Trab. Lab. Invest. biol. Univ. Madr.* **15**, 367.

Rio-Hortega, P. del (1919). El 'tercer elemento' de los centros nerviosos. 1. La microglia en estudo normal. *Boln. Soc. esp. Biol.* **9**, 68.

Rio-Hortega, P. del (1921). Estudios sobre la neuroglia. La glia de escasas radiaciones (oligodendroglia). *Boln. R. Soc. esp. Hist. nat.* **21**, 63.

Rogers, A. W. (1967). *Techniques of Autoradiography.* Amsterdam: Elsevier.

Romeis, B. (1924). *Taschenbuch der Mikroskopischen Technik,* 11th ed. München: Oldenbourg.

Romeis, B. (1968). *Mikroskopische Technik,* 16th ed. München: Oldenbourg.

Rosenthal, M. & Traut, H. F. (1951). Mucolytic action of papain for cell concentration in diagnosis of gastric cancer. *Cancer, N.Y.* **4**, 147.

Russell, Dorothy S. (1939). *Histological Techniques for Intracranial Tumours.* London: Oxford University Press.

Russell, Dorothy S., Krayenbühl, H. & Cairns, H. (1937). The wet film technique in the histological diagnosis of intracranial tumours: a rapid method. *J. Path. Bact.* **45**, 501.

Ryder, J. A. (1887). *Queen's Micro. Bulletin* **IV**, 43 (cited in *Jl R. microsc. Soc.*, 1888, p. 512).

Sabatini, D. D., Bensch, K. & Barrnett, R. J. (1963). Cytochemistry and electron microscopy; the preservation of cellular ultrastructure and enzymatic activity by aldehyde fixation. *J. Cell Biol.* **17**, 19.

Schmorl, G. (1907). *Die pathologisch-histologischen Untersuchungsmethoden,* 4th ed. Leipzig: Vogel.

Schmorl, G. (1918). *Die pathologisch-histologischen Untersuchungsmethoden,* 8th ed. Leipzig: Vogel.

Schmorl, G. (1934). *Die pathologisch-histologischen Untersuchungsmethoden,* 16th ed. Ed. Geipel, P. Berlin: Vogel.

Schubert, M. & Hamerman, D. (1956). Metachromasia; chemical theory and histochemical use. *J. Histochem. Cytochem.* **4**, 159.

Schultz, A. (1924). Eine Methode des mikrochemischen Cholesterinnachweises am Gewebsschnitt. *Zentbl. allg. Path. path. Anat.* **35**, 314.

Schultze, M. & Rudneff, M. (1865). Weitere Mittheilungen über die Einwirkung der Ueberosmiumsäure auf thierische Gewebe. *Arch. mikrosk. Anat. EntwMech.* **1**, 298.

SCOTT, H. R. (1952). Rapid staining of beta cell granules in pancreatic islets. *Stain Technol.* **27**, 267.

SCOTT, S. G. (1912). On successive double staining for histological purposes. *J. Path. Bact.* **16**, 390.

SEARS, W. G. (1958). *Anatomy and Physiology for Nurses*, 3rd ed. London: Arnold.

SHORR, E. (1941). A new technic for staining vaginal smears: III, a single differential stain. *Science, N.Y.* **94**, 545.

SILLS, B. (1953). Dry method for conserving and transporting cytological smears. *J. Am. med. Ass.* **151**, 230.

SILLS, B. & GARRET, M. (1957). Mailing of fixed and dried cytological smears. *J. Am. med. Ass.* **165**, 2219.

SILVERTON, R. E. & ANDERSON, M. J. (1961). *Handbook of Medical Laboratory Formulae.* London: Butterworths.

SLIDDERS, W. (1961). The OFG and BrAB-OFG methods for staining the adenohypophysis. *J. Path. Bact.* **82**, 532.

SMITH, A. (1962). The use of frozen sections in oral histology. *J. med. Lab. Technol.* **19**, 26 and 89.

SMITH, MARION C. (1951). The use of Marchi staining in the later stages of human tract degeneration. *J. Neurol. Neurosurg. Psychiat.* **14**, 222.

SMITH, MARION C. (1956). The recognition and prevention of artefacts of the Marchi method. *J. Neurol. Neurosurg. Psychiat.* **19**, 74.

SMITH, MARION C., STRICH, SABINA J. & SHARP, P. (1956). The value of the Marchi method for staining tissue stored in formalin for prolonged periods. *J. Neurol. Neurosurg. Psychiat.* **19**, 62.

SOUTHGATE, H. W. (1927). Note on preparing mucicarmine. *J. Path. Bact.* **30**, 729.

SPATZ, MARIA (1960). Bismarck brown as a selective stain for mast cells. *Am. J. clin. Path.* **34**, 285.

STEEDMAN, H. F. (1950). Alcian blue 8GS: a new stain for mucin. *Q. Jl microsc. Sci.* **91**, 477.

STEEDMAN, H. F. (1960). *Section Cutting in Microscopy.* Oxford: Blackwell.

STEWART SMITH, G. (1943). A danger attending the use of ammoniacal solutions of silver. *J. Path. Bact.* **55**, 227.

SWANK, R. L. & DAVENPORT, H. A. (1935). Chlorate-osmic-formalin method for staining degenerating myelin. *Stain Technol.* **10**, 87.

SYMMERS, W. ST. C. (1968). Aspects of the contributions of histopathology to the study of deep-seated fungal infections. In *Systemic Mycoses*, ed. Wolstenholme, G. E. W. & Porter, Ruth, London: Churchill.

TIRMANN, J. (1898). Ueber den Uebergang des Eisens in die Milch. *Görbersdorfer Veröffentlichungen* **2**, 101.

TOMPSETT, D. H. (1956). *Anatomical Techniques.* Edinburgh: Livingstone.

TWORT, F. W. (1924). An improved neutral red light green double stain, for staining animal parasites, micro-organisms and tissues. *J. St. Med.* **32**, 351.

UNIVERSITIES FEDERATION OF ANIMAL WELFARE (1967). *UFAW Handbook on the Care and Management of Laboratory Animals,* 3rd ed. Edinburgh: Livingstone.

UNNA, P. G. (1902). Eine Modifikation der Pappenheimschen Färbung auf Granoplasma. *Mh. prakt. Derm.* **35**, 76.

UZMAN, L. L. (1956). Histochemical localization of copper with rubeanic acid. *Lab. Invest.* **5**, 299.

VASSAR, P. S. & CULLING, C. F. A. (1959). Fluorescent stains, with special reference to amyloid and connective tissue. *Archs Path.* **68**, 487.

VERHOEFF, F. H. (1908). Some new staining methods of wide applicability. Including a rapid differential stain for elastic tissue. *J. Am. med. Ass.* **50**, 876.

VOLK, B. W. & POPPER, H. (1944). Microscopic demonstration of fat in urine and stool by means of fluorescence microscopy. *Am. J. clin. Path.* **14**, 234.

WADE, H. W. (1957). A modification of the Fite formaldehyde (Fite I) method for staining acid-fast bacilli in paraffin sections. *Stain Technol.* **32**, 287.

WALLINGTON, E. A. (1955). Secondary fixation as a routine procedure. *J. med. Lab. Technol.* **13**, 53.

WALLINGTON, E. A. (1965). The explosive properties of ammoniacal-silver solutions. *J. med. Lab. Tech.* **22**, 220.

WEIGERT, C. (1884a). Addendum to 'Ueber veränderungen der Clarke'schen Säulen bei Tabes dorsalis' by H. Lissauer. *Fortschr. Med.* **2**, 120.

WEIGERT, C. (1884b). Ausführliche Beschreibung der in No. 2 dieser Zeitschrift erwähnten neuen Färbungsmethode für das Centralnervensystem. *Fortschr. Med.* **2**, 190.

WEIGERT, C. (1885). Eine Verbesserung der Haematoxylin-Blutlaugensalzmethode für das Centralnervensystem. *Fortschr. Med.* **3**, 236.

WEIGERT, C. (1898). Ueber eine Methode zur Färbung elastischer Fasern. *Zentbl. allg. Path. path. Anat.* **9**, 289.

WEIGERT, K. (1904). Eine kleine Verbesserung der Hämatoxylin-van Gieson-methode. *Z. wiss. Mikrosk.* **21**, 1.

WENTWORTH, J. E. (1938). A new method of preserving museum

specimens in their natural colours. *Bull. int. Ass. Mus.* **18**, 53.

WENTWORTH, J. E. (1939). The hydrosulphite method of preserving museum specimens. *Bull. int. Ass. med. Mus.* **19**, 79.

WENTWORTH, J. E. (1957). Hydrosulphite method of museum mounting. *J. med. Lab. Technol.* **14**, 193.

WIED, G. L. & MANGLANO, J. I. (1962). A comparative study of the Papanicolaou technic and the acridine-orange fluorescence method. *Acta cytol.* **6**, 554.

WRIGHT, G. P. (1958). *An Introduction to Pathology*, 3rd ed. London: Longmans.

YATES, P. O. & HUTCHINSON, E. C. (1961). *Cerebral Infarction: the Role of Stenosis of the Extracranial Cerebral Arteries* (M.R.C. special report No. 300). London: H.M. Stationery Office.

ZENKER, K. (1894). Chromkali-Sublimat-Eisessig als Fixirungsmittel. *Münch. med. Wschr.* **41**, 532.

ZIEHL, F. (1882). Zur Färbung des Tuberkelbacillus. *Dt. med. Wschr.* **8**, 451.

Suppliers

THE companies in the following list are recommended from personal experience of their products or service. No attempt has been made to compile a comprehensive list of suppliers.

Bulk chemicals

CARBON TETRACHLORIDE

Honeywell and Stein, Devonshire House, Mayfair Place, London W.1.

ETHANOL, METHANOL AND INDUSTRIAL METHYLATED SPIRIT

B.P. Chemicals, Dagenham Dock, Essex.

FORMALIN

Synthite Ltd., Ryders Green, West Bromwich, Staffordshire.

TRICHLOROETHYLENE

Robert Womersley and Son Ltd., 27 River Road, Barking, Essex.

XYLENE

Dorman Long Chemicals Ltd., Port Clarence, Co. Durham.

Chemicals

Baird and Tatlock, Freshwater Road, Chadwell Heath, Essex.
British Drug House Chemicals Ltd., Poole, Dorset.
Hopkin and Williams Ltd., Freshwater Road, Chadwell Heath, Essex.
Koch-Light Laboratories Ltd., Poyle Estate, Colnbrook, Buckinghamshire.
May and Baker, Dagenham, Essex.

Equipment

AUTOMATIC KNIFE SHARPENERS

Shandon-Elliott, Shandon Scientific Company Ltd., 65 Pound Lane, London N.W.10.

AUTOMATIC PROCESSING MACHINES AND AUTOMATIC STAINING MACHINES

Hendry Relays and Electrical Equipment Ltd., Bath Road, Slough, Buckinghamshire.

Shandon-Elliott, Shandon Scientific Company Ltd., 65 Pound Lane, London N.W.10.

CRYOSTATS

Bright Instrument Company Ltd., Clifton Road, St. Peter's Road, Huntingdon.

FILING CABINETS

Slide Master, 1 Leeke Street, London, W.C.1.

INCUBATORS, OVENS AND CENTRIFUGES

The Baird and Tatlock Group, Freshwater Road, Chadwell Heath, Essex.

Griffin and George Ltd., Ealing Road, Alperton, Wembley, Middlesex.

Measuring and Scientific Equipment Ltd., 25–28 Buckingham Gate, London S.W.1.

MICROSCOPES

Gillett and Sibert, 417 Battersea Park Road, London S.W.11.

Ernst Leitz, Wetzlar, West Germany. *UK Agent* E. Leitz (Instruments) Ltd., 30 Mortimer Street, London W.1.

Nikon, Nippon Kogaku K.K., Chuo-Ku, Tokyo, Japan. *UK Agent* The Projectina Company Ltd., 8 Montgomerie Terrace, Skelmorlie, Ayrshire.

C. Reichert Optische Werke AG., A1171 Wien, Austria. *UK Agent* Shandon Scientific Company Ltd., 65 Pound Lane, London N.W.10.

Vickers Ltd., Vickers Instruments, Haxby Road, York.

W. Watson and Sons Ltd., Barnet, Hertfordshire.

Wild Heerbrugg AG., Heerbrugg, Switzerland. *UK Agent* Wild Heerbrugg (UK) Ltd., 49–51 Church Street, Maidstone, Kent.

Carl Zeiss, 7082 Oberkochen, Wurttenburg, Western Germany. *UK Agent* Carl Zeiss, Degenhardt and Company Ltd., Carl Zeiss House, 31–36 Foley Street, London W.1.

MICROTOMES, KNIVES AND ACCESSORIES

Cambridge Scientific Instruments Ltd., Chesterton Road, Cambridge.

Jung AG., Heidelberg, Western Germany. *UK Agent* Glen Creston, The Red House, 37 The Broadway, Stanmore, Middlesex.

Ernst Leitz, Wetzlar, West Germany. *UK Agent* E. Leitz (Instruments) Ltd., 30 Mortimer Street, London W.1.

Measuring and Scientific Equipment Ltd., 25–28 Buckingham Gate, London S.W.1.

C. Reichert Optische Werke AG., A1171 Wien, Austria. *UK Agent* Shandon Scientific Company Ltd., 65 Pound Lane, London N.W.10.

MOUNTING BATHS

Electrothermal Engineering Ltd., 270 Neville Road, London E.7.

Raymond A. Lamb, 12 The Viaduct, Ealing Road, Alperton, Middlesex.

Luckham Ltd., Victoria Gardens, Burgess Hill, Sussex.

THERMO-ELECTRIC MODULES.

De La Rue Frigistor Ltd., Canal Estate, Station Road, Langley, Buckinghamshire.

WAX DISPENSERS

Hendry Relays and Electrical Equipment Ltd., Bath Road, Slough, Buckinghamshire.

Raymond A. Lamb, 12 The Viaduct, Ealing Road, Alperton, Middlesex.

Lipshaw Manufacturing Company, 7446 Central Avenue, Detroit, Michigan, U.S.A. *UK Agent* Schuco International London Ltd., Halliwick Court Place, Woodhouse Road, London N.12.

General histological suppliers

George T. Gurr Ltd., 14 Carlisle Road, The Hyde, London N.W.9.

Arnold R. Horwell Ltd., 2 Grangeway, Kilburn High Road, London N.W.6.

Raymond A. Lamb, 12 The Viaduct, Ealing Road, Alperton, Middlesex.

Solmedia Ltd., 31 Orford Road, London E.17.

General cytological supplier

Ortho Diagnostics, Raritan, New Jersey 08869, U.S.A. *UK Agent* Ortho Pharmaceutical Ltd., Saunderton, High Wycombe, Buckinghamshire.

Histological Dyes

British Drug House Chemicals Ltd., Poole, Dorset.

George T. Gurr Ltd., 14 Carlisle Road, The Hyde, London N.W.9.

Hopkin and Williams Ltd., Freshwater Road, Chadwell Heath, Essex.

Raymond A. Lamb, 12 The Viaduct, Ealing Road, Alperton, Middlesex.

E. Merck AG, 61 Darmstadt, Germany. *UK Agent* Anderman and Company Ltd., Battlebridge House, 87–95 Tooley Street, London S.E.1.

Miscellaneous histological supplies

ARCTIC SPRAY

Electronic Chemicals Ltd., 30 Notting Hill Gate, London W.11.

CARP

Tufnall Ltd., Perry Bar, Birmingham.

CHROMOPAQUE

Damancy and Company Ltd., Sandycroft, Deeside, Flintshire.

DENTAL WAX

Dental Manufacturing Company, Alston Road, Barnet, Hertfordshire.

DEXTRAN

Fisons Pharmaceuticals Ltd., Loughborough, Leicestershire.

DISPOSABLE PLASTIC CONTAINERS

A. W. Gregory and Company Ltd., Glynde House, Glynde Street, London S.E.4.

Sterilin Ltd., 9–11 The Quadrant, Richmond, Surrey.

EMBEDDING MOULDS

Mast Laboratories, 38 Queensland Street, Liverpool.

Peel-A-Way Scientific, 1800D Floradale Avenue, South El Monte, California, U.S.A.

Tissue-Tek, Lab-Tek Plastics Company, Westmont, Illinois, U.S.A.

FILING BOXES FOR WAX BLOCKS

N. Sale and Company Ltd., 130 New Bedford Road, Luton, Bedfordshire.

FILING CARDS FOR SLIDES

Burrall Bros. Ltd., Wisbech, Cambridgeshire.

GLUTARALDEHYDE

TAAB Laboratories, 52 Kidmore End Road, Emmer Green, Reading, Berkshire.

LONG RAZOR BLADES

Gillette Surgical Industries, Great West Road, Isleworth, Middlesex.

MEMBRANE FILTER HOLDERS

A. Gallenkamp and Company Ltd., P.O. Box 290, Christopher Street, London E.C.2.

Gelman Instrument Company, P.O. Box 1448, Ann Arbor, Michigan, U.S.A. *UK Agent* Hawksley and Sons Ltd., 12 Peter Road, Lancing, Sussex.

Hemming's Filters, Beaumaris Instrument Company Ltd., Rosemary Lane, Beaumaris, Anglesey.

Millipore Corporation, Bedford, Massachusetts 01730, U.S.A. *UK Agent* Millipore (UK) Ltd., Heron House, 109 Wembley Hill Road, Wembley, Middlesex.

2 D

MEMBRANE FILTERS

Gelman Instrument Company, P.O. Box 1448, Ann Arbor, Michigan, U.S.A. *UK Agent* Hawksley and Sons Ltd., 12 Peter Road, Lancing, Sussex.

Millipore Corporation, Bedford, Massachusetts 01730, U.S.A. *UK Agent* Millipore (UK) Ltd., Heron House, 109 Wembley Hill Road, Wembley, Middlesex.

Oxoid Ltd., Southwark Bridge Road, London S.E.1.

PERSPEX MUSEUM JARS

The 'Visijar' Laboratories, 149 London Road, Croydon, Surrey.

SLIDES AND COVERSLIPS

Chance Bros. Ltd., Glassworks, Smethwick 40, Birmingham.

STRIPPING FILM AND EMULSION

Kodak Ltd., Box 33, Swallowdale Lane, Hemel Hempstead, Hertfordshire.

Dyes

(With acknowledgements to Hopkin and Williams Ltd. and G. T. Gurr Ltd.)

Dye (and common alternative name)	Colour index (2nd ed.) Number and name		Approximate solubility in g/100 ml.	
			Water	*Alcohol*
Acridine orange	46005	basic orange 14	sol.	sol.
Alcian blue 8GX	74240	ingrain blue 1	5	1·6
Alizarin red S	58005	mordant red 3	7·5	0·15
Aniline blue	42755	acid blue 22	sol.	slight
(*soluble blue 3M or 2R; water blue*)				
Auramine O	41000	basic yellow 2	0·7	4·5
Azophloxine	18050	acid red 1	3	slight
Azure A	52005		sol.	sol.
Azure C			sol.	sol.
Biebrich scarlet	26905	acid red 66	sol.	0·05
Bismarck brown	21000	basic brown 1	1·3	1·1
(*vesuvin*)				
Brilliant crystal scarlet 6R	16250	acid red 44	3	0·5
(*ponceau 6R; crystal ponceau 6R*)				
Carmine	75470	natural red 4	sol.	slight
Chlorantine fast red	28160	direct red 81	sol.	slight
Chromotrope 2R	16570	acid red 29	19	0·15
Congo red	22120	direct red 28	sol.	0·2
Cresyl violet			sol.	slight
(*cresyl fast violet; cresyl echt violet; cresyl fast violet acetate*)				
Crystal violet	42555	basic violet 3	1·7	13
(*gentian violet*)				
Eosin, yellowish, water and alcohol soluble	45380	acid red 87	44	2
(*eosin Y*)				
Erythrosin B	45430	acid red 51	11	2
Fast blue RR salt	37155	azoic diazo 24	sol.	—
Fast garnet GBC salt	37210	azoic diazo 4	5	—
Fast green FCF	42053	food green 3	16	0·35
Fast red B salt	37125	azoic diazo 5	20	—
Fast red ITR salt	37150	azoic diazo 42	6	—
(*Brentamine fast red LTR*)				
Fast red TR salt	37085	azoic diazo 11	20	—
Fuchsin, acid	42685	acid violet 19	20	0·25
Fuchsin, basic	42510	basic violet 14	0·4	8
Gallocyanin	51030	mordant blue 10	insol.	slight
Haematoxylin	75290	natural black 1 and 2	1·5	more than 30
Light green	42095	acid green 5	20	0·8
Luxol fast blue		solvent blue 38	v. slight	sol.
Martius yellow	10315	acid yellow 24	4·5	0·15
(*naphthol yellow*)				

Dye (and common alternative name)	Colour index (2nd ed.) Number and name		Approximate solubility in g/100 ml.	
			Water	Alcohol
Methasol fast blue	74360	solvent blue 25	v. slight	sol.
Methyl blue	42780	acid blue 93	sol.	slight
Methyl green	42585	basic blue 20	sol.	insol.
Methyl violet	42535	basic violet 1	3	15
Methylene blue	52015	basic blue 9	3·5	1·5
Neutral red	50040	basic red 5	5·5	2·5
Oil red O	26125	solvent red 27	insol.	0·5
Orange G	16230	acid orange 10	10	0·2
Phloxine B	45410	acid red 92	50	9
Phosphine 3R	46045	basic orange 15	sol.	sol.
Picric acid	10305		1·2	8
Ponceau 2R (ponceau de xylidine)	16150	acid red 26	6	0·1
Ponceau S	27195	acid red 112	1·2	insol.
Pyronin Y (pyronin G)	45005		9	0·6
Rhodamine B	45170	basic violet 10	0·8	1·5
Safranin	50240	basic red 2	5·5	3·5
Solochrome cyanin RS (Eriochrome cyanine R)	43820	mordant blue 3	sol.	sol.
Sudan III	26100	solvent red 23	insol.	0·2
Sudan IV (scarlet R; Scharlach R)	26105	solvent red 24	insol.	0·2
Sudan black B	26150	solvent black 3	insol.	1·13
Tartrazine	19140	food yellow 4 acid yellow 23	11	0·1*
Thioflavine T	49005	basic yellow 1	sol.	sol.
Thionin	52000		0·25	0·25
Toluidine blue	52040	basic blue 17	3·8	0·5
Victoria blue R	44040	basic blue 11	0·5	4

* Commonly used as a saturated solution in cellosolve (0·3%).

Index

ROBERT CUNNINGHAM AND SONS LTD, ALVA